Pediatric Endocrinology

Editor

ANDREA KELLY

ENDOCRINOLOGY AND METABOLISM CLINICS OF NORTH AMERICA

www.endo.theclinics.com

Consulting Editor
ADRIANA G. IOACHIMESCU

December 2020 • Volume 49 • Number 4

ELSEVIER

1600 John F. Kennedy Boulevard ● Suite 1800 ● Philadelphia, Pennsylvania, 19103-2899

http://www.theclinics.com

ENDOCRINOLOGY AND METABOLISM CLINICS OF NORTH AMERICA Volume 49, Number 4
December 2020 ISSN 0889-8529, ISBN 13: 978-0-323-75911-3

Editor: Katerina Heidhausen
Developmental Editor: Nicole Congleton

Endocrinology and Metabolism Clinics of North America (ISSN 0889-8529) is published quarterly by Elsevier Inc., 360 Park Avenue South, New York, NY 10010-1710. Months of issue are March, June, September, and December. Periodicals postage paid at New York, NY and additional mailing offices. Subscription prices are USD 375.00 per year for US individuals, USD 799.00 per year for US institutions, USD 100.00 per year for US students and residents, USD 454.00 per year for Canadian individuals, USD 988.00 per year for Canadian institutions, USD 497.00 per year for international individuals, USD 988.00 per year for international institutions, USD 100.00 per year for Canadian students/residents, and USD 245.00 per year for international students/residents. To receive student/resident rate, orders must be accompanied by name of affiliated institution, date of term, and the signature of program/residency coordinator on institution letterhead. Orders will be billed at individual rate until proof of status is received. Foreign air speed delivery is included in all *Clinics* subscription prices. All prices are subject to change without notice. **POSTMASTER:** Send address changes to *Endocrinology and Metabolism Clinics of North America*, Elsevier Health Sciences Division, Subscription Customer Service, 3251 Riverport Lane, Maryland Heights, MO 63043. **Customer Service: Telephone: 1-800-654-2452** (U.S. and Canada); **1-314-447-8871** (outside U.S. and Canada). **Fax: 1-314-447-8029. E-mail: journalscustomerservice-usa@elsevier.com (for print support); journalsonlinesupport-usa@elsevier.com (for online support).**

Reprints. For copies of 100 or more, of articles in this publication, please contact the Commercial Rights Department, Elsevier Inc., 360 Park Avenue South, New York, NY 10010-1710; phone: +1-212-633-3874; fax: +1-212-633-3820; E-mail: reprints@elsevier.com.

Endocrinology and Metabolism Clinics of North America is covered in *MEDLINE/PubMed (Index Medicus), EMBASE/Excerpta Medica, Current Contents/Clinical Medicine, Current Contents/Life Sciences, Science Citation Index, ISI/BIOMED, BIOSIS,* and *Chemical Abstracts.*

Contributors

CONSULTING EDITOR

ADRIANA G. IOACHIMESCU, MD, PhD, FACE
Professor, Departments of Medicine: Endocrinology and Metabolism, and Neurosurgery, Emory University, Emory University School of Medicine, Atlanta, Georgia, USA

EDITOR

ANDREA KELLY, MD, MSCE
Attending Physician, Children's Hospital of Philadelphia, Professor of Pediatrics, CE, Perelman School of Medicine, University of Pennsylvania, Philadelphia, Pennsylvania, USA

AUTHORS

DAVID B. ALLEN, MD
Professor of Pediatrics, Head, Division of Pediatric Endocrinology and Diabetes, Department of Pediatrics, University of Wisconsin-Madison School of Medicine and Public Health, Madison, Wisconsin, USA

ANDREW J. BAUER, MD
Division of Endocrinology and Diabetes, Director, Thyroid Center, Children's Hospital of Philadelphia, Professor, Department of Pediatrics, Perelman School of Medicine, University of Pennsylvania, Philadelphia, Pennsylvania, USA

JOSEPH M. BRAUN, RN, MSPH, PhD
Associate Professor, Department of Epidemiology, Brown University School of Public Health, Providence, Rhode Island, USA

DIANA L. COUSMINER, PhD
Center for Spatial and Functional Genomics, Division of Human Genetics, Department of Pediatrics, Children's Hospital of Philadelphia, Department of Genetics, Perelman School of Medicine, University of Pennsylvania, Philadelphia, Pennsylvania, USA

KAREN E. EFFINGER, MD, MS
Assistant Professor of Pediatrics, Division of Hematology/Oncology/BMT, Department of Pediatrics, Emory University, Aflac Cancer and Blood Disorders Center, Children's Healthcare of Atlanta, Atlanta, Georgia, USA

ERICA A. EUGSTER, MD
Division of Pediatric Endocrinology, Professor, Department of Pediatrics, Riley Hospital for Children at IU Health, Indiana University School of Medicine, Indianapolis, Indiana, USA

SOBENNA A. GEORGE, MD
Assistant Professor of Pediatrics, Division of Endocrinology, Department of Pediatrics, Emory University, Atlanta, Georgia, USA

ANISHA GOHIL, DO
Assistant Professor of Clinical Pediatrics, Division of Pediatric Endocrinology, Department of Pediatrics, Riley Hospital for Children at IU Health, Indiana University School of Medicine, Indianapolis, Indiana, USA

STRUAN F.A. GRANT, PhD
Center for Spatial and Functional Genomics, Division of Human Genetics, Department of Pediatrics, Children's Hospital of Philadelphia, Department of Genetics, Perelman School of Medicine, University of Pennsylvania, Philadelphia, Pennsylvania, USA

LORRAINE E. LEVITT KATZ, MD
Professor, Division of Endocrinology and Diabetes, Department of Pediatrics, Children's Hospital of Philadelphia, Professor, Department of Pediatrics, Perelman School of Medicine, University of Pennsylvania, Philadelphia, Pennsylvania, USA

MARISSA KILBERG, MD, MSEd
Division of Endocrinology and Diabetes, Children's Hospital of Philadelphia, Philadelphia, Pennsylvania, USA

VICTOR N. KONJI, PhD
Research Associate, The Ottawa Pediatric Bone Health Research Group, Children's Hospital of Eastern Ontario Research Institute, Ottawa, Ontario, Canada

SHANA McCORMACK, MD, MTR
Division of Endocrinology and Diabetes, Children's Hospital of Philadelphia, Philadelphia, Pennsylvania, USA

LILLIAN R. MEACHAM, MD
Professor of Pediatrics, Division of Endocrinology, Department of Pediatrics, Emory University, Division of Hematology/Oncology/BMT, Department of Pediatrics, Emory University, Aflac Cancer and Blood Disorders Center, Children's Healthcare of Atlanta, Atlanta, Georgia, USA

SARA E. PINNEY, MD, MTR
Division of Endocrinology and Diabetes, Children's Hospital of Philadelphia, Philadelphia, Pennsylvania, USA

MELISSA S. PUTMAN, MD, MSc
Assistant Professor of Pediatrics, Harvard Medical School, Diabetes Research Center, Massachusetts General Hospital, Boston, Massachusetts, USA

STEVEN J. RUSSELL, MD, PhD
Associate Professor of Medicine, Harvard Medical School, Diabetes Research Center, Massachusetts General Hospital, Boston, Massachusetts, USA

TALIA ALYSSA SAVIC HITT, MD, MPH
Pediatric Endocrine Fellow, Division of Endocrinology and Diabetes, Department of Pediatrics, Children's Hospital of Philadelphia, Philadelphia, Pennsylvania, USA

CLARA G. SEARS, PhD
Postdoctoral Research Associate, Department of Epidemiology, Brown University School of Public Health, Providence, Rhode Island, USA

JORDAN S. SHERWOOD, MD
Instructor in Pediatrics, Harvard Medical School, Diabetes Research Center, Massachusetts General Hospital, Boston, Massachusetts, USA

JACLYN TAMAROFF, MD
Division of Endocrinology and Diabetes, Children's Hospital of Philadelphia, Philadelphia, Pennsylvania, USA

LEANNE M. WARD, MD, FRCPC, FAAP
Pediatric Endocrinologist, Division of Endocrinology and Metabolism, Children's Hospital of Eastern Ontario, Professor of Pediatrics, Tier 1 Research Chair in Pediatric Bone Health, University of Ottawa, Ottawa, Ontario, Canada

DAVID R. WEBER, MD, MSCE
Adjunct Professor of Pediatrics, Department of Pediatrics - Endocrinology, Golisano Children's Hospital, University of Rochester, Rochester, New York, USA

Contents

Many children with chronic disease are now surviving into adulthood. As a result, there is a growing interest in optimizing bone health early in the disease course with the dual goals of improving quality of life during childhood and reducing life-long fracture risk. Risk factors for impaired bone health in these children include immobility, nutritional deficiency, exposure to bone toxic therapies, hormonal deficiencies affecting growth and pubertal development, and chronic inflammation. This review focuses on the chronic diseases of childhood most commonly associated with impaired bone health. Recent research findings and clinical practice recommendations, when available, for specific disorders are summarized.

Asthma is the most common chronic inflammatory disease of children, and inhaled corticosteroids (ICSs) are the most effective and commonly used treatment of persistent asthma. ICSs currently approved for and commonly used by children with asthma include beclomethasone dipropionate, budesonide, fluticasone propionate, mometasone furoate, ciclesonide, and triamcinolone acetonide. This article reviews 4 areas critical to understanding potential adverse endocrine outcomes of ICSs and placing them in proper perspective: (1) influence of drug/delivery device properties on systemic steroid burden; (2) adrenal insufficiency during ICS treatment; (3) growth effects of ICS and asthma itself; and (4) bone mineral accretion during ICS therapy.

There has been a rapid advancement in the pace of development of new diabetes technologies and therapies for the management of type 1 diabetes over the past decade. The Diabetes Control and Complications Trial conclusively established that tight glycemic control with intensive insulin therapy decreases the rates of diabetes complications in proportion to glycemic control, and diabetes technologies have accordingly been developed to help patients reach these goals. In this review, the authors discuss new diabetes therapeutics and technologies, including new insulin analogues, insulin pumps, continuous glucose monitoring systems, and automated insulin delivery systems.

Pediatric type 2 diabetes mellitus (T2DM) is increasing in incidence, with risk factors including obesity, puberty, family history of T2DM in a first-degree or second-degree relative, history of small-for-gestational-age at birth, child of a gestational diabetes pregnancy, minority racial group, and lower socioeconomic status. The pathophysiology of T2DM consists of insulin resistance and progression to pancreatic beta-cell failure, which is more rapid in pediatric T2DM compared with adult T2DM. Treatment options are limited. Treatment failure and nonadherence rates are high in pediatric T2DM; therefore, early diagnosis and treatment and new pharmacologic options and/or effective behavioral interventions are needed.

hormonal functions during early life. These disruptions may alter development during late childhood and adolescence. This article discusses the potential effects of phthalate exposure on adiposity, puberty, and neurodevelopment during late childhood and adolescence. It also highlights studies of behavioral interventions to reduce phthalate exposures and the roles of health care professionals and policy makers in preventing phthalate exposure.

ENDOCRINOLOGY AND METABOLISM CLINICS OF NORTH AMERICA

SERIES OF RELATED INTEREST

Medical Clinics
https://www.medical.theclinics.com
Primary Care: Clinics in Office Practice
https://www.primarycare.theclinics.com/

Preface

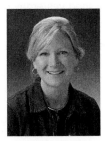

Andrea Kelly, MD, MSCE
Editor

The past decade has witnessed tremendous advances in both our understanding and our treatment of many endocrine disorders. Similarly, the care of youth with chronic medical conditions has accelerated. While some therapeutic successes celebrate the capacity to reverse or even avert development of endocrine complications, other triumphs are accompanied by the emergence of endocrine comorbidities. For some childhood disorders, the jury remains undecided as to whether endocrine comorbidities are prevented or merely delayed. Complicating these judgments, the extent to which endocrine issues arise primarily or even secondarily is at least partly explained by both protective and risk-conferring environmental and genetic modifiers. Harnessing these latter genetic factors for therapeutic benefit is on the horizon while the mechanisms underlying many endocrine comorbidities may be clarified in the wake of new therapeutic strategies.

Recognizing the role of the endocrinologist in managing endocrine sequelae of nonendocrine disease, this Pediatric Endocrinology issue of *Endocrinology and Metabolism Clinics of North America* includes reviews on endocrine late effects arising in survivors of childhood cancer and those occurring with exogenous glucocorticoid use. We also review the many forms of diabetes that fall under the umbrella of non-Type 1 and non-Type 2 diabetes and which often represent secondary manifestations of nonendocrine diseases. Accordingly, the exciting novel interventions aimed at more "typical" diabetes but with potential extension to atypical diabetes forms are presented. In addition, bone health in chronic childhood disease and strategies for characterizing bone health in these situations is examined. Precocious puberty and delayed puberty often occur in isolation and are common complications of chronic childhood conditions for which they may be the presenting symptom; thus, this issue includes new mechanistic insights and therapeutic approaches to pubertal disorders.

Acknowledging that conditions traditionally considered confined to adulthood are increasingly common in youth but with distinct determinants and courses, this issue includes discussions of type 2 diabetes and thyroid cancer in youth. Finally, attesting to the role of environmental and genetic contributors, endocrine disruptors and the role of genetic variants in complex endocrine traits are presented.

Endocrinol Metab Clin N Am 49 (2020) xiii–xiv
https://doi.org/10.1016/j.ecl.2020.10.001
0889-8529/20/© 2020 Published by Elsevier Inc.

endo.theclinics.com

Many of these reviews highlight the relevance of endocrine disorders to long-term nonendocrine sequelae and underscore James Joyce's words, "I am tomorrow, or some future day, what I establish today. I am today what I established yesterday or some previous day." Here's to altering the future today. Enjoy.

Andrea Kelly, MD, MSCE
Children's Hospital of Philadelphia
Perelman School of Medicine of
University of Pennsylvania
Room 14363
Roberts Building
2716 South Street
Philadelphia, PA 19146, USA

E-mail address:
KELLYA@email.chop.edu

Endocrine Sequelae in Childhood Cancer Survivors

Sobenna A. George, MD[a],*, Karen E. Effinger, MD, MS[b,c], Lillian R. Meacham, MD[a,b,c]

KEYWORDS

- Childhood cancer survivors • Endocrine late effects • Surveillance • Endocrinopathy

KEY POINTS

- Endocrine late effects are common after certain childhood cancer treatments and can present long after therapy completion.
- Childhood cancer survivors require lifelong surveillance for late effects.
- The Children's Oncology Group Long-Term Follow-Up Guidelines provide oncologists and primary care providers with surveillance guidelines for late effects and suggested thresholds for referral to an endocrinologist.
- Endocrinologists should be aware of special considerations for the management of endocrinopathies in childhood cancer survivors.

INTRODUCTION

The incidence of childhood cancer in the United States has increased by 0.7% per year since 1975.[1] It is estimated that approximately 16,850 new cases of cancer among children aged 0 to 19 years will be diagnosed in 2020.[1] The incidence of specific cancer types differs with age (**Fig. 1**). In young children, leukemia is the most common cancer, whereas central nervous system (CNS) tumors are most common in adolescents.[2] Although the incidence of childhood cancer is increasing, more children are surviving cancer and living longer because of cooperative group clinical trials, advances in multimodal therapy and targeted therapeutic agents, and improved supportive care. The 5-year childhood cancer survival rate has increased from 63% in the mid-1970s to greater than 85% in recent years.[2]

Although childhood cancer survival rates are increasing, cancer treatment can be associated with undesirable late effects that may present decades after the completion of therapy.[3,4] In a cohort of approximately 1700 childhood cancer survivors (CCS),

[a] Division of Endocrinology, Department of Pediatrics, Emory University, Atlanta, GA, USA;
[b] Division of Hematology/Oncology/BMT, Department of Pediatrics, Emory University, 2015 Uppergate Drive Northeast, 4th Floor, Atlanta, GA 30322, USA; [c] Aflac Cancer and Blood Disorders Center, Children's Healthcare of Atlanta, Atlanta, GA, USA
* Corresponding author. Center for Advanced Pediatrics, 1400 Tullie Road, Suite 8243, Atlanta, GA 30329.
E-mail address: sgeorg4@emory.edu

Endocrinol Metab Clin N Am 49 (2020) 565–587
https://doi.org/10.1016/j.ecl.2020.07.001
0889-8529/20/© 2020 Elsevier Inc. All rights reserved.
endo.theclinics.com

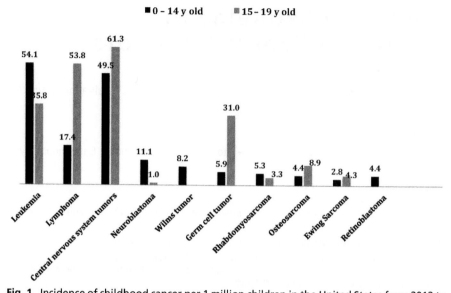

Fig. 1. Incidence of childhood cancer per 1 million children in the United States from 2012 to 2016. (*Data from* Howlader N, Noone AM, Krapcho M, Miller D, Brest A, Yu M, Ruhl J, Tatalovich Z, Mariotto A, Lewis DR, Chen HS, Feuer EJ, Cronin KA (eds). SEER Cancer Statistics Review, 1975-2016, National Cancer Institute. Bethesda, MD, https://seer.cancer.gov/csr/1975_2016/, based on November 2018 SEER data submission, posted to the SEER web site, April 2019.)

the estimated cumulative prevalence of any chronic health condition was 95.5% by age 45 years, with the pulmonary (65.2%), auditory (62.1%), and endocrine-reproductive (62%) systems most commonly affected.[3] Using data from the Childhood Cancer Survivor Study (CCSS), Mostoufi-Moab and colleagues[5] described self-reported endocrinopathies by cancer type in adult survivors of childhood cancer treated between 1970 and 1986. Survivors of Hodgkin lymphoma reported the most endocrine late effects (60%), followed by survivors of CNS tumors (54%), leukemia (46%), soft tissue sarcoma (41%), non-Hodgkin lymphoma (40%), neuroblastoma (32%), Wilms tumor (29%), and bone cancer (28%).[5] Although current therapies are intended to minimize late effects, many of the agents used in previous eras are still used. Furthermore, newer therapeutic agents may have off-target effects that lead to endocrinopathies. Although the distribution and frequency of endocrine late effects in CCS have changed over time, endocrine dysfunction is still common. It is crucial that CCS receive lifelong surveillance because early detection and prompt treatment of late effects can improve health and quality of life.[6,7]

This article (1) summarizes the endocrine late effects that can result from childhood cancer treatments, (2) provides endocrinologists with an understanding of the national surveillance guidelines for endocrine late effects that are being used in pediatric oncology long-term follow-up, and (3) provides clinical considerations that are key to the management of endocrinopathies in CCS.

CANCER TREATMENTS AND ASSOCIATED ENDOCRINE LATE EFFECTS

Many endocrinopathies have been associated with specific chemotherapy, radiation, and surgical modalities used to treat childhood cancer (**Table 1**). Some

Table 1
Cancer treatments and associated endocrine late effects

Endocrine Toxic Cancer Treatment[a]	Pituitary Hormone Deficiencies					Pituitary Hormone Excess	Non-pituitary Related							
	GH	ACTH	FSH/LH	TSH	PRL	CPP	Non-GHD Short Stature	Primary Hypothyroidism	Hyperthyroidism	Thyroid Nodules	Gonadal Dysfunction	DM	Obesity	Low BMD
Chemotherapy														
Traditional alkylators	—	—	—	—	—	—	—	—	—	—	X	—	—	—
Heavy metals	—	—	—	—	—	—	—	—	—	—	X	—	—	—
Glucocorticoids	—	X	—	—	—	—	X	—	—	—	—	—	X	X
Antimetabolites[b]	—	—	—	—	—	—	—	—	—	—	—	—	—	X
Radiation[c]														
Head/brain	X	X	X	X	X	X	—	X	X	X	—	—	X	—
Neck	—	—	—	—	—	—	—	X	X	X	—	—	—	—
Chest	—	—	—	—	—	—	X	—	—	—	—	—	—	—
Abdomen	—	—	—	—	—	—	X	—	—	—	X	X	—	—
Pelvis	—	—	—	—	—	—	—	—	—	—	X	—	—	—
Testicular	—	—	—	—	—	—	—	—	—	—	X	—	—	—
Cervical spine	—	—	—	—	—	—	—	X	X	X	—	—	—	—
Sacral spine	—	—	—	—	—	—	—	—	—	—	X	—	—	—
Whole spine	—	—	—	—	—	—	X	X	X	X	X	—	—	—
TBI	X	—	X	—	—	—	X	X	—	X	X	X	—	—

(continued on next page)

Table 1
(continued)

Endocrine Toxic Cancer Treatment[a]	Pituitary Hormone Deficiencies					Pituitary Hormone Excess	Associated Endocrine Late Effects			Non-pituitary Related				
	GH	ACTH	FSH/LH	TSH	PRL	CPP	Short Stature Non-GHD	Primary Hypothyroidism	Hyperthyroidism	Thyroid Nodules	Gonadal Dysfunction	DM	Obesity	Low BMD
Targeted Therapeutic Agents														
I-131-MIBG[d]	—	—	—	—	—	—	—	X	—	X	+	—	—	—
TKI	—	—	—	—	—	+	+	+	+	—	—	—	—	—
Immune checkpoint inhibitors	—	+	+	+	—	—	—	+	+	—	—	—	—	—
Retinoids	—	—	—	—	—	—	+	—	—	—	—	—	—	—
Hedgehog pathway inhibitors	—	—	—	—	—	—	+	—	—	—	—	—	—	—
Angiogenesis inhibitors[e]	—	—	—	—	—	—	—	—	—	—	+	—	—	—

X, endocrine disorders recognized in national guidelines or commonly accepted disorders; +, emerging data on endocrine late effects; —, no data.

Abbreviations: ACTH, adrenocorticotropic hormone; ADH, antidiuretic hormone; BMD, bone mineral density; CPP, central precocious puberty; DM, diabetes mellitus; FSH, follicle-stimulating hormone; GH, growth hormone; GHD, growth hormone deficiency; I-131-MIBG, iodine-131-metaiodobenzylguanidine; LH, luteinizing hormone; PRL, hyperprolactinemia; TBI, total body irradiation; TKI, tyrosine kinase inhibitors; TSH, thyroid-stimulating hormone.

[a] Tumors and surgical resection can directly damage organs, leading to endocrinopathies such as diabetes insipidus and hypothalamic obesity.

[b] Methotrexate only.

[c] Based on conventional radiation therapy. Newer techniques and proton beam radiation are expected to have less scatter and cause less damage.

[d] Based on systemic therapeutic dosing.

[e] Bevacizumab only.

associations are clearly evidence based, whereas others, such as those with targeted therapeutic agents, are just starting to emerge in the medical literature. When details regarding past cancer treatment are known, risk for endocrine late effects can be determined through the use of long-term follow-up guidelines such as those produced by the Children's Oncology Group.[6] However, this information may be hard to discern for many survivors who have limited access to their previous medical records and lack detailed information about their cancer treatment. For this population of patients, their risk for endocrine dysfunction can be surmised based on knowledge of typical endocrine toxic modalities used for the treatment of specific childhood cancers (**Table 2**).

Chemotherapy

Chemotherapy is the backbone of treatment of most childhood cancers. Several agents are associated with endocrine late effects, particularly gonadal dysfunction and low bone mineral density (BMD).

Traditional alkylators

Traditional alkylators are gonadotoxic in both male and female patients.[6] Dosing for most traditional alkylator agents can be converted to cyclophosphamide equivalent doses (CED) in order to calculate cumulative dosing and estimate gonadotoxicity.[8] Green and colleagues[9] assessed semen parameters in 214 adult male CCS with a history of alkylator exposure without radiation exposure. Approximately 50% of survivors had oligospermia or azoospermia, with higher CED associated with low sperm counts. Survivors with azoospermia had an average CED exposure of 10,830 mg/m^2 (standard deviation [SD], 7274), whereas those with oligospermia had an average CED exposure of 8480 mg/m^2 (SD, 4264) and those with normospermia had an average CED of 6626 mg/m^2 (SD, 3576). Overall, 89% of survivors who received less than 4000 mg/m^2 CED had normal sperm counts.[9] In men, reproductive germ cells are more prone to damage from alkylators than Leydig cells.[10] When Leydig cell damage is present, it is more often subclinical, resulting in increased luteinizing hormone (LH) but normal testosterone levels.[10]

In women, alkylators have been associated with premature ovarian insufficiency (POI). POI is characterized by decreased ovarian hormone production and menopausal follicle-stimulating hormone (FSH) levels. It can result in delayed puberty, lack of pubertal progression, irregular menses, cardiovascular disease, and decreased BMD.[11] POI is more commonly observed in survivors who received a CED greater than or equal to 8000 mg/m^2.[11] In girls, an older age at treatment increases the risk for gonadal dysfunction.[6,12] Studies have also shown that there is a dose-dependent effect of alkylators on the development of diminished ovarian reserve (DOR). DOR is a subclinical reduction in the primordial follicle pool that may eventually progress to POI.[13,14] The timing of POI aligns with the relative gonadotoxicity of treatment. After a high level of gonadotoxicity, acute ovarian failure can occur within 5 years, but, after lower levels of exposure, POI may occur years to decades later.[15,16]

Heavy metals

Like traditional alkylating agents, heavy metals can be gonadotoxic in both men and women.[6,17,18]

Glucocorticoids

Exposure to exogenous glucocorticoids as treatment of acute lymphoblastic leukemia, CNS tumors, or graft-versus-host disease (GVHD) after hematopoietic stem

Table 2
Cancer treatments that cause endocrine late effects and examples of types of cancers that are treated by those agents

Cancer Treatment	Examples of Cancer Treatment	Childhood Cancers Where Treatment Is Commonly Used
Chemotherapy		
Traditional alkylators	Busulfan, carmustine, chlorambucil, cyclophosphamide, ifosfamide, lomustine, mechlorethamine, melphalan, procarbazine, thiotepa, dacarbazine, temozolomide	Leukemia, lymphoma, neuroblastoma, Wilms tumor, CNS tumors, Ewing sarcoma, osteosarcoma, rhabdomyosarcoma, conditioning for HSCT
Heavy metals	Carboplatin, cisplatin	Osteosarcoma, neuroblastoma, CNS tumors, retinoblastoma, germ cell tumor, hepatoblastoma
Glucocorticoids	Dexamethasone, prednisone	Leukemia, lymphoma, CNS tumors, Langerhans cell histiocytosis
Antimetabolites	Methotrexate[a]	Leukemia, lymphoma, osteosarcoma, Langerhans cell histiocytosis
Radiation[b]		
Head/brain	—	Leukemia, CNS tumors, retinoblastoma, rhabdomyosarcoma, neuroblastoma
Neck	—	Lymphoma
Chest	—	Lymphoma, neuroblastoma, Wilms tumor, Ewing sarcoma, rhabdomyosarcoma
Abdomen	—	Lymphoma, neuroblastoma, Wilms tumor, rhabdomyosarcoma
Pelvis	—	Rhabdomyosarcoma, Ewing sarcoma
Testicular	—	Leukemia
Whole spine	—	CNS tumors
TBI	—	Conditioning for HSCT

Emerging Therapies		
I-131-MIBG	—	Neuroblastoma
TKI	Imatinib mesylate, dasatinib, nilotinib	Leukemia
Immune checkpoint inhibitors	Ipilimumab, nivolumab, pembrolizumab	Melanoma
Retinoids	Tretinoin, isotretinoin	Leukemia, neuroblastoma
Hedgehog pathway inhibitors	Vismodegib	CNS tumors
Angiogenesis inhibitors	Bevacizumab[c]	CNS tumors, relapsed solid tumors
Surgical Resection		
Suprasellar tumor resection	—	CNS tumors
Gonadectomy	—	Germ cell tumor
Thyroidectomy	—	Thyroid cancer

Abbreviations: HSCT, hematopoietic stem cell transplantation.
[a] Reported endocrine late effects are specific to methotrexate.
[b] Based on primary tumor location. Common tumors located in these regions are listed.
[c] Reported endocrine late effects are specific to bevacizumab.

cell transplant (HSCT) can result in several endocrine late effects. Abrupt discontinuation of therapeutic glucocorticoids has been associated with iatrogenic adrenal insufficiency caused by suppression of the hypothalamic-pituitary-adrenal (HPA) axis. In a large Cochrane Review, recovery of the HPA axis took weeks to months after the cessation of steroid therapy in children with leukemia.[19] Glucocorticoids can also cause low BMD by decreasing osteoblast bone formation.[20] One study of 346 adult CCS found that 45% were osteopenic, with steroid exposure identified as a risk factor.[21] Short stature from steroid therapy may be caused by direct damage to growth plates, reduced proliferation of chondrocytes, and a reduction in endogenous growth hormone (GH) release.[20]

Antimetabolites
Methotrexate, but not other antimetabolites, has been associated with increased osteoclast and decreased osteoblast activities leading to low BMD.[20]

Radiation

Risk for radiation-associated endocrine late effects is based on the dose to the endocrine organ exposed as the target of the therapy, from inclusion in the radiation field, or because of radiation scatter. The total body irradiation (TBI) dose used for conditioning before HSCT should be considered when calculating the total radiation exposure to any endocrine organ. For example, if a patient received 10 Gy of neck radiation and 10 Gy of TBI, the total dose to the thyroid would be 20 Gy.

Pituitary/hypothalamus
Cranial radiation therapy (CRT) and TBI can result in central endocrinopathies. Chemaitilly and colleagues[22] reported that, in a cohort of adult CCS who had hypothalamus/pituitary radiation exposure as part of their cancer treatment, 50% had at least 1 anterior pituitary hormone deficiency and 11% had multiple pituitary hormone deficiencies. GH deficiency (GHD) is the most common, and often the first, hormone deficiency to develop.[23] GHD occurs in about 13% of CCS[24] and is seen after CRT doses greater than or equal to 18 Gy.[23] The risk of GHD is dose and time dependent. Merchant and colleagues[25] predicted that survivors would develop GHD 12 months after receiving greater than 60 Gy of CRT but 60 months after receiving 15 to 20 Gy of CRT. TBI alone can result in GHD but does not typically result in other central endocrinopathies.[23] Gonadotropin, thyroid-stimulating hormone (TSH), and adrenocorticotropic hormone (ACTH) deficiencies are associated with CRT greater than or equal to 30 Gy.[23] LH and FSH deficiencies have been reported in 10.8% of CCS, whereas TSH deficiency has been found in 2.6% to 14.9% of CCS.[23] In a study by Brignardello and colleagues,[26] ACTH deficiency was detected in about 1% of adult CCS. Hypothalamic damage from radiation exposure can also result in central precocious puberty (CPP), which has been reported in 11.9% to 15.2% of CCS after greater than 18 Gy of CRT.[23] The risk for CPP is higher in women, young children, and in patients with an increased body mass index.[23] Chemaitilly and colleagues[27] retrospectively assessed 80 young survivors with a history of CNS tumors and/or CRT exposure who had developed CPP. Fifteen of these survivors (19%) subsequently developed LH/FSH deficiencies, an average of 4.1 years (SD, 3.3 years) after the discontinuation of gonadotropin-releasing hormone agonist therapy. Risk factors were not identified.[27] Hyperprolactinemia can be seen after hypothalamic radiation doses greater than or equal to 50 Gy.[6,23] In addition, survivors exposed to CRT greater than or equal to 18 Gy are more likely to be obese.[18]

Thyroid

Radiation to the head, brain, neck, and cervical spine, including TBI, can expose the thyroid gland and increase the risk of hypothyroidism, hyperthyroidism, thyroid nodules, and thyroid cancer. Primary hypothyroidism occurs in 13% to 26% of CCS.[24,28] The risk is greater in women and in survivors who received greater than or equal to 10 Gy of radiation to the thyroid gland, with even higher risk in those who received greater than or equal to 20 Gy.[6] CCS who receive greater than or equal to 20 Gy of radiation to the thyroid gland, especially greater than or equal to 30 Gy, are at risk for hyperthyroidism.[6] Thyroid nodules are common in CCS, with a subset being malignant.[28] In 1 study of 120 CCS, thyroid nodules were found in 22% of survivors. Eleven percent of these nodules were malignant.[28]

Vertebrae

Chest, abdominal, and spinal radiation and TBI may be directly toxic to vertebral growth plates. This damage can result in poor spinal and linear growth.[29]

Pancreas

Exposure of the pancreas to radiation (abdominal and TBI) can result in diabetes mellitus (DM). Abdominal radiation is thought to damage the tail of the pancreas (where islets of Langerhans are most concentrated) leading to pancreatic endocrine insufficiency, whereas TBI may cause DM through hyperinsulinemia and insulin resistance.[30] The prevalence of DM in CCS has been reported to be 2.5%, which is almost 50% higher compared with rates in siblings of survivors.[31] The risk of DM is higher in CCS who were young at diagnosis, received abdominal or total body irradiation, and currently have an increased body mass index.[31] Using participants from the CCSS, Friedman and colleagues[32] assessed 4568 CCS who were exposed to abdominal radiation. Compared with those who received less than 10 Gy to the pancreas tail, the relative risk of DM was 5.81 (95% confidence interval [CI], 2.33–14.53), 5.81 (95% CI, 1.85–18.25), and 8.62 (95% CI, 2.64–28.14) in survivors who received 10.0 to 19.9 Gy, 20.0 to 29.9 Gy, and greater than or equal to 30 Gy, respectively, to the pancreas tail.

Ovaries/uterus

Radiation fields including the sacral spine, pelvis, and abdomen as well as TBI can result in ovarian damage and dysfunction. Age at the time of exposure affects sensitivity to damage, with younger age at radiation exposure being protective. Ovarian radiation exposure of greater than or equal to 10 Gy in prepubertal girls but greater than or equal to 5 Gy in pubertal girls can result in ovarian dysfunction.[6] To protect the ovaries from the deleterious effects of radiation, techniques such as shielding and transposition can be used.[33] Radiation of greater than or equal to 30 Gy with uterine exposure can also compromise the uterine vascular supply, leading to increased risk of miscarriage, fetal growth restriction, and premature birth.[6]

Testes

Testicular radiation and TBI can result in testicular dysfunction. Germ and Sertoli cells are more sensitive to radiation damage than Leydig cells. Permanent azoospermia can occur with testicular radiation doses greater than or equal to 6 Gy and testosterone deficiency after greater than or equal to 12 Gy.[6] Although TBI can impair spermatogenesis, it is rarely associated with Leydig cell damage.[17] Similar to approaches in women, techniques such as testicular shielding and transposition can be used in men to decrease radiation exposure.[17]

Targeted Therapeutic Agents

Data are beginning to emerge on endocrine toxicities associated with the use of novel targeted therapeutic agents.

I-131-metaiodobenzylguanidine

After metabolism of I-131-metaiodobenzylguanidine (I-131-MIBG), it dissociates and can concentrate in the thyroid gland, leading to hypothyroidism, thyroid nodules, and thyroid cancer.[34] Pretreatment with potassium iodide, which blocks the uptake of I-131, was thought to be protective, but this may not be true.[34] A case report of POI after exposure to I-131-MIBG has raised suspicions that I-131-MIBG may be gonadotoxic as well.[35]

Tyrosine kinase inhibitors

Tyrosine kinase inhibitors (TKIs), especially imatinib mesylate, have been associated with height impairment,[29] although the mechanism of poor growth is not well elucidated. Theories include impaired GH signaling and/or direct skeletal toxicity.[29] In addition, TKI use may result in thyroid dysfunction caused by inflammation, poor iodine uptake, or impairment of the vascular supply of the thyroid gland.[34]

Immune checkpoint inhibitors

Ipilimumab is a monoclonal antibody against cytotoxic T lymphocyte antigen 4 (CTLA-4). It has been associated with autoimmune hypophysitis, which can result in pituitary hormone deficiencies, especially TSH, ACTH, FSH, and LH deficiencies, although the mechanism is unknown. Nivolumab and pembrolizumab are monoclonal antibodies against the programmed death-1 (PD-1) protein that have been linked to both hypothyroidism and transient hyperthyroidism when used as monotherapy or in combination with an anti–CTLA-4 agent.[36]

Retinoids and hedgehog pathway inhibitors

Retinoids and hedgehog pathway inhibitors are independently thought to impair linear growth through premature fusion of growth plates.[29,37]

Angiogenesis inhibitors

Bevacizumab is an angiogenesis inhibitor that is a monoclonal antibody against vascular endothelial growth factor. It may compromise the ovary's vascular supply, leading to impaired folliculogenesis.[38] This effect has not been studied in other angiogenesis inhibitors.

Tumor Location or Surgical Resection

Suprasellar tumors and/or their resection can cause direct damage to the hypothalamus and/or pituitary, leading to endocrine late effects. In 1 study, nearly 30% of CCS with CPP had a history of a hypothalamic/pituitary tumor.[27] Hyperprolactinemia can be caused by pituitary stalk interruption by tumor mass effect or surgical transection. TSH and gonadotropin deficiencies have been reported in survivors of optic gliomas.[39] Antidiuretic hormone (ADH) deficiency is observed in less than 1% of CCS, but is more prevalent in the setting of Langerhans cell histiocytosis, germinoma, or craniopharyngioma.[5,40] In addition, hypothalamic obesity is common in patients after surgical resection of a craniopharyngioma, occurring in 30% to 77% of that population.[40]

Hematopoietic Stem Cell Transplant

HSCT is used to treat high-risk leukemia and refractory cancers. Long-term toxicity from HSCT is related to high-dose chemotherapy, radiation exposure, GVHD, and/

or treatment of GVHD. In addition to the endocrine toxicities attributed to these treatments, patients who undergo HSCT are at risk for low BMD.[6]

SURVEILLANCE FOR ENDOCRINE LATE EFFECTS IN CHILDHOOD CANCER SURVIVORS

Endocrine late effects may occur many years to decades after the completion of cancer therapy.[5] Lifelong surveillance is therefore needed. The Children's Oncology Group (COG), supported by the National Cancer Institute, is a clinical trials group of more than 200 centers across North America, Europe, Australia, and New Zealand focused on pediatric cancer research. The COG provides long-term follow-up (LTFU) guidelines that are updated every few years and are available online with open public access.[6] These guidelines provide screening recommendations for potential late effects in CCS. The guidelines are devised by experts and are based on scientific literature and, in some scenarios, expert consensus. The guidelines are organized by cancer treatment exposure and help health care providers to (1) identify CCS who are at risk for late effects, (2) screen for late effects, and (3) determine when specialty care should be pursued. Of note, these guidelines do not provide surveillance recommendations for late effects from therapies that lack clear supportive data in the medical literature; therefore, more recently discovered late effects and/or emerging cancer therapies are not likely to be included in the guidelines.

The COG LTFU guidelines are especially useful for oncologists or primary care providers who see patients in long-term follow-up clinics. Consistent application of these guidelines aids in prompt detection of late effects and timely referral to specialists, such as endocrinologists, when needed.[6] **Table 3** summarizes endocrine late effects in CCS outlined in the most recent COG LTFU guidelines[6] and also highlights the recommended thresholds for referral of CCS from oncology/survivor clinics to endocrinologists, according to these guidelines.

MANAGEMENT OF ENDOCRINE LATE EFFECTS IN CHILDHOOD CANCER SURVIVORS

In general, the clinical manifestations, diagnosis, and treatment of endocrinopathies are similar for CCS and the general population. However, there are some unique clinical management features for endocrine late effects that should be considered when providing care for CCS (**Table 4**).

Poor Growth

Many factors other than GHD affect linear growth in CCS, including skeletal radiation, steroid therapy, and other cancer treatments that prematurely close the growth plates. Coexistence of other endocrinopathies, precocious puberty, and hypothyroidism can make assessment of growth challenging. GH stimulation tests using GH-releasing hormone should be avoided in patients with underlying hypothalamic damage because results can be falsely reassuring.[23]

The decision to treat GHD in CCS should include discussions between the endocrinologist and oncologist. The general consensus is that GH therapy can be considered in CCS who are disease free for a year or more after the completion of cancer treatment.[41] Data support that CCS are (1) not at increased risk for primary cancer recurrence, and (2) in general not at increased risk for secondary neoplasms related to GH treatment.[41] GH therapy is not indicated in patients with high-risk tumors or active cancer and should be considered with caution in patients with cancer predisposition syndromes.[41] Patients who have skeletal asymmetries caused by direct radiation toxicity, such as a small cranium or shortened spine, should be counseled that these differences may be exacerbated by GH treatment because of differential effects in

Table 3
Surveillance guidelines for endocrine late effects per Children's Oncology Group Long-Term Follow-Up Guidelines, version 5.0[a]

Endocrine Late Effect	Surveillance Recommendations		Guideline Recommendations for When to Refer to an Endocrinologist
	Risk Factors	How to Screen	
GHD	Radiation (head/brain, TBI)	Every 6 mo until growth complete, then yearly: • Height, weight, BMI, nutritional status Every 6 mo until sexually mature: • Tanner staging If poor growth consider: • Thyroid function tests, bone age	• Received radiation dose $\geq$30 Gy[b] • Poor growth for age or stage of puberty as shown by decline in growth velocity and change in percentile ranking on growth chart • Weight <third percentile
ACTH deficiency	Radiation (head/brain)	Yearly: • Assess for failure to thrive, anorexia, dehydration, hypoglycemia, lethargy, hypotension • 8 AM cortisol if received $\geq$30 Gy (if not followed by an endocrinologist)	• Received radiation dose $\geq$30 Gy[b] • 8 AM cortisol <13 μg/dL or <365 nmol/L
LH/FSH deficiency	Radiation (head/brain, TBI)	Yearly: • Assessment of sexual function, pubertal progression, and menstrual history • Assessment of growth, Tanner stage, and testicular volume If pubertal delay/arrest, irregular menses, or symptoms of sex hormone deficiency, consider: • FSH, LH, testosterone (boys), estradiol (girls)	• Received radiation dose $\geq$30 Gy[b] • Delayed puberty • Abnormal hormone levels • Hormone replacement therapy

TSH deficiency	Radiation (head/brain)	Yearly • Assessment of symptoms of hypothyroidism • Height, weight, hair, skin, and thyroid examination • TSH, free T4	• Received radiation dose $\geq$30 Gy[b] • For thyroid hormone replacement
ADH deficiency	Brain surgery	Yearly assessment for: • Polyuria and polydipsia If symptomatic consider: • Na, K, Cl, CO_2, serum and urine osmolarity • Assess for other pituitary hormone deficiencies	• For medical management of DI
Hyperprolactinemia	Radiation (head/brain)	Yearly assessment of: • Libido, galactorrhea, menstrual history If decreased libido, galactorrhea, and/or amenorrhea, consider: • Prolactin level (head CT if increased)	Evidence of: • Hyperprolactinemia • Galactorrhea
CPP	Radiation (head/brain)	Yearly until sexually mature: • Height, weight, Tanner staging, testicular volume (boys) If rapid growth or pubertal progression, consider: • FSH, LH, testosterone (boys), estradiol (girls), bone age	• Puberty <9 y old in boys and <8 y old in girls

(continued on next page)

Table 3
(continued)

Endocrine Late Effect	Surveillance Recommendations		Guideline Recommendations for When to Refer to an Endocrinologist
	Risk Factors	How to Screen	
Non-GHD short stature	Any radiation (including TBI)	Yearly: • Height, weight • Sitting height (if prior trunk irradiation) • Limb length (if extremity irradiation)	• Not specified
Primary hypothyroidism	Radiation (head/brain, neck, cervical/whole spine, TBI), MIBG, thyroidectomy	Yearly: • Assess for symptoms of hypothyroidism • Height, weight, hair, skin, and thyroid examination • TSH, free T4	• For thyroid hormone replacement (immediately if postthyroidectomy)
Hyperthyroidism	Radiation (head/brain, neck, cervical/whole spine)	Yearly: • Assess for symptoms of hyperthyroidism • Eye, skin, thyroid, cardiac, and neurologic examination • TSH, free T4	• For medical management of hyperthyroidism
Thyroid nodules/cancer	Radiation (head/brain, neck, cervical/whole spine, TBI)	Yearly: • Thyroid examination If palpable thyroid nodule, consider: • Ultrasonography ± FNA	• Further management of nodules

| Female gonadal dysfunction | Traditional alkylators, heavy metals, radiation (pelvis, sacral/whole spine, TBI), oophorectomy | Yearly:
• Assessment of onset and tempo of puberty, menstrual patterns, sexual function, symptoms of menopause, and medication use
• Assess growth and Tanner stage until mature
If pubertal delay, irregular menses, symptoms of sex hormone deficiency, consider:
• FSH, estradiol
To assess ovarian reserve, consider:
• AMH | • No pubertal signs by 13 y old
• No pubertal progression
• Irregular menses
• Menopausal symptoms
• Ovarian hormone deficiency |

(continued on next page)

Table 3
(continued)

Endocrine Late Effect	Surveillance Recommendations		Guideline Recommendations for When to Refer to an Endocrinologist
	Risk Factors	How to Screen	
Male gonadal dysfunction	Traditional alkylators, heavy metals, radiation (testicular, TBI), orchiectomy	Yearly: • Assess onset and tempo of puberty, sexual function, and medication use • Assess growth, Tanner stage, and testicular volume until mature If pubertal delay, poor growth, symptoms of sex hormone deficiency, consider: • Early morning testosterone If seeking fertility information, consider: • Semen analysis (optimal) • FSH and inhibin B are alternative assessments if the patient is unable or unwilling to provide semen sample	• No pubertal signs by 14 y old • No pubertal progression • Decline in growth velocity • Low testosterone levels

Condition	Risk factors	Surveillance	Notes
DM	Radiation (abdomen, TBI)	Every 2 y: • Fasting blood sugar or HbA1c If positive, consider evaluation of other comorbidities: • Dyslipidemia, HTN, overweight/obesity	• For further evaluation/diagnosis of DM
Obesity	Radiation (head/brain), brain surgery	Yearly: • Height, weight, BMI	• If pituitary hormone deficiencies also present
Low BMD	Methotrexate, glucocorticoids, HSCT	Baseline DXA (adjusted for height) and then as needed	History of: • Osteoporosis • Multiple fractures

Abbreviations: AMH, antimullerian hormone; BMI, body mass index; Cl, chloride; CO_2, bicarbonate; CT, computed tomography; DI, diabetes insipidus; DXA, dual energy X-ray absorptiometry; FNA, fine-needle aspiration; HbA1c, hemoglobin A1c; HTN, hypertension; T4, thyroxine.

[a] Children's Oncology Group. Long-Term Follow-Up Guidelines for Survivors of Childhood, Adolescent and Young Adult Cancers, Version 5.0. Monrovia, CA: Children's Oncology Group; October 2018; Available online: www.survivorshipguidelines.org.

[b] Radiation with hypothalamus/pituitary exposure at doses greater than or equal to 30 Gy increases the risk for multiple pituitary hormone deficiencies, warranting a referral to an endocrinologist.

Table 4
Special considerations regarding endocrine late effects in childhood cancer survivors

Endocrine Late Effect	Clinical Pearls
Poor growth	• Spinal irradiation can cause poor spinal growth, scoliosis, and kyphosis, resulting in a shortened upper body segment • Radiation exposure of a lower limb can cause limb length discrepancy • Cranial irradiation can result in hypoplasia and decreased head circumference • Precocious puberty can mask poor growth • Retinoic acid and hedgehog inhibitors cause premature closure of growth plates • GH stimulation tests with GHRH are not reliable in patients with underlying hypothalamic damage • Delay GH therapy until >1 y after cancer treatment if no evidence of recurrence (consult with oncologist before beginning GH therapy) • GH therapy does not increase the risk of primary cancer recurrence. • There are limited data on the risk of secondary neoplasms in CCS treated with GH • Be mindful of cancer predisposition syndromes when considering GH therapy • GH therapy can exacerbate skeletal dysmorphism because of direct radiation toxicity
Adrenal insufficiency	• Iatrogenic AI can be seen after steroid use for chronic GVHD • Iatrogenic AI can be seen after use of the appetite simulant megestrol acetate (Megace) • Endocrinologists should work closely with oncologists to develop a steroid wean plan and a plan to test adrenal axis recovery
Female gonadal dysfunction	• Hormone and oocyte production are equally sensitive to the damaging effects of cancer treatment • Low AMH level is an indicator of DOR • Menopausal FSH is diagnostic of POI but is a late indicator of ovarian damage • Fertility preservation should be considered before and potentially after the completion of gonadotoxic cancer therapy • Ovarian stimulation and oocyte cryopreservation can be offered to at-risk pubertal girls • Ovarian tissue cryopreservation may be available to prepubertal and pubertal girls
Male gonadal dysfunction	• Germ/Sertoli cells are more sensitive to the gonadotoxic effects of cancer therapy than Leydig cells • Leydig cell function and testosterone production may be preserved even in the face of decreased testicular volume and turgor • Normal virilization should not be used as reassurance that spermatogenesis is unaffected • Semen analysis should be used for fertility status assessment • Sperm count recovery may take several years after the completion of cancer treatment

(continued on next page)

Endocrine Late Effect	Clinical Pearls
Table 4 **(continued)**	
	• Fertility preservation should be offered before the start of gonadotoxic therapy • Pubertal boys can undergo semen cryopreservation • Testicular tissue cryopreservation can be offered in prepubertal boys (experimental)
ADH deficiency	• Common in patients with Langerhans cell histiocytosis • Adipsic patients require a daily fluid prescription to prevent extreme hypernatremia
Primary hypothyroidism	• Radiation therapy that exposes both the hypothalamus/pituitary and the thyroid gland may have a mixed picture of central and primary hypothyroidism • Maintaining a low/normal TSH level may decrease risk for thyroid cancer after radiation exposure
Low BMD	• Not typically associated with an increased risk of fractures compared with siblings

Abbreviations: AI, adrenal insufficiency; GHRH, growth hormone releasing hormone.

growth of irradiated and nonirradiated bones. For example, in a survivor with a history of spinal radiation, GH therapy may result in disproportionate growth with extremity lengthening without improvement in spinal height because of damage to the vertebral growth plates.

Adrenal Insufficiency

In addition to exogenous glucocorticoid use, survivors may experience adrenal insufficiency after the use of the appetite stimulant, megestrol acetate (Megace).[42] This drug is a synthetic progestin that can bind to the glucocorticoid receptor and suppress pituitary ACTH release. Once steroid or megestrol acetate therapy is no longer needed, it may be beneficial for endocrinologists to provide guidelines for the timing and tempo of a steroid wean before performing an ACTH stimulation test to assess for HPA axis recovery. During the steroid wean, CCS should be instructed in maintenance and stress glucocorticoid replacement, and when injectable steroid or emergency room care is needed in order to avoid adrenal crises.

Female Gonadal Dysfunction

Referral to a reproductive endocrinologist for potential fertility preservation therapy should be considered ideally before and possibly after gonadotoxic therapy.[33] Gonadotropin-releasing hormone (GnRH) agonists are often used in pubertal girls to cease menses during cancer treatment. It is thought that the resultant less metabolically active ovaries may be protected from gonadotoxic treatments.[33] However, definitive data are lacking on its effectiveness as a fertoprotectant and GnRH agonists should not be offered as such. Cryopreservation of oocytes is standard of care in pubertal girls who are at risk for infertility and can delay cancer treatment of ovarian stimulation and oocyte harvest. Ovarian tissue cryopreservation is less commonly available but can be performed in both pubertal and prepubertal girls. After cancer treatment, the ovarian tissue can be reimplanted in the survivors if there is no risk for reintroduction of cancer cells that might be harbored in the ovary. Time-limited resumption of ovarian hormone production and follicular maturation has been documented in transplanted tissue.[33] The window of opportunity to pursue fertility preservation therapy might be limited in survivors because of the onset of POI.

Male Gonadal Dysfunction

Most male CCS experience normal pubertal development; however, after gonadotoxic therapy, testicular volume and turgor are typically decreased. Testicular size is not a reliable indicator of testicular hormone production, and normal testosterone levels should not be equated with fertility status. Semen analysis is the most reliable assessment of fertility status after cancer therapy; however, it can take several years for sperm counts to recover after completion of cancer treatment.[43] Sperm cryopreservation in at-risk pubertal boys before cancer therapy is a priority given that 46% of male CCS self-report infertility.[44] Testicular tissue cryopreservation in prepubertal boys with the goal of future autotransplant is still considered experimental.[45]

Antidiuretic Hormone Deficiency

Some patients with ADH deficiency may also be adipsic because of damage to hypothalamic osmoreceptors from the tumor location or from surgical resection. These patients with a disrupted thirst mechanism are at an increased risk of significant hypernatremia. They require a daily fluid prescription to ensure that their sodium levels stay in a safe range.[46]

Primary Hypothyroidism

Risk factors for primary and secondary hypothyroidism are similar in CCS. Patients may have elements of both forms of thyroid disease concurrently. Maintaining a low TSH level may minimize the risk of thyroid cancer.[34]

Low Bone Mineral Density

BMD z scores should be corrected for height. Although CCS may have low BMD, they are not at increased risk for fractures compared with their siblings.[47]

SUMMARY

Endocrine late effects are common in CCS and may emerge years to decades after exposure to cancer treatment. Health care providers need to be informed about long-term surveillance strategies in at-risk survivors. The COG LTFU guidelines are easily accessible and provide comprehensive recommendations for the screening of treatment-related endocrinopathies in CCS. Ultimately, routine screening, early detection of late effects, and appropriate referral to an endocrinologist can result in prompt treatment of endocrinopathies and reduced morbidity in survivors.

FINANCIAL DISCLOSURE

S.A. George, K.E. Effinger, and L.R. Meacham have no conflicts of interest and no external funding.

REFERENCES

1. Siegel RL, Miller KD, Jemal A. Cancer statistics, 2020. CA Cancer J Clin 2020; 70(1):7–30.
2. Howlader NNA, Krapcho M, Miller D, et al. SEER cancer statistics review, 1974-2016. Bethesda, MD: National Cancer Institute; 2019. https://seer.cancer.gov/csr/1975_2016/.

3. Hudson MM, Ness KK, Gurney JG, et al. Clinical ascertainment of health outcomes among adults treated for childhood cancer. JAMA 2013;309(22):2371–81.
4. Oeffinger KC, Mertens AC, Sklar CA, et al. Chronic health conditions in adult survivors of childhood cancer. N Engl J Med 2006;355(15):1572–82.
5. Mostoufi-Moab S, Seidel K, Leisenring WM, et al. Endocrine abnormalities in aging survivors of childhood cancer: a report from the childhood cancer survivor study. J Clin Oncol 2016;34(27):3240–7.
6. Children's Oncology Group. Long-term follow-up guidelines for survivors of childhood, adolescent and young adult cancers, version 5.0. Monrovia (CA): Children's Oncology Group; 2018. Available at: www.survivorshipguidelines.org.
7. Oeffinger KC, Hudson MM, Landier W. Survivorship: childhood cancer survivors. Prim Care 2009;36(4):743–80.
8. Green DM, Nolan VG, Goodman PJ, et al. The cyclophosphamide equivalent dose as an approach for quantifying alkylating agent exposure: a report from the Childhood Cancer Survivor Study. Pediatr Blood Cancer 2014;61(1):53–67.
9. Green DM, Liu W, Kutteh WH, et al. Cumulative alkylating agent exposure and semen parameters in adult survivors of childhood cancer: a report from the St Jude Lifetime Cohort Study. Lancet Oncol 2014;15(11):1215–23.
10. Chemaitilly W, Liu Q, van Iersel L, et al. Leydig cell function in male survivors of childhood cancer: a report from the St Jude Lifetime Cohort Study. J Clin Oncol 2019;37(32):3018–31.
11. Chemaitilly W, Li Z, Krasin MJ, et al. Premature ovarian insufficiency in childhood cancer survivors: a report from the St. Jude Lifetime Cohort. J Clin Endocrinol Metab 2017;102(7):2242–50.
12. Sklar CA, Mertens AC, Mitby P, et al. Premature menopause in survivors of childhood cancer: a report from the childhood cancer survivor study. J Natl Cancer Inst 2006;98(13):890–6.
13. Wallace WH, Kelsey TW. Human ovarian reserve from conception to the menopause. PLoS One 2010;5(1):e8772.
14. Sowers MR, Eyvazzadeh AD, McConnell D, et al. Anti-mullerian hormone and inhibin B in the definition of ovarian aging and the menopause transition. J Clin Endocrinol Metab 2008;93(9):3478–83.
15. Green DM, Sklar CA, Boice JD, et al. Ovarian failure and reproductive outcomes after childhood cancer treatment: results from the Childhood Cancer Survivor Study. J Clin Oncol 2009;27(14):2374–81.
16. Wallace WH, Thomson AB, Saran F, et al. Predicting age of ovarian failure after radiation to a field that includes the ovaries. Int J Radiat Oncol Biol Phys 2005; 62(3):738–44.
17. Chemaitilly W, Sklar CA. Childhood cancer treatments and associated endocrine late effects: a concise guide for the pediatric endocrinologist. Horm Res Paediatr 2019;91(2):74–82.
18. Yu C. Endocrine consequences of childhood cancer therapy and transition considerations. Pediatr Ann 2019;48(8):e326–32.
19. Rensen N, Gemke RJ, van Dalen EC, et al. Hypothalamic-pituitary-adrenal (HPA) axis suppression after treatment with glucocorticoid therapy for childhood acute lymphoblastic leukaemia. Cochrane Database Syst Rev 2017;(11):Cd008727.
20. van Leeuwen BL, Kamps WA, Jansen HW, et al. The effect of chemotherapy on the growing skeleton. Cancer Treat Rev 2000;26(5):363–76.
21. den Hoed MA, Klap BC, te Winkel ML, et al. Bone mineral density after childhood cancer in 346 long-term adult survivors of childhood cancer. Osteoporos Int 2015;26(2):521–9.

22. Chemaitilly W, Li Z, Huang S, et al. Anterior hypopituitarism in adult survivors of childhood cancers treated with cranial radiotherapy: a report from the St Jude Lifetime Cohort study. J Clin Oncol 2015;33(5):492–500.

23. Sklar CA, Antal Z, Chemaitilly W, et al. Hypothalamic-pituitary and growth disorders in survivors of childhood cancer: an endocrine society clinical practice guideline. J Clin Endocrinol Metab 2018;103(8):2761–84.

24. Chemaitilly W, Cohen LE, Mostoufi-Moab S, et al. Endocrine late effects in childhood cancer survivors. J Clin Oncol 2018;36(21):2153–9.

25. Merchant TE, Rose SR, Bosley C, et al. Growth hormone secretion after conformal radiation therapy in pediatric patients with localized brain tumors. J Clin Oncol 2011;29(36):4776–80.

26. Brignardello E, Felicetti F, Castiglione A, et al. Endocrine health conditions in adult survivors of childhood cancer: the need for specialized adult-focused follow-up clinics. Eur J Endocrinol 2013;168(3):465–72.

27. Chemaitilly W, Merchant TE, Li Z, et al. Central precocious puberty following the diagnosis and treatment of paediatric cancer and central nervous system tumours: presentation and long-term outcomes. Clin Endocrinol 2016;84(3):361–71.

28. Caglar AA, Oguz A, Pinarli FG, et al. Thyroid abnormalities in survivors of childhood cancer. J Clin Res Pediatr Endocrinol 2014;6(3):144–51.

29. Antal Z, Balachandar S. Growth disturbances in childhood cancer survivors. Horm Res Paediatr 2019;91(2):83–92.

30. Friedman DN, Tonorezos ES, Cohen P. Diabetes and metabolic syndrome in survivors of childhood cancer. Horm Res Paediatr 2019;91(2):118–27.

31. Meacham LR, Sklar CA, Li S, et al. Diabetes mellitus in long-term survivors of childhood cancer. Increased risk associated with radiation therapy: a report for the childhood cancer survivor study. Arch Intern Med 2009;169(15):1381–8.

32. Friedman DN, Moskowitz CS, Hilden P, et al. Radiation dose and volume to the pancreas and subsequent risk of diabetes mellitus. J Natl Cancer Inst 2019;112(5):525–32.

33. ACOG Committee Opinion No. 747: gynecologic issues in children and adolescent cancer patients and survivors. Obstet Gynecol 2018;132(2):e67–77.

34. Waguespack SG. Thyroid sequelae of pediatric cancer therapy. Horm Res Paediatr 2019;91(2):104–17.

35. Clement SC, Kraal KC, van Eck-Smit BL, et al. Primary ovarian insufficiency in children after treatment with 131I-metaiodobenzylguanidine for neuroblastoma: report of the first two cases. J Clin Endocrinol Metab 2014;99(1):E112–6.

36. Chang LS, Barroso-Sousa R, Tolaney SM, et al. Endocrine toxicity of cancer immunotherapy targeting immune checkpoints. Endocr Rev 2019;40(1):17–65.

37. Robinson GW, Kaste SC, Chemaitilly W, et al. Irreversible growth plate fusions in children with medulloblastoma treated with a targeted hedgehog pathway inhibitor. Oncotarget 2017;8(41):69295–302.

38. Imai A, Ichigo S, Matsunami K, et al. Ovarian function following targeted anti-angiogenic therapy with bevacizumab. Mol Clin Oncol 2017;6(6):807–10.

39. Gan HW, Phipps K, Aquilina K, et al. Neuroendocrine morbidity after pediatric optic gliomas: a longitudinal analysis of 166 children over 30 years. J Clin Endocrinol Metab 2015;100(10):3787–99.

40. Rose SR, Horne VE, Howell J, et al. Late endocrine effects of childhood cancer. Nat Rev Endocrinol 2016;12(6):319–36.

41. Raman S, Grimberg A, Waguespack SG, et al. Risk of neoplasia in pediatric patients receiving growth hormone therapy–a report from the pediatric endocrine

society drug and therapeutics committee. J Clin Endocrinol Metab 2015;100(6): 2192–203.

42. Meacham LR, Mazewski C, Krawiecki N. Mechanism of transient adrenal insufficiency with megestrol acetate treatment of cachexia in children with cancer. J Pediatr Hematol Oncol 2003;25(5):414–7.

43. Okada K, Fujisawa M. Recovery of Spermatogenesis Following Cancer Treatment with Cytotoxic Chemotherapy and Radiotherapy. World J Mens Health 2019; 37(2):166–74.

44. Wasilewski-Masker K, Seidel KD, Leisenring W, et al. Male infertility in long-term survivors of pediatric cancer: a report from the childhood cancer survivor study. J Cancer Surviv 2014;8(3):437–47.

45. Osterberg EC, Ramasamy R, Masson P, et al. Current practices in fertility preservation in male cancer patients. Urol Ann 2014;6(1):13–7.

46. Arima H, Wakabayashi T, Nagatani T, et al. Adipsia increases risk of death in patients with central diabetes insipidus. Endocr J 2014;61(2):143–8.

47. Wilson CL, Dilley K, Ness KK, et al. Fractures among long-term survivors of childhood cancer: a report from the Childhood Cancer Survivor Study. Cancer 2012; 118(23):5920–8.

Pediatric Thyroid Cancer
Genetics, Therapeutics and Outcome

Andrew J. Bauer, MD[a,b,*]

KEYWORDS

- Thyroid nodule • Thyroid cancer • Pediatric • Child • Adolescent • Papillary
- Follicular • Medullary

KEY POINTS

- Ultrasonography characteristics of the nodule should be used to decide whether a nodule should undergo fine-needle aspiration.
- In most patients, differentiated thyroid cancer is sporadic. In contrast, most pediatric patients with medullary thyroid cancer have multiple endocrine neoplasia type 2.
- Knowledge of the oncogenic driver mutation can aid in diagnosis, help stratify surgery, and be used to select systemic therapy for patients that present with morbidly advanced disease or develop progressive disease refractory to traditional therapy.
- Most pediatric patients with thyroid cancer have excellent prognosis. The goal of treating pediatric patients with thyroid cancer is to optimize outcome and reduce complications.

INTRODUCTION

Most patients with thyroid cancer are asymptomatic at the time of diagnosis even in the presence of regional or distant metastasis. More than 85% of childhood thyroid carcinomas are papillary thyroid cancer (PTC), with the remainder divided between follicular thyroid cancer (FTC) and medullary thyroid cancer (MTC), and most MTC associated with multiple endocrine neoplasia type 2 (MEN2).[1] This article reviews the cause, the clinical evaluation, the treatment, and the outcome of thyroid cancer in pediatrics.

CAUSE AND GENETICS OF DIFFERENTIATED THYROID CARCINOMA

In most pediatric patients with differentiated thyroid cancer (DTC), both PTC and FTC, the cancer is sporadic and it arises from a de novo somatic oncogenic alteration. In a

[a] Division of Endocrinology and Diabetes, The Thyroid Center, Children's Hospital of Philadelphia, 3500 Civic Center Boulevard, Buerger Center, 12-149, Philadelphia, PA 19104, USA;
[b] Department of Pediatrics, The Perelman School of Medicine, The University of Pennsylvania, 415 Curie Boulevard, Philadelphia, PA 19104, USA
* Division of Endocrinology and Diabetes, The Thyroid Center, Children's Hospital of Philadelphia, 3500 Civic Center Boulevard, Buerger Center, 12-149, Philadelphia, PA 19104.
E-mail address: bauera@chop.edu

Endocrinol Metab Clin N Am 49 (2020) 589–611
https://doi.org/10.1016/j.ecl.2020.08.001
0889-8529/20/© 2020 Elsevier Inc. All rights reserved.

smaller number of patients, there is an identifiable risk factor, including ionizing radiation (inhaled, ingested, or external beam) in PTC or genetic predisposition in patients with PTC, FTC, or MTC.

Radiation treatment of nonthyroid malignancy is the most common identifiable cause associated with developing PTC with increased risk, and decreased latency, associated with exposure to ionizing radiation before 10 years of age.[2–4] The overall standard incidence ratio for radiation-induced DTC ranges from 5-fold to 70-fold, with the risk limited to patients less than 16 years of age at the time of exposure.[5] The higher proliferative cellular activity in the thyroid of children or adolescents compared with adults is thought to explain the disparate effect that all forms of radiation have on radiation-induced thyroid tumorigenesis.[3]

Genetic predisposition is the second most common identifiable risk factor for the development of thyroid cancer. Predisposition can be divided into 2 broad categories: nonsyndromic (familial thyroid cancer that is not associated with a clinical phenotype and not associated with an increased risk of developing additional, nonthyroid tumors) and syndromic (thyroid cancer associated with other tumors). The former, often referred to as familial nonmedullary thyroid cancer (FNMTC), is defined by the presence of 2 or more first-degree relatives with either PTC or FTC with the inheritance pattern most consistent with an autosomal dominant mode of transmission.[6,7] Compared with sporadic DTC, FNMTC presents at a younger age and shows clinical anticipation between generations, in which subsequent generation family members may present with earlier and more invasive disease.[8] To date, a single, reliable germline locus has not been identified, necessitating thyroid ultrasonography (US) monitoring of other first-degree family members.[9,10]

Syndromic forms of thyroid cancer are associated with germline mutations in several genes, with resultant increased risk for thyroid cancer, other nonthyroid neoplasms, and phenotypic findings on physical examination. The syndromic, familial thyroid cancer predisposition syndromes are inherited in an autosomal dominant pattern and include PTEN hamartoma tumor syndrome (PHTS), familial adenomatous polyposis (FAP), DICER1 syndrome, Carney complex (CNC), and MEN2 (**Table 1**). The risk of developing thyroid cancer in syndromic DTC is approximately 10% in FAP,[11] 16% in DICER1-related disorders,[12] and 35% in PTEN hamartoma tumor syndrome.[13] In DICER1, treatment of pleuropulmonary blastoma is associated with an increased risk of developing thyroid nodules and DTC before adolescence.[14] In general, syndromic DTC is typically associated with indolent behavior and the cancers are less invasive. However, in both CNC[15] and DICER1,[16] fatal outcomes associated with poorly differentiated thyroid cancer have been reported.

For the remaining, and larger number of, patients, DTC develops sporadically, without an identifiable risk factor. In these patients, thyroid tumorigenesis and progression are most commonly associated with somatic point mutations in BRAF, RAS, DICER1, and PTEN, as well as gene fusions involving the rearranged during transfection (RET), neurotropic tropomyosin receptor kinase (NTRK) tyrosine kinases, and anaplastic lymphoma kinase (ALK) with resultant constitutive activation of the mitogen-activated protein kinase (MAPK) and phosphatidylinositol 3-kinase (PI3K) protein kinase B (AKT) signaling pathways.[17,18] With uncommon exceptions, these genetic alterations are mutually exclusive events, and a fairly predictable relationship exists between oncogenic genotype and histopathologic phenotype, with (1) RET/PTC and NTRK rearrangements and BRAF point mutations common in PTC; (2) paired-box gene 8 (PAX8)–peroxisome proliferator–activated receptor gamma (PPARγ) rearrangement and DICER1 mutations common in FTC; and (3) RAS, DICER1, and PTEN mutations found across the spectrum of thyroid tumors, from benign follicular

Table 1
Familial thyroid cancer predisposition syndromes with additional clinical features

Predisposition Syndrome	Gene (Chromosome) with GeneReviews Link	Thyroid Phenotype	Other Features
PHTS • Cowden syndrome, Bannayan-Riley-Ruvalcaba syndrome	PTEN (10q23) https://www.ncbi.nlm.nih.gov/books/NBK1488/	• Thyroid adenomas and multinodular goiter • Thyroid carcinoma (PTC and FTC)	• Macrocephaly (95% or more) • Mucocutaneous lesions; papillomatous papules, trichilemmomas, acral keratoses, pigmented macules of the glans penis • Breast cancer (women only) • Endometrial carcinoma/uterine fibroids • Genitourinary tumors • Autism
DICER1 syndrome DICER1 pleuropulmonary blastoma familial tumor predisposition syndrome	DICER1 (14q32.13) https://www.ncbi.nlm.nih.gov/books/NBK196157/	• Multinodular goiter • Thyroid carcinoma (PTC, FTC, and poorly differentiated thyroid carcinoma/rare)	• Pleuropulmonary blastoma • Sertoli-Leydig cell ovarian tumor • Cystic nephroma • Wilms tumor • Botryoid embryonal rhabdomyosarcoma • Eye and nose tumors • Pituitary blastoma
APC-associated polyposis FAP	APC (5q21-q22) https://www.ncbi.nlm.nih.gov/books/NBK1345/	• PTC, cribriform-morular variant	• Adrenocortical tumors • Colorectal polyps/colorectal carcinoma • Osteomas • Desmoid tumors • Pancreas adenocarcinomas • Medulloblastoma • Hepatoblastoma

(continued on next page)

Table 1
(continued)

Predisposition Syndrome	Gene (Chromosome) with GeneReviews Link	Thyroid Phenotype	Other Features
Carney complex	*PRKAR1A* (17q24.2) and chromosome locus 2p16 (unknown gene) https://www.ncbi.nlm.nih.gov/books/NBK1286/	• Thyroid adenomas • Thyroid carcinoma (PTC FTC, and poorly differentiated thyroid carcinoma/rare)	• Mammosomatotroph • Growth hormone–secreting pituitary adenoma • Primary pigmented nodular adrenocortical disease • Large-cell calcifying Sertoli cell tumors • Spotty skin pigmentation (lentigines) • Blue nevi • Cardiac, cutaneous, or breast myxomas • Psammomatous melanotic schwannoma
MEN2A	*RET* (10q11.2) https://www.ncbi.nlm.nih.gov/books/NBK1257/	• Medullary thyroid carcinoma	• Pheochromocytoma • Parathyroid adenoma/hyperplasia • Codon-specific variants with cutaneous lichen amyloidosis and Hirschsprung disease

| MEN2B | *RET* (10q11.2) | • Medullary thyroid carcinoma | Infancy
• Absent tears in infancy (alacrima)
• Feeding difficulties and constipation
• Hypotonia
Later onset
• Pheochromocytoma
• Mucosal neuromas: lips, tongue, and eyelids
• Distinctive facies with enlarged lips
• Skeletal abnormalities; joint laxity, slipped capital femoral epiphysis, pes cavus
• Ganglioneuromatosis of the gastrointestinal tract
• Marfanoid body habitus |

Data from Adam MP, Ardinger HH, Pagon RA et al. GeneReviews [Internet]. Seattle, WA: University of Washington, Seattle; 1993-2020. https://www.ncbi.nlm.nih.gov/books/NBK1116/. Accessed July 28, 2020.

adenomas to follicular-variant PTC (fvPTC), FTC, and poorly differentiated thyroid carcinoma.[15,16,18] In pediatrics, *RET/PTC* and *NTRK*-fusion genes are associated with an increased risk of invasive disease, although there are no data to suggest that these alterations are associated with increased disease-specific mortality.[17,18] In children, *BRAF* mutations do not seem to be associated with an increased risk of radioactive iodine (RAI)–refractory disease, an association that is common in adults.[17] A summary of the most common oncogenes and their association with thyroid cancer variants and clinical behavior is provided in **Table 2**.

CAUSE AND GENETICS OF MEDULLARY THYROID CARCINOMA

MTC is a malignancy that originates from the parafollicular C cells of the thyroid gland rather than the follicular cells, the origin of DTC.[19] Thus, in contrast with follicular cell–derived thyroid tumors, MTC cells are not responsive to thyroid-stimulating hormone (TSH), are not responsive to RAI therapy secondary to a lack of expression of the sodium-iodine symporter, and do not produce thyroglobulin (Tg). C cells produce calcitonin (Ctn) and carcinoembryonic antigen (CEA), both of which serve as tumor markers of MTC. With rare exceptions, MTC in children and adolescents is associated with MEN2, an autosomal dominant tumor predisposition syndrome associated with activating germline mutations in the *RET* protooncogene, designated as either MEN2A or MEN2B depending on the specific mutation.[20,21] Sporadic MTC is uncommon in the pediatric population and, similar to adults, is most commonly associated with somatic mutations of *RET* or *RAS*, with data from adults suggesting a higher rate of lymph node metastasis and decreased survival associated with *RET*-associated sporadic MTC.[19,22]

DIAGNOSTIC EVALUATION OF THYROID NODULE
Physical Examination

Physical findings related to genetic syndromes should be evaluated and recorded. PHTS is associated with macrocephaly, small benign cutaneous neoplasms on the face and neck (trichilemmomas), lipomas, and freckling of the glans penis.[23–25] Carney complex[26] and FAP[27] are associated with lentigines and MEN2B is associated with alacrima (an inability or decreased ability to produce tears); marfanoid facies (typically noted around 5 years of age); and oral mucosal neuromas, most commonly of the lips and tongue.[28]

A complete thyroid examination includes inspection and palpation of the thyroid gland as well as the lateral neck cervical lymph nodes (https://www.youtube.com/watch?v=Z9norsLPKfU). The presence of a thyroid nodule with cervical lymphadenopathy is a significant predictor for malignancy, especially if the lymph nodes are firm, immobile, and located in levels III (mid) and IV (lower) regions of the lateral neck.[29,30] In contrast, rubbery, mobile, and symmetric level II (under the mandible) lymph nodes are a common finding in otherwise healthy pediatric patients despite these lymph nodes being larger on physical and US examination.

Laboratory Evaluation

In general, there are no laboratory tests or values that can help discern the risk that a thyroid nodule is more likely to be benign or malignant. The 1 exception is that a suppressed TSH level is often associated with an autonomously functioning thyroid nodule, a nodule that carries a lower risk of malignancy in both adult and pediatric patients (1%–10%).[31] A serum Ctn level should be obtained if the patient has a family history of MEN2, clinical features suggestive of MEN2B, or if the cytology is suspicion

Table 2
Oncogenic mutation with correlation to histology and invasive potential, recommended surgical approach, and potential systemic therapy for neoadjuvant or adjuvant therapy

Somatic Driver Mutation	Histology	Invasive Potential[a]	Surgical Approach	Multikinase Inhibitor[b]	Systemic Therapy (Clinical Trials #)
Gene Fusion					
RET fusions and mutations	PTC	High	Thyroidectomy with central neck lymph node dissection; lateral neck dissection based on US and FNA	Lenvatinib Sorafenib	BLU-667 (NCT03037385) LOXO-292 (NCT03157128; NCT03899792)
	MTC	Based on RET codon	Based on calcitonin level, imaging, FNA	Vandetanib Cabozantinib	
NTRK fusion	PTC	High	Thyroidectomy with central neck lymph node dissection; lateral neck dissection based on US and FNA	Lenvatinib Sorafenib	Larotrectinib (all ages) Entrectinib (12 y and older)
ALK fusion[c]	PTC	High	Thyroidectomy with central neck lymph node dissection; lateral neck dissection based on US and FNA	Lenvatinib Sorafenib	Crizotinib (NCT02034981) Ceritinib (NCT02289144) Alectinib (NCT03194893) Ensartinib (NCT03155620)
	MTC	Limited cases	Based on calcitonin level, imaging, FNA	Vandetanib Cabozantinib	
Point Mutation					
BRAFV600E	PTC	Intermediate	Thyroidectomy with central neck lymph node dissection; lateral neck dissection based on US and FNA	Lenvatinib Sorafenib	Vemurafenib (NCT03155620) Dabrafenib with trametinib

(continued on next page)

Table 2
(continued)

Somatic Driver Mutation	Histology	Invasive Potential[a]	Surgical Approach	Multikinase Inhibitor[b]	Systemic Therapy (Clinical Trials #)
RAS[c] PTEN DICER1[c] PAX8/PPARg[c]	PTC, FTC, and benign	Low	Lobectomy if unilateral disease Consider thyroidectomy if thyroid cancer predisposition syndrome or autoimmune thyroiditis	Lenvatinib Sorafenib	No current medical therapy
TSHR GNAS	Benign	Not applicable	Lobectomy	Not applicable	Not applicable
TERT, EIF1X, CTNNB1, AKT1, others	PTC and FTC	Limited data in pediatrics			

Abbreviations: FNA, fine-needle aspiration; TSHR, thyroid-stimulating hormone receptor.
[a] Invasive potential: (1) low, intrathyroidal; (2) intermediate, intrathyroidal and N1a; (3) high, intrathyroidal, N1a/N1b and M1.
[b] Multikinase inhibitors are selected based on thyroid cancer variant (DTC vs MTC) not oncogene. NCT01876784 and NCT03690388 are ongoing studies of re-fractory DTC.
[c] May be associated with poorly differentiated thyroid cancer; rare in pediatrics.

for MTC.[32] Clinicians should be aware that, in infants and young children, there is a normal physiologic increase in Ctn level, with values as high as 35 ng/L before 6 months of age that decrease into the adult range by approximately 3 years of age.[33]

Radiologic Imaging

Thyroid and neck US is the best radiologic modality to assess thyroid tissue morphology and lymph node status. Both the American Thyroid Association (ATA) adult thyroid nodule pictorial risk classification system and the Thyroid Imaging Reporting and Data System (TI-RADS) in children and adolescents may be used as a construct paradigm to stratify the nodules that should undergo further evaluation with fine-needle aspiration (FNA).[34] The US report should describe the background echogenicity of the thyroid parenchyma as well as the size, location, composition (solid, cystic, or spongiform), echogenicity (hypoechoic, isoechoic, or hyperechoic), shape (taller than wide on transverse imaging), margins (regular, infiltrative, microlobulated, or macrolobulated, and the presence or absence of extrathyroidal extension [ETE]), and the presence of echogenic foci in the nodules. Cystic composition is the single most reliable feature for assessing the risk of malignancy, with cystic composition greater than 75% associated with lower risk.[35,36] In patients with a thyroid nodule, US evaluation of the lateral neck should be performed looking for the presence of abnormal lymph nodes. Abnormal US features of lymph nodes that are consistent with thyroid cancer metastasis include rounded shape, increased echogenicity with loss of the hilum, cystic composition, echogenic foci, and increased peripheral blood flow on Doppler imaging.[37]

Most adult criteria for selecting nodules for FNA apply to children and adolescents, with the following exceptions: (1) US features and clinical context should be considered rather than size to select nodules for FNA[38]; and (2) a widely invasive form of PTC, called diffuse sclerosing variant PTC (dsvPTC), presents with nonnodular, diffuse infiltration of the thyroid associated with diffuse microcalcifications throughout the gland, a snowstorm appearance on US.[39–41] dsvPTC is commonly associated with macroscopic metastasis to lateral neck lymph nodes as well as increased thyroglobulin antibody or anti-thyroglobulin (TgAb) level.[40,42] The nonnodular appearance and the presence of increased TgAb level may mimic autoimmune hypothyroidism; however, the diffuse echogenic foci and abnormal lateral neck lymph node should help distinguish between these two conditions.

There is ongoing debate whether patients at increased risk for developing thyroid cancer should undergo monitoring by thyroid US or by physical examination. For oncology survivors treated with radiation, the most recent recommendation suggests that patients and families should be counseled about the options for surveillance but that US detects tumors at an earlier state of growth and invasiveness.[43] In familial thyroid cancer predisposition syndromes (PHTS, DICER1, and FAP), thyroid surveillance by US is recommended. However, the approach to evaluation and treatment of thyroid nodules must be considered within the context of the generally indolent behavior of DTC-predisposition syndromes.

The risk of performing thyroid US is minimal when clinicians experienced in reading thyroid US images and managing pediatric thyroid nodular disease are involved in the process. Complication from thyroid nodule aspiration are extraordinarily low and the rate of permanent complications from thyroid surgery should be less than 3% to 5% if performed by a high-volume thyroid surgeon.[44] Thus, in populations at increased risk of developing DTC, the benefit of pursuing thyroid US monitoring seems to outweigh the risk of the procedure.

Fine-Needle Aspiration

As in adults, The Bethesda System for Reporting Thyroid Cytopathology (TBSRTC) is used to classify the FNA results in pediatrics with equal sensitivity, specificity, and overall accuracy.[36,45] However, although the results of the FNA are similarly used to stratify an appropriate management plan, there seems to be an increased risk of malignancy for pediatric patients with benign and indeterminate cytology. In adults, benign cytology is associated with a 0% to 3% risk of malignancy, whereas, in pediatrics, the risk of malignancy may be as high as 10%.[46] For nodules with TBSRTC category III (atypia of undetermined significance or follicular lesion of undetermined significance), category IV (follicular neoplasm), or category V (suspicious for malignancy) the risk of malignancy may be as high as 28%, 58%, and 100%, respectively.[46]

For patients with nondiagnostic cytology (TBSRTC category 1), repeat FNA may be considered but there should be a 3-month delay between FNAs to avoid potential post-FNA reactive cellular atypia.[47] Cytologic confirmation of sample adequacy at the bedside can decrease the rate of nondiagnostic results. Nodules that are category V and VI (suspicious for malignancy and malignant) correlate with a near 100% risk of PTC.[46]

In an effort to decrease reliance on diagnostic surgery, there is increasing use of supplemental molecular profile testing in pediatrics following the more widespread use of oncogene panels and gene-expression classifier testing in adults. Based on current data, oncogene panels are the only test that have clinical utility to predict an increased risk for malignancy in patients less than 19 years of age.[46] In children, the presence of a thyroid oncogene mutation or fusion ($BRAF^{V600E}$, RET/PTC, NTRK fusion, and others) in an indeterminate FNA specimen is associated with a near-100% likelihood of PTC.[48,49] The presence of other mutations and fusions, including RAS, DICER1, and PTEN, is associated with both benign and malignant disease, and, until additional molecular markers are available, diagnostic lobectomy for unilateral nodules with indeterminate oncogenes is still the best approach to determining the malignant potential (see **Table 2**).[17] For nodules with indeterminate oncogenes, or without an identifiable oncogene, microRNA testing may provide further preoperative risk stratification for identifying malignancy.[50]

SURGICAL MANAGEMENT

Thyroid surgery should be performed by a high-volume thyroid surgeon, defined as a surgeon who performs 30 or more cervical endocrine procedures annually within the age group of the patient undergoing surgery, in an effort to minimize the risk of operative complications.[38,44,51] Although the exact number of surgeries performed annually may not reflect the quality of the surgeon, it increases the likelihood that the surgeon understands the disease process in pediatric patients and is familiar with age-specific treatment recommendations. Even in the pediatric setting, the goal should be to minimize the risk of permanent surgical complications to less than 1% to 3%.[52]

Complete and accurate preoperative radiologic imaging, with FNA confirmation of at least 1 abnormal lymph node per cervical level of the neck, is critical to optimize the surgical plan and reduce the risk of an incomplete dissection that may necessitate a second operative procedure. PTC typically follows a predictable pattern of metastasis from the thyroid to the central neck (level VI) followed by spread to the lateral neck (levels II; III; IV; and, rarely, V). In general, neck US is adequate for preoperative planning. Anatomic imaging with computed tomography (CT) or MRI may be added to assess for areas not easily visualized by US.[53]

The use of intraoperative parathyroid hormone levels helps to identify patients at risk of hypoparathyroidism and to ensure early administration of calcium and calcitriol in an effort to avoid symptomatic hypocalcemia.[54] The perioperative calcium and phosphorus levels must be monitored to ensure stable values before discharge from the inpatient setting.[54,55] Early identification of hypoparathyroidism with subsequent initiation of calcitriol and calcium decreases the risk of symptomatic hypocalcemia, as well as the duration of postoperative hospitalization.[52,54,55]

Papillary Thyroid Cancer

The ATA pediatric guidelines recommend that most children with PTC undergo total or near-total thyroidectomy.[38] This recommendation is based on data showing an increased risk of bilateral disease in children, including a recent report of 172 children and adolescents where up to 40% had bilateral disease, with 23% (40 of 172) not detected on preoperative thyroid US.[56] These findings corroborate previous reports showing a lower risk of recurrence in children undergoing thyroidectomy compared with lobectomy, 6% versus 30%, respectively, over 4 decades of observation.[57]

However, lobectomy may suffice to achieve surgical remission in a subgroup of patients with noninvasive or low-invasive disease. US findings consistent with a lower risk of invasion include solid nodules that are not taller than wide on transverse imaging with smooth margins and no evidence of microcalcifications or lymphadenopathy.[58] Cytology of these lesions is often indeterminate (TBSRTC III or IV), with the final histology revealing encapsulated fvPTC,[59] minimally invasive FTC (miFTC),[38,60] or the recently designated noninvasive follicular thyroid neoplasm with papillarylike nuclear features.[61]

Prophylactic central neck lymph node dissection should be considered in pediatric patients undergoing surgery for nodules with cytology suspicious for, or consistent with, PTC (Bethesda category V and VI) secondary to a high risk of central neck (level VI) metastasis.[38] In addition, the ATA pediatric risk levels are designed to use the data obtained from the central neck lymph node dissection to stratify patients into 3 levels of persistent postoperative disease (low, intermediate, and high) for selection of patients that may benefit from RAI therapy.[38]

A therapeutic central neck dissection should be performed in all children found to have central and/or lateral neck lymph node metastases on preoperative evaluation. Lateral neck dissections should only be performed in the presence of FNA-proven metastatic lateral neck disease. When nodal dissection is performed, a complete dissection of the affected compartment should be performed, rather than "berry picking."[38]

Follicular Thyroid Cancer

In contrast with PTC, FTC is typically unifocal and shows hematogenous rather than lymphatic metastasis. Pediatric FTC is diagnosed in 10% or less of pediatric patients with DTC. FTC may develop as part of PHTS. Thus, clinicians should have a high index of suspicion in children with FTC, particularly in those with macrocephaly, lipoma, freckling of the glans penis, or a suggestive family history.[23,25,62]

FTC is typically subdivided into miFTC and widely invasive FTC (wiFTC). miFTC is defined as FTC with microscopic or no capsular invasion and/or limited vascular invasion, less than 4 vessels in or adjacent to the tumor capsule.[60] wiFTC is defined as FTC with widespread capsular invasion, widespread vascular invasion, or tumor extension into adjacent, surrounding tissue. Invasion of 4 or more vessels is associated with an increased risk of distant metastases and poorer prognosis.[63–65]

Similar to adult patients, children ultimately diagnosed with FTC typically have indeterminate FNA cytology (TBSRTC III or IV). Thus, the most initially undergo diagnostic lobectomy with consideration of total thyroidectomy for patients with underlying thyroid disease, bilateral nodules, or a known diagnosis of a thyroid tumor predisposition syndrome, such as PHTS. Frozen section cannot be used to rule out FTC because the diagnosis is based on complete histologic examination of the nodule capsule to determine whether the nodule is a follicular adenoma (no evidence of invasion) or follicular carcinoma (evidence of capsular and vascular invasion).[66] For minimally invasive FTC, lobectomy is considered sufficient to achieve surgical remission. For widely invasive FTC, completion thyroidectomy should be performed along with a postoperative RAI diagnostic whole-body scan (DxWBS) to assess for evidence of distant metastasis, most commonly to the lung or bone.[67,68]

Medullary Thyroid Cancer

For patients with MEN2, the ATA divides the germline *RET* mutations into 3 risk categories for developing MTC (highest risk, high risk, and moderate risk) and bases the recommended age for initial screening, as well as the timing of prophylactic thyroidectomy, to coincide with the goal of achieving surgical remission.[19] Total thyroidectomy is recommended as follows: within the first year of life for carriers of the highest-risk mutation (MEN2B, codon 918), at or before age 5 years for those with a high-risk mutation (MEN2A, codons 634 and 883), and for all other moderate-risk mutations when the serum Ctn level shows an increasing upward trend or at any time the parents or patient do not wish to continue with laboratory surveillance.[19] For patients with moderate-risk mutations, the course from C-cell hyperplasia to MTC may be indolent, with MTC not developing until the third, fourth, or later decades of life. Thyroid US is useful to detect the location of a thyroid nodule and to assess for regional lymph node disease. However, it is not as sensitive as serum Ctn to determine the timing of thyroidectomy to optimize surgical remission.[69] As a general rule, thyroidectomy should be scheduled once the Ctn level shows an upward trend above the normal range. A central lymph node dissection is recommended in children whose basal Ctn level is greater than 40 ng/L and in all patients that display central or lateral neck lymph node metastasis.[19,70]

In contrast with MEN2A, mutations in codon 918 (MEN2B) are more often de novo. Thus, recognition of the early clinical signs and symptoms is critically important in order to diagnose the syndrome before MTC metastasis, which may occur before 1 year of age or, more commonly, before 4 years of age.[71,72] The earliest clinical signs and symptoms of MEN2B include alacrima (the inability, or decreased ability, to make tears), constipation (associated with intestinal ganglioneuromatosis), and hypotonia (feeding difficulties with failure to thrive, club feet, hip dislocation).[28] The more classically defining symptoms, including oral and lip mucosal neuromas and elongated, marfanoid facies, are not clinically evident until school age, around 5 years of age.[28,73]

MEDICAL THERAPY
Radioactive Iodine Therapy

RAI is a highly effective, targeted medical therapy to treat persistent postsurgical disease. Over the past 5 decades, there has been a near 2-fold increase in the number of patients receiving RAI without any impact on the excellent (~98%) 20-year disease-specific survival.[74] Although there is a paucity of long-term prospective data to define the lifetime risk of RAI administered during childhood and adolescence, with increased awareness of the potential short-term and long-term risks of ^{131}I therapy there are renewed efforts to identify which patients may (ATA pediatric intermediate and high risk) or may not (ATA pediatric low risk) benefit from ^{131}I therapy.[38,75,76]

Although there is no staging system for children and adolescents with PTC secondary to the extremely low disease-specific mortality, the American Joint Committee on Cancer (AJCC) tumor, nodes, metastases (TNM) classification system[77] is used to describe the extent of disease and stratify which patients may or may not benefit from RAI. The following is an updated version of the ATA pediatric risk levels with proposed adjustments based on recent data (**Table 3**).[38,58,78]

1. ATA pediatric low risk is defined by disease grossly confined to the thyroid with N0 (no lymph node metastasis) or less than or equal to 5 metastatic lymph nodes from the central neck (N1a).[58,78] It is difficult to assess the risk of persistent lymph node disease in patients who have no lymph nodes resected (Nx). However, the risk may be considered low if the primary tumor had no invasive potential (ie, miFTC), low-invasive potential (ie, Enc-fvPTC), or was a DTC with a low-invasive somatic oncogene (ie, *RAS*, *DICER1*, or *PTEN*).
2. ATA pediatric intermediate risk is defined by the presence of ETE (microscopic or gross); unilateral or lateral neck lymph node metastasis (N1b); or 6 to 10 metastatic lymph nodes (extensive N1a). The addition of ETE to the intermediate risk level is important if a central neck lymph node dissection was not performed because ETE has been shown to be associated with an increased risk for lymph node metastasis.[58] Clinicians should be aware that microETE was removed as a criterion for T3 tumors in the eighth edition of the AJCC TNM classification system. The synoptic pathology report must be reviewed in order to identify whether microETE was present in order to accurately interpret the risk of postoperative persistent disease.[77]
3. ATA pediatric high risk is defined by regionally extensive disease, including bilateral N1b, greater than 10 metastatic lymph nodes, and patients with distant metastasis (M1) being considered high risk for persistent postoperative disease.

For ATA low-risk patients, clinicians may consider following the TSH-suppressed Tg level with repeat neck US instead of pursuing a stimulated Tg level with DxWBS in the immediate postoperative time frame. A stimulated Tg and DxWBS can be performed

Table 3		
Proposed update to the American Thyroid Association postsurgical risk levels to guide selection for radioactive iodine therapy		
ATA Pediatric Risk Level	**Definition**	**Initial Postoperative Evaluation**
Low risk	Disease confined to the thyroid gland and N0 or N1a with ≤5 metastatic lymph nodes[a]	TSH-suppressed Tg
Intermediate risk	Presence of extrathyroidal extension or unilateral N1b or 6–10 metastatic lymph nodes	TSH-stimulated (>30 mIU/L) Tg and RAI DxWBS
High risk	Bilateral N1b or >10 metastatic lymph nodes or distant metastasis (M1)	TSH-stimulated (>30 mIU/L) Tg and RAI DxWBS

Abbreviations: N0, no metastatic lymph nodes; N1a, metastasis to lymph nodes limited to the central neck (level VI); N1b, metastasis to lymph nodes in the lateral neck (levels II, III, and/or IV).
[a] See text for discussion of the risk associated with Nx (no lymph nodes removed).

at a later time if there is an unexpected increased and/or increasing Tg level and no evidence of disease based on US and/or anatomic imaging (CT or MRI).[38,75,76]

For intermediate-risk and high-risk patients, a TSH-stimulated Tg level and a ^{123}I-DxWBS are recommended to search for residual or metastatic disease.[38] The use of ^{123}I is favored rather than ^{131}I because of superior imaging quality and prevention of stunning.[79]

The decision to administer ^{131}I therapy should be based on the TSH-stimulated Tg level as well as the data obtained from the ^{123}I-DxWBS. A TSH-stimulated Tg level 2 ng/mL has a 94.9% predictive value for the absence of postsurgical disease.[80] If TSH-stimulated Tg level is 2 to 10 ng/mL, ^{131}I therapy should be considered for patients with thyroid bed uptake; invasive histology, including dsvPTC, solid-variant PTC (sPTC), and widely invasive fvPTC (wi-fvPTC); evidence of gross ETE; extranodal extension; or in patients with extensive regional metastasis (extensive N1a or any N1b disease). If the TSH-stimulated Tg level is greater than 10 ng/mL, ^{131}I therapy is indicated. Repeat surgery before administration of ^{131}I should be pursued if there is evidence of persistent, macroscopic disease noted during this initial postoperative time frame because there is reduced efficacy for RAI ablation of lymph nodes larger than 1 cm.[32] The addition of single-photon emission CT with integrated conventional CT may provide more accurate anatomic localization to differentiate metastatic regional lymph node from remnant thyroid tissue.[81]

Therapeutic ^{131}I can be dosed empirically or based on bone marrow dose-limited dosimetry. There are 2 formulas to decide on empiric dosing: (1) given as a fraction of a child's weight compared with an average-sized adult (kilograms divided by 70 kg) multiplied by a typical adult dose used to treat similar disease extent,[82,83] or (2) based on millicuries/weight with a typical range between 1.0 and 3.0 mCi/Kg based on the presence of regional or distant disease.[84] Dosimetry should be considered in younger children (<10 years), those with diffuse pulmonary metastases, and those who received radiation therapy for other malignancies.[85] A posttreatment whole-body scan should be obtained 5 to 7 days after all ^{131}I treatments and is associated with a greater sensitivity for detecting persistent disease compared with the DxWBS.[86]

Even with efforts to limit the delivered activity and frequency of RAI, long-term follow-up studies are needed to confirm or refute previous reports on the risk of developing RAI-induced, second primary malignancies (SPMs).[57,74,87,88] Although the overall numbers are small, many of the SPMs are in iodine-avid glands (ie, salivary glands) or in nonavid tissues passively exposed to ^{131}I during physiologic clearance (bone marrow, colon, bladder, and others).[57,89] Thus, the challenge is to determine whether the SPM is RAI related or associated with risk factors that led to development of the thyroid malignancy. Clinicians should not fear the use of RAI. However, there is an obligation to differentiate patients who may benefit from ^{131}I therapy from patients in whom the risks of RAI outweigh the benefit. In pediatrics, the goals of achieving remission and avoiding recurrence must be balanced with the risk of complications of therapy.

PERSISTENT AND RECURRENT DISEASE

Cervical lymph nodes are the most common location for residual and recurrent PTC.[90–92] If macroscopic cervical disease is identified by imaging and confirmed via FNA, surgery is preferable to ^{131}I therapy.[93,94] Children with iodine-avid, small-volume cervical disease can be considered for therapeutic ^{131}I therapy depending on the individual risk/benefit ratio as well as the absence or presence of distant metastasis.[95]

US-guided percutaneous ethanol or radiofrequency ablation may be considered as nonsurgical treatment options in patients with a limited number of neck metastasis (1 or 2 lymph nodes) depending on the location and size of the lymph nodes.[95–97] The therapeutic success rates of ethanol injection and radiofrequency ablation have been reported to be between 70% and 98%, with decreased to absent blood flow and reduced posttreatment size of the lymph node 3 to 6 months after the procedure defining successful ablation.[95,96,98]

The lungs are the most common site for persistent or recurrent disease distal metastasis. In contrast with adults, children and adolescents with pulmonary metastasis have low disease-specific mortality, most likely secondary to the pulmonary lesions maintaining RAI avidity.[99,100] Retreatment of ^{131}I-avid pulmonary metastases should be considered in children who have shown previous improvement but continue to have persistent disease based on cross-sectional imaging obtained more than 1 to 2 years after the last RAI treatment, and sooner if there is evidence of disease progression on serial imaging obtained on a 6-month interval. The timing of additional ^{131}I should be at least 12 months from the previous treatment, with several studies showing a continuous decline in serum Tg levels for 18 to 24 months, or longer, following the previous RAI therapy.[100,101] However, up to one-third of children with significant pulmonary disease may develop stable, persistent, or progressive disease that does not respond to repeated doses of [131]I.[99]

Systemic Therapy for Radioactive Iodine–Refractory Differentiated Thyroid Cancer

A small proportion of children and adolescents develop progressive DTC that is refractory to ^{131}I therapy. RAI refractory (RAIR) is defined by the (1) absence of initial RAI uptake in metastasis; (2) absence of RAI uptake in metastasis after treatment with RAI; (3) presence of RAI uptake in some metastasis, but absence in others; and (4) progression despite RAI uptake in metastasis.[102] The main criteria for initiation of systemic therapy in adults are (1) large tumor burden with tumors larger than 1 to 2 cm, (2) Response Evaluation Criteria in Solid Tumors (RECIST) progressive disease over 12 months, and (3) symptomatic disease and risk of local complications.[102,103] There are no pediatric age-specific definitions for RAIR or criteria for when to initiate systemic therapy.

Over the last decade, there has been an increasing number of oral systemic therapies that have been incorporated into clinical practice for adults with similar disease. These agents target tyrosine kinase receptors or constitutively activated protein kinases in the MAPK and PI3K signaling pathways.[104] The multitargeted tyrosine kinase inhibitors (TKIs) target the vascular endothelial growth factor receptors as well as other tyrosine kinase receptors, including the epithelial growth factor receptor, fibroblast growth factor receptor, platelet-derived growth factor receptor, and RET. There are currently 4 MKIs that have received US Food and Drug Administration (FDA) approval for the treatment of advanced thyroid cancer: sorafenib and lenvatinib for DTC, and vandetanib and cabozantinib for MTC.[105] These agents are not tumoricidal but they have been shown to slow progression and to decrease tumor burden for many patients. However, in adults, the effect is often transient and many patients experience side effects, including hypertension, diarrhea, anorexia with weight loss, dermatitis, and fatigue.[105] Within pediatrics, there are several case reports where MKIs have been used; however, the data are limited and there is no consensus with regard to the timing to initiate therapy or in the selection of which oral chemotherapeutic agent should be used.[106,107]

The newer oncogene-specific targeted inhibitors have increased efficacy and less toxicity compared with the multityrosine inhibitors. Several of these agents have been in clinical use for several years, repurposed from other cancers with similar molecular alterations. The most effective of these molecular targeted inhibitors have shown remarkable clinical efficacy with regression in tumors harboring *RET*, *NTRK*, and *ALK* fusion genes and the *BRAF^V600E* mutation.[105] Larotrectinib (LOXO-101) is a selective *NTRK* inhibitor that has been approved for use in pediatric patients. The Children's Oncology Group (COG) recently opened a phase II study with larotrectinib (ADVL1823, NCT03834961) for children with previously untreated tropomyosin receptor kinase (TRK) fusion solid tumors, including thyroid cancer. This prospective study provides an opportunity to define the benefits and risks of medical therapy for children and adolescents with thyroid cancer for whom surgery caries a high risk of morbidity. In addition, the National Cancer Institute and COG Pediatric Molecular Analysis for Therapy Choice (MATCH) (NCT03155620) is a phase II study that offers access to several agents based on knowledge of the oncogenic driver mutation, including BRAF alterations (vemurafenib), ALK fusions (ensartinib), and soon to include RET mutations/fusions (LOXO 292).

Systemic Therapy for Medullary Thyroid Cancer

For patients with MTC with symptomatic or progressive metastatic disease that is not amenable to surgery, systemic treatment with receptor tyrosine kinase inhibitors or oncogene-specific targeted therapies against *RET* may be indicated (see **Table 2**). The same criteria used for initiation of systemic therapy, described earlier, should be followed for patients with MTC within the context that most patients with metastatic MTC do not achieve remission from disease. Vandetanib and cabozantinib have been FDA approved for the treatment of adults with progressive, metastatic MTC.[104,108] Limited data suggest that vandetanib is effective and well tolerated in children with advanced MTC in the setting of MEN2B.[109] The selective *RET* inhibitors (BLU-667 and LOXO-292) are currently in clinical trials, with preliminary data showing very favorable response with few side effects.[105]

FUTURE DIRECTIONS

Knowledge of the somatic oncogene driver mutation is becoming increasingly important for the diagnosis of thyroid nodules with indeterminate cytology as well as for the prediction of clinical behavior, response to therapy, and for the selection of systemic therapy.[17,18] **Table 2** summarizes a proposed oncogene-directed surgical approach, as well as potential multikinase inhibitors and oncogene-specific targeted therapy that could be used as neoadjuvant or adjuvant therapy. For patients that present with morbidly invasive disease, including evidence of recurrent laryngeal nerve paralysis, encasement of great vessels, or evidence of aerodigestive tract invasion, or with pulmonary metastasis associated with hypoxia, neoadjuvant systemic therapy should be considered. For patients with DTC, surgery and RAI should be pursued once the patient achieves improved clinical status associated with systemic therapy–induced tumor regression. For patients with MTC, surgery may be deferred if the systemic therapy is associated with significant regression because it is unlikely to achieve surgical remission once MTC metastasizes. For patients with progressive DTC or MTC that is not surgically resectable, or in patients with RAI-refractory DTC, adjuvant systemic therapy should be considered based on anatomic progression.

With the potential for significant side effects, and limited experience in using these agents in children and adolescents, multicenter collaborative studies are needed to better define the timing for initiation, selection of drug, monitoring, and adjustment of therapy so that outcome can be optimized while minimizing the risk of side effects and adverse events.[38,105,110]

DISCLOSURE

The author has no financial disclosures that affect the content of this article. The author has received an honorarium from Hexal AG to review abstracts for EndoToday (2019).

REFERENCES

1. Dermody S, Walls A, Harley EH Jr. Pediatric thyroid cancer: An update from the SEER database 2007-2012. Int J Pediatr Otorhinolaryngol 2016;89:121–6.
2. Meadows AT, Friedman DL, Neglia JP, et al. Second neoplasms in survivors of childhood cancer: findings from the Childhood Cancer Survivor Study cohort. J Clin Oncol 2009;27(14):2356–62.
3. Ron E, Lubin JH, Shore RE, et al. Thyroid cancer after exposure to external radiation: a pooled analysis of seven studies. Radiat Res 1995;141(3):259–77.
4. Ronckers CM, Sigurdson AJ, Stovall M, et al. Thyroid cancer in childhood cancer survivors: a detailed evaluation of radiation dose response and its modifiers. Radiat Res 2006;166(4):618–28.
5. Shuz J, (Chair) TKSC, Ahn HS, et al. Thyroid health monitoring after nuclear accidents. Lyon (France): World Health Organization; 2018.
6. Charkes ND. On the prevalence of familial nonmedullary thyroid cancer in multiply affected kindreds. Thyroid 2006;16(2):181–6.
7. Mazeh H, Benavidez J, Poehls JL, et al. In patients with thyroid cancer of follicular cell origin, a family history of nonmedullary thyroid cancer in one first-degree relative is associated with more aggressive disease. Thyroid 2012; 22(1):3–8.
8. Capezzone M, Marchisotta S, Cantara S, et al. Familial non-medullary thyroid carcinoma displays the features of clinical anticipation suggestive of a distinct biological entity. Endocr Relat Cancer 2008;15(4):1075–81.
9. Bauer AJ. Clinical behavior and genetics of nonsyndromic, familial nonmedullary thyroid cancer. Front Horm Res 2013;41:141–8.
10. Bauer AJ. Thyroid nodules and differentiated thyroid cancer. Endocr Dev 2014; 26:183–201.
11. Jasperson KW, Patel SG, Ahnen DJ. APC-Associated Polyposis Conditions. 1998 Dec 18 [updated 2017 Feb 2]. In: Adam MP, Ardinger HH, Pagon RA, et al, editors. GeneReviews® [Internet]. Seattle (WA): University of Washington, Seattle; 1993–2020. PMID: 20301519.
12. Khan NE, Bauer AJ, Schultz KAP, et al. Quantification of thyroid cancer and multinodular goiter risk in the DICER1 syndrome: a family-based cohort study. J Clin Endocrinol Metab 2017;102(5):1614–22.
13. Eng C. PTEN Hamartoma Tumor Syndrome. 2001 Nov 29 [updated 2016 Jun 2]. In: Adam MP, Ardinger HH, Pagon RA, et a, editors. GeneReviews® [Internet]. Seattle (WA): University of Washington, Seattle; 1993–2020. PMID: 20301661.
14. Schultz KAP, Williams GM, Kamihara J, et al. DICER1 and associated conditions: identification of at-risk individuals and recommended surveillance strategies. Clin Cancer Res 2018;24(10):2251–61.
15. Carney JA, Lyssikatos C, Seethala RR, et al. The spectrum of thyroid gland pathology in carney complex: the importance of follicular carcinoma. Am J Surg Pathol 2018;42(5):587–94.

16. Chernock RD, Rivera B, Borrelli N, et al. Poorly differentiated thyroid carcinoma of childhood and adolescence: a distinct entity characterized by DICER1 mutations. Mod Pathol 2020;33(7):1264–74.

17. Bauer AJ. Molecular genetics of thyroid cancer in children and adolescents. Endocrinol Metab Clin North Am 2017;46(2):389–403.

18. Paulson VA, Rudzinski ER, Hawkins DS. Thyroid cancer in the pediatric population. Genes (Basel) 2019;10(9):723.

19. Wells SA Jr, Asa SL, Dralle H, et al. Revised American Thyroid Association guidelines for the management of medullary thyroid carcinoma. Thyroid 2015; 25(6):567–610.

20. Waguespack SG, Rich TA, Perrier ND, et al. Management of medullary thyroid carcinoma and MEN2 syndromes in childhood. Nat Rev Endocrinol 2011; 7(10):596–607.

21. Margraf RL, Crockett DK, Krautscheid PM, et al. Multiple endocrine neoplasia type 2 RET protooncogene database: repository of MEN2-associated RET sequence variation and reference for genotype/phenotype correlations. Hum Mutat 2009;30(4):548–56.

22. Fussey JM, Vaidya B, Kim D, et al. The role of molecular genetics in the clinical management of sporadic medullary thyroid carcinoma: A systematic review. Clin Endocrinol (Oxf) 2019;91(6):697–707.

23. Pilarski R, Burt R, Kohlman W, et al. Cowden syndrome and the PTEN hamartoma tumor syndrome: systematic review and revised diagnostic criteria. J Natl Cancer Inst 2013;105(21):1607–16.

24. Lauper JM, Krause A, Vaughan TL, et al. Spectrum and risk of neoplasia in Werner syndrome: a systematic review. PLoS One 2013;8(4):e59709.

25. Bubien V, Bonnet F, Brouste V, et al. High cumulative risks of cancer in patients with PTEN hamartoma tumour syndrome. J Med Genet 2013;50(4):255–63.

26. Bertherat J, Horvath A, Groussin L, et al. Mutations in regulatory subunit type 1A of cyclic adenosine 5'-monophosphate-dependent protein kinase (PRKAR1A): phenotype analysis in 353 patients and 80 different genotypes. J Clin Endocrinol Metab 2009;94(6):2085–91.

27. Septer S, Slowik V, Morgan R, et al. Thyroid cancer complicating familial adenomatous polyposis: mutation spectrum of at-risk individuals. Hered Cancer Clin Pract 2013;11(1):13.

28. Wray CJ, Rich TA, Waguespack SG, et al. Failure to recognize multiple endocrine neoplasia 2B: more common than we think? Ann Surg Oncol 2008;15(1): 293–301.

29. Buryk MA, Simons JP, Picarsic J, et al. Can malignant thyroid nodules be distinguished from benign thyroid nodules in children and adolescents by clinical characteristics? A review of 89 pediatric patients with thyroid nodules. Thyroid 2015;25(4):392–400.

30. Papendieck P, Gruneiro-Papendieck L, Venara M, et al. Differentiated thyroid cancer in children: prevalence and predictors in a large cohort with thyroid nodules followed prospectively. J Pediatr 2015;167(1):199–201.

31. Ly S, Frates MC, Benson CB, et al. Features and outcome of autonomous thyroid nodules in children: 31 consecutive patients seen at a single center. J Clin Endocrinol Metab 2016;101(10):3856–62.

32. Haugen BR, Alexander EK, Bible KC, et al. 2015 American Thyroid Association Management Guidelines for Adult Patients with Thyroid Nodules and Differentiated Thyroid Cancer: The American Thyroid Association Guidelines Task Force

on Thyroid Nodules and Differentiated Thyroid Cancer. Thyroid 2016;26(1): 1–133.

33. Castagna MG, Fugazzola L, Maino F, et al. Reference range of serum calcitonin in pediatric population. J Clin Endocrinol Metab 2015;100(5):1780–4.

34. Martinez-Rios C, Daneman A, Bajno L, et al. Utility of adult-based ultrasound malignancy risk stratifications in pediatric thyroid nodules. Pediatr Radiol 2018;48(1):74–84.

35. Gannon AW, Langer JE, Bellah R, et al. Diagnostic accuracy of ultrasound with color flow doppler in children with thyroid nodules. J Clin Endocrinol Metab 2018;103(5):1958–65.

36. Gupta A, Ly S, Castroneves LA, et al. A standardized assessment of thyroid nodules in children confirms higher cancer prevalence than in adults. J Clin Endocrinol Metab 2013;98(8):3238–45.

37. Leboulleux S, Girard E, Rose M, et al. Ultrasound criteria of malignancy for cervical lymph nodes in patients followed up for differentiated thyroid cancer. J Clin Endocrinol Metab 2007;92(9):3590–4.

38. Francis GL, Waguespack SG, Bauer AJ, et al. Management guidelines for children with thyroid nodules and differentiated thyroid cancer. Thyroid 2015;25(7): 716–59.

39. Akaishi J, Sugino K, Kameyama K, et al. Clinicopathologic features and outcomes in patients with diffuse sclerosing variant of papillary thyroid carcinoma. World J Surg 2015;39(7):1728–35.

40. Koo JS, Hong S, Park CS. Diffuse sclerosing variant is a major subtype of papillary thyroid carcinoma in the young. Thyroid 2009;19(11):1225–31.

41. Lee JY, Shin JH, Han BK, et al. Diffuse sclerosing variant of papillary carcinoma of the thyroid: imaging and cytologic findings. Thyroid 2007;17(6):567–73.

42. Chen CC, Chen WC, Peng SL, et al. Diffuse sclerosing variant of thyroid papillary carcinoma: diagnostic challenges occur with Hashimoto's thyroiditis. J Formos Med Assoc 2013;112(6):358–62.

43. Clement SC, Kremer LCM, Verburg FA, et al. Balancing the benefits and harms of thyroid cancer surveillance in survivors of Childhood, adolescent and young adult cancer: Recommendations from the international Late Effects of Childhood Cancer Guideline Harmonization Group in collaboration with the PanCare-SurFup Consortium. Cancer Treat Rev 2018;63:28–39.

44. Adam MA, Thomas S, Youngwirth L, et al. Is there a minimum number of thyroidectomies a surgeon should perform to optimize patient outcomes? Ann Surg 2017;265(2):402–7.

45. Mussa A, De Andrea M, Motta M, et al. Predictors of malignancy in children with thyroid nodules. J Pediatr 2015;167(4):886–92.e1.

46. Bauer AJ. Thyroid nodules in children and adolescents. Curr Opin Endocrinol Diabetes Obes 2019;26(5):266–74.

47. Baloch ZW, LiVolsi VA. Post fine-needle aspiration histologic alterations of thyroid revisited. Am J Clin Pathol 1999;112(3):311–6.

48. Buryk MA, Monaco SE, Witchel SF, et al. Preoperative cytology with molecular analysis to help guide surgery for pediatric thyroid nodules. Int J Pediatr Otorhinolaryngol 2013;77(10):1697–700.

49. Monaco SE, Pantanowitz L, Khalbuss WE, et al. Cytomorphological and molecular genetic findings in pediatric thyroid fine-needle aspiration. Cancer Cytopathol 2012;120(5):342–50.

50. Franco AT, Labourier E, Ablordeppey KK, et al. miRNA expression can classify pediatric thyroid lesions and increases the diagnostic yield of mutation testing. Pediatr Blood Cancer 2020;67(6):e28276.

51. Sosa JA, Tuggle CT, Wang TS, et al. Clinical and economic outcomes of thyroid and parathyroid surgery in children. J Clin Endocrinol Metab 2008;93(8): 3058–65.

52. Baumgarten HD, Bauer AJ, Isaza A, et al. Surgical management of pediatric thyroid disease: Complication rates after thyroidectomy at the Children's Hospital of Philadelphia high-volume Pediatric Thyroid Center. J Pediatr Surg 2019;54(10): 1969–75.

53. Yeh MW, Bauer AJ, Bernet VA, et al. American Thyroid Association statement on preoperative imaging for thyroid cancer surgery. Thyroid 2015;25(1):3–14.

54. Tsai SD, Mostoufi-Moab S, Bauer S, et al. Clinical utility of intraoperative parathyroid hormone measurement in children and adolescents undergoing total thyroidectomy. Front Endocrinol (Lausanne) 2019;10:760.

55. Patel NA, Bly RA, Adams S, et al. A clinical pathway for the postoperative management of hypocalcemia after pediatric thyroidectomy reduces blood draws. Int J Pediatr Otorhinolaryngol 2018;105:132–7.

56. Baumgarten H, Jenks CM, Isaza A, et al. Bilateral papillary thyroid cancer in children: Risk factors and frequency of postoperative diagnosis. J Pediatr Surg 2020;55(6):1117–22.

57. Hay ID, Gonzalez-Losada T, Reinalda MS, et al. Long-term outcome in 215 children and adolescents with papillary thyroid cancer treated during 1940 through 2008. World J Surg 2010;34(6):1192–202.

58. Jain NK, Mostoufi-Moab S, Hawkes CP, et al. Extrathyroidal extension is an important predictor of regional lymph node metastasis in pediatric differentiated thyroid cancer. Thyroid 2020;30(7):1037–43.

59. Samuels SL, Surrey LF, Hawkes CP, et al. Characteristics of follicular variant papillary thyroid carcinoma in a pediatric cohort. J Clin Endocrinol Metab 2018;103(4):1639–48.

60. Dionigi G, Kraimps JL, Schmid KW, et al. Minimally invasive follicular thyroid cancer (MIFTC)–a consensus report of the European Society of Endocrine Surgeons (ESES). Langenbecks Arch Surg 2014;399(2):165–84.

61. Nikiforov YE, Baloch ZW, Hodak SP, et al. Change in diagnostic criteria for noninvasive follicular thyroid neoplasm with papillarylike nuclear features. JAMA Oncol 2018;4(8):1125–6.

62. Smith JR, Marqusee E, Webb S, et al. Thyroid nodules and cancer in children with PTEN hamartoma tumor syndrome. J Clin Endocrinol Metab 2011; 96(1):34–7.

63. Ito Y, Hirokawa M, Masuoka H, et al. Prognostic factors of minimally invasive follicular thyroid carcinoma: extensive vascular invasion significantly affects patient prognosis. Endocr J 2013;60(5):637–42.

64. Kim HJ, Sung JY, Oh YL, et al. Association of vascular invasion with increased mortality in patients with minimally invasive follicular thyroid carcinoma but not widely invasive follicular thyroid carcinoma. Head Neck 2014;36(12):1695–700.

65. O'Neill CJ, Vaughan L, Learoyd DL, et al. Management of follicular thyroid carcinoma should be individualised based on degree of capsular and vascular invasion. Eur J Surg Oncol 2011;37(2):181–5.

66. LiVolsi VA, Baloch ZW. Use and abuse of frozen section in the diagnosis of follicular thyroid lesions. Endocr Pathol 2005;16(4):285–93.

67. Sugino K, Ito K, Nagahama M, et al. Prognosis and prognostic factors for distant metastases and tumor mortality in follicular thyroid carcinoma. Thyroid 2011; 21(7):751–7.
68. Lin JD, Chao TC, Chen ST, et al. Operative strategy for follicular thyroid cancer in risk groups stratified by pTNM staging. Surg Oncol 2007;16(2):107–13.
69. Morris LF, Waguespack SG, Edeiken-Monroe BS, et al. Ultrasonography should not guide the timing of thyroidectomy in pediatric patients diagnosed with multiple endocrine neoplasia syndrome 2A through genetic screening. Ann Surg Oncol 2013;20(1):53–9.
70. Machens A, Schneyer U, Holzhausen HJ, et al. Prospects of remission in medullary thyroid carcinoma according to basal calcitonin level. J Clin Endocrinol Metab 2005;90(4):2029–34.
71. Brauckhoff M, Machens A, Lorenz K, et al. Surgical curability of medullary thyroid cancer in multiple endocrine neoplasia 2B: a changing perspective. Ann Surg 2014;259(4):800–6.
72. Castinetti F, Waguespack SG, Machens A, et al. Natural history, treatment, and long-term follow up of patients with multiple endocrine neoplasia type 2B: an international, multicentre, retrospective study. Lancet Diabetes Endocrinol 2019; 7(3):213–20.
73. Brauckhoff M, Machens A, Hess S, et al. Premonitory symptoms preceding metastatic medullary thyroid cancer in MEN 2B: An exploratory analysis. Surgery 2008;144(6):1044–50 [discussion: 1050–3].
74. Marti JL, Jain KS, Morris LG. Increased risk of second primary malignancy in pediatric and young adult patients treated with radioactive iodine for differentiated thyroid cancer. Thyroid 2015;25(6):681–7.
75. Lazar L, Lebenthal Y, Segal K, et al. Pediatric thyroid cancer: postoperative classifications and response to initial therapy as prognostic factors. J Clin Endocrinol Metab 2016;101(5):1970–9.
76. Pires B, Alves-Junior PA, Bordallo MA, et al. Prognostic factors for early and long-term remission in pediatric differentiated thyroid cancer: the role of gender, age, clinical presentation and the newly proposed American Thyroid Association risk stratification system. Thyroid 2016;26(10):1480–7.
77. Tuttle RMM, Haugen BRM, Perrier N. The Updated AJCC/TNM Staging System for Differentiated and Anaplastic Thyroid Cancer (8th edition): What changed and why? Thyroid 2017;27(6):751–6.
78. Jeon MJ, Kim YN, Sung TY, et al. Practical initial risk stratification based on lymph node metastases in pediatric and adolescent differentiated thyroid cancer. Thyroid 2018;28(2):193–200.
79. Schoelwer MJ, Zimmerman D, Shore RM, et al. The use of 123i in diagnostic radioactive iodine scans in children with differentiated thyroid carcinoma. Thyroid 2015;25(8):935–41.
80. Lee JI, Chung YJ, Cho BY, et al. Postoperative-stimulated serum thyroglobulin measured at the time of 131I ablation is useful for the prediction of disease status in patients with differentiated thyroid carcinoma. Surgery 2013;153(6): 828–35.
81. Xue YL, Qiu ZL, Song HJ, et al. Value of (1)(3)(1)I SPECT/CT for the evaluation of differentiated thyroid cancer: a systematic review of the literature. Eur J Nucl Med Mol Imaging 2013;40(5):768–78.
82. Hung W, Sarlis NJ. Current controversies in the management of pediatric patients with well-differentiated nonmedullary thyroid cancer: a review. Thyroid 2002;12(8):683–702.

83. Dinauer C, Francis GL. Thyroid cancer in children. Endocrinol Metab Clin North Am 2007;36(3):779–806, vii.

84. Jarzab B, Handkiewicz-Junak D, Wloch J. Juvenile differentiated thyroid carcinoma and the role of radioiodine in its treatment: a qualitative review. Endocr Relat Cancer 2005;12(4):773–803.

85. Lassmann M, Hanscheid H, Verburg FA, et al. The use of dosimetry in the treatment of differentiated thyroid cancer. Q J Nucl Med Mol Imaging 2011;55(2): 107–15.

86. Urhan M, Dadparvar S, Mavi A, et al. Iodine-123 as a diagnostic imaging agent in differentiated thyroid carcinoma: a comparison with iodine-131 post-treatment scanning and serum thyroglobulin measurement. Eur J Nucl Med Mol Imaging 2007;34(7):1012–7.

87. Brown AP, Chen J, Hitchcock YJ, et al. The risk of second primary malignancies up to three decades after the treatment of differentiated thyroid cancer. J Clin Endocrinol Metab 2008;93(2):504–15.

88. Lee YA, Jung HW, Kim HY, et al. Pediatric patients with multifocal papillary thyroid cancer have higher recurrence rates than adult patients: a retrospective analysis of a large pediatric thyroid cancer cohort over 33 years. J Clin Endocrinol Metab 2015;100(4):1619–29.

89. Klubo-Gwiezdzinska J, Van Nostrand D, Burman KD, et al. Salivary gland malignancy and radioiodine therapy for thyroid cancer. Thyroid 2010;20(6):647–51.

90. Hay ID, Hutchinson ME, Gonzalez-Losada T, et al. Papillary thyroid microcarcinoma: a study of 900 cases observed in a 60-year period. Surgery 2008;144(6): 980–7 [discussion: 987–8].

91. Chow SM, Law SC, Mendenhall WM, et al. Differentiated thyroid carcinoma in childhood and adolescence-clinical course and role of radioiodine. Pediatr Blood Cancer 2004;42(2):176–83.

92. Handkiewicz-Junak D, Wloch J, Roskosz J, et al. Total thyroidectomy and adjuvant radioiodine treatment independently decrease locoregional recurrence risk in childhood and adolescent differentiated thyroid cancer. J Nucl Med 2007; 48(6):879–88.

93. Clayman GL, Agarwal G, Edeiken BS, et al. Long-term outcome of comprehensive central compartment dissection in patients with recurrent/persistent papillary thyroid carcinoma. Thyroid 2011;21(12):1309–16.

94. Clayman GL, Shellenberger TD, Ginsberg LE, et al. Approach and safety of comprehensive central compartment dissection in patients with recurrent papillary thyroid carcinoma. Head Neck 2009;31(9):1152–63.

95. Hay ID, Lee RA, Davidge-Pitts C, et al. Long-term outcome of ultrasound-guided percutaneous ethanol ablation of selected "recurrent" neck nodal metastases in 25 patients with TNM stages III or IVA papillary thyroid carcinoma previously treated by surgery and 131I therapy. Surgery 2013;154(6):1448–54 [discussion: 1454–5].

96. Shin JE, Baek JH, Lee JH. Radiofrequency and ethanol ablation for the treatment of recurrent thyroid cancers: current status and challenges. Curr Opin Oncol 2013;25(1):14–9.

97. Heilo A, Sigstad E, Fagerlid KH, et al. Efficacy of ultrasound-guided percutaneous ethanol injection treatment in patients with a limited number of metastatic cervical lymph nodes from papillary thyroid carcinoma. J Clin Endocrinol Metab 2011;96(9):2750–5.

98. Kim SY, Kim SM, Chang H, et al. Long-term outcomes of ethanol injection therapy for locally recurrent papillary thyroid cancer. Eur Arch Otorhinolaryngol 2017;274(9):3497–501.
99. Pawelczak M, David R, Franklin B, et al. Outcomes of children and adolescents with well-differentiated thyroid carcinoma and pulmonary metastases following (1)(3)(1)I treatment: a systematic review. Thyroid 2010;20(10):1095–101.
100. Biko J, Reiners C, Kreissl MC, et al. Favourable course of disease after incomplete remission on (131)I therapy in children with pulmonary metastases of papillary thyroid carcinoma: 10 years follow-up. Eur J Nucl Med Mol Imaging 2011;38(4):651–5.
101. Padovani RP, Robenshtok E, Brokhin M, et al. Even without additional therapy, serum thyroglobulin concentrations often decline for years after total thyroidectomy and radioactive remnant ablation in patients with differentiated thyroid cancer. Thyroid 2012;22(8):778–83.
102. Berdelou A, Lamartina L, Klain M, et al. Treatment of refractory thyroid cancer. Endocr Relat Cancer 2018;25(4):R209–23.
103. Eisenhauer EA, Therasse P, Bogaerts J, et al. New response evaluation criteria in solid tumours: revised RECIST guideline (version 1.1). Eur J Cancer 2009; 45(2):228–47.
104. Covell LL, Ganti AK. Treatment of advanced thyroid cancer: role of molecularly targeted therapies. Target Oncol 2015;10(3):311–24.
105. Rao SN, Cabanillas ME. Navigating systemic therapy in advanced thyroid carcinoma: from standard of care to personalized therapy and beyond. J Endocr Soc 2018;2(10):1109–30.
106. Mahajan P, Dawrant J, Kheradpour A, et al. Response to lenvatinib in children with papillary thyroid carcinoma. Thyroid 2018;28(11):1450–4.
107. Waguespack SG, Sherman SI, Williams MD, et al. The successful use of sorafenib to treat pediatric papillary thyroid carcinoma. Thyroid 2009;19(4):407–12.
108. Weitzman SP, Cabanillas ME. The treatment landscape in thyroid cancer: a focus on cabozantinib. Cancer Manag Res 2015;7:265–78.
109. Fox E, Widemann BC, Chuk MK, et al. Vandetanib in children and adolescents with multiple endocrine neoplasia type 2B associated medullary thyroid carcinoma. Clin Cancer Res 2013;19(15):4239–48.
110. Tuttle RM, Brose MS, Grande E, et al. Novel concepts for initiating multitargeted kinase inhibitors in radioactive iodine refractory differentiated thyroid cancer. Best Pract Res Clin Endocrinol Metab 2017;31(3):295–305.

Advances in the Bone Health Assessment of Children

Leanne M. Ward, MD, FRCPC, FAAP[a],*, Victor N. Konji, PhD[b]

KEYWORDS

• Children • DXA • QCT • pQCT • HR-pQCT • Morphometry • Fractures

KEY POINTS

• Advances in bone assessment techniques, such as low-radiation quantitative computed tomography, provide the ability to measure size-independent cortical and trabecular volumetric bone mineral density, bone and muscle geometry, and estimates of bone strength. These have been useful in understanding bone development, disease mechanisms, and responses to bone-active interventions.

• Numerous skeletal sites can now be measured, which overcomes challenges in patient positioning and surgical hardware placement, and which allows the clinician to select the most logical part of the skeleton to monitor in response to bone health threats or interventions.

• Dual energy x-ray absorptiometry–based vertebral fracture assessment holds promise for more widespread vertebral fracture screening in high-risk populations, such as children with primary osteoporosis and glucocorticoid-treated diseases.

• Bone marrow fat is an endocrine-active tissue that merits further study of its role in bone strength and disease.

INTRODUCTION

Pediatric bone diseases present with a variety of signs and symptoms. Although some diagnoses may be straightforward based on history and physical examination, other presentations require more extensive bone assessments. In addition, clinical follow-up, research studies, and drug trials are predicated on strong bone health assessment

Funding Sources: Dr L.M. Ward has been supported by Tier 1 and Tier 2 Research Chair Awards from the University of Ottawa, the Children's Hospital of Eastern Ontario Departments of Pediatrics and Surgery, and the Children's Hospital of Eastern Ontario Research Institute. The STeroid-induced Osteoporosis in the Pediatric Population (STOPP) study was funded by the Canadian Institutes of Health Research (Funding Reference Number 64285).
[a] Division of Endocrinology and Metabolism, Children's Hospital of Eastern Ontario, University of Ottawa, 401 Smyth Road, Ottawa, Ontario K1H 8L1, Canada; [b] The Ottawa Pediatric Bone Health Research Group, Children's Hospital of Eastern Ontario Research Institute, 401 Smyth Road, Ottawa, Ontario K1H 8L1, Canada
* Corresponding author.
E-mail address: Lward@cheo.on.ca

Endocrinol Metab Clin N Am 49 (2020) 613–636
https://doi.org/10.1016/j.ecl.2020.07.005
0889-8529/20/© 2020 Elsevier Inc. All rights reserved.

endo.theclinics.com

methods, which include use of appropriate reference data and knowledge about ca-veats or pitfalls in their interpretation.

For many years, dual energy x-ray absorptiometry (DXA), radiography, and biochemical tests were the only methods available to characterize a child's skeletal phenotype (with the exception of trans-iliac bone biopsies, which have been around for decades but only in highly specialized centers). Over time, the use of DXA has expanded to include an increasing number of skeletal sites, and additional imaging techniques have allowed 3-dimensional quantification of cortical and trabecular volu-metric bone mineral density (vBMD), as well as muscle-bone geometry, skeletal archi-tecture, and estimates of bone strength. The spine has been a particular focus of recent developments in children, including standardization of methodologies for verte-bral fracture identification, quantification of vertebral body reshaping, and the low-radiation vertebral fracture assessment (VFA) method by DXA.

Here the authors describe advances in techniques that are currently available for children with bone diseases. In addition, they provide their skeletal site–specific appli-cations, give examples of ways in which various techniques help diagnose and care for children with bone disorders, and highlight how these methods shed light on prin-ciples of bone development and underlying mechanisms of bone diseases.

AN OVERVIEW OF BONE HEALTH ASSESSMENT TECHNIQUES IN CHILDREN

Bone health assessment methods that are currently used in children fall into 2 broad categories: (1) static (imaging) techniques, including radiography, radiom-etry, DXA, central (axial) and peripheral quantitative computed tomography (QCT), and MRI; and (2) dynamic techniques, including bone turnover markers and trans-iliac histomorphometry (**Fig. 1**). Most bone imaging and quantification

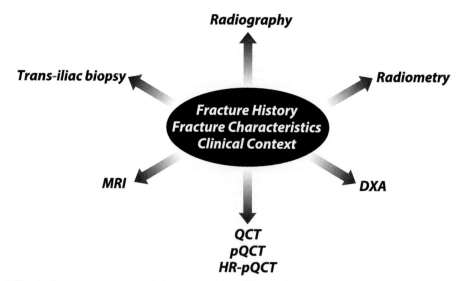

Fig. 1. Bone assessment techniques used in children for routine clinical care and/or in research studies. DXA, dual energy x-ray absorptiometry; HR-pQCT, high-resolution pQCT; MRI, magnetic resonance imaging; pQCT, peripheral quantitative computed tomography; QCT, quantitative computed tomography.

Bone Imaging and Quantification Techniques

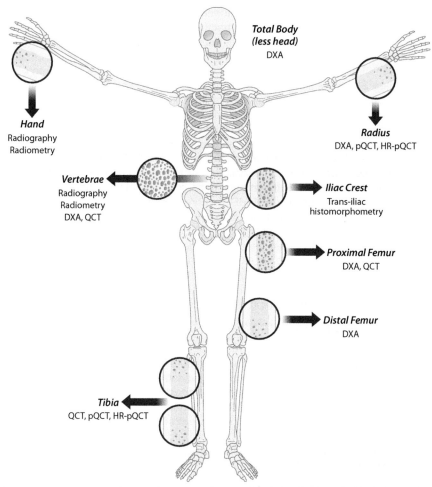

Fig. 2. Bone imaging and quantification techniques by skeletal site. DXA, dual energy x-ray absorptiometry; HR-pQCT, high-resolution peripheral quantitative computed tomography; pQCT, peripheral quantitative computed tomography; QCT, quantitative peripheral computed tomography. QCT can technically be applied to any skeletal site; the published sites are listed here. For MRI, see text.

techniques are skeletal site-specific (**Fig. 2**), which can be useful depending on the clinical situation.

Dual Energy X-Ray Absorptiometry

DXA is the most widely used quantitative bone imaging method in clinical practice. As a 2-dimensional projection of a 3-dimensional structure, it does not measure true bone density in mass/volume, but rather areal BMD (aBMD) in g/cm^2. That aBMD is a composite of bone mass and size is evident when serial aBMD measurements are mapped out relative to the healthy average on a normative curve, such as provided by the DXA machine manufacturer. These trajectories show increases that mimic changes in height and weight on a growth curve. Although true bone density will be underestimated in short children, small bone size relative to healthy peers is nevertheless an important predictor of bone strength.[1] Furthermore, aBMD predicts clinically relevant endpoints, such as prevalent vertebral fractures in children with leukemia at diagnosis,[2] and incident vertebral fractures at future timepoints in the same population.[3]

The most common site of DXA measurement in children is the spine (L1 to L4 or L2 to L4), given the rapid scan time and ease of positioning at this site relative to other skeletal sites. Skilled pediatric DXA technologists are able to achieve informative lumbar spine DXA scans even in the first year of life. Forearm, proximal femur, and lateral distal femur (LDF) are additional sites of measurement, with recent guidelines published for their use in select groups of children.[4]

Different normative databases generate different BMD Z-scores for a given child, as discussed in detail elsewhere.[5] Therefore, use of absolute BMD Z-score thresholds as part of an osteoporosis definition in children, or to trigger certain care pathways in osteoporosis diagnosis or treatment algorithms, is challenging. In addition, children can demonstrate bone fragility at BMD Z-scores greater than −2.0, which means that reserving the diagnosis of osteoporosis in at-risk children for those with Z-scores lower than −2.0 may fail to identify some children in a timely fashion. In practical terms, DXA-based BMD is best used as a trajectory, to chart gains and declines over time in relationship to the child's clinical status (fracture history, status of the underlying disease), accounting for changes in anthropometry/pubertal development. The latter is important, considering the contributions of linear growth failure, weight loss, or delayed puberty to declining BMD Z-scores.

Radiography and Radiometry

Radiography, the technique of taking radiographs in order to obtain a picture of the skeleton, and radiometry, the technique of using radiographs to measure individual bones within the skeleton, are long-standing, fundamental methods that continue to hold a place in the assessment of children with bone diseases. At the spine, semiquantitative and qualitative methods help identify vertebral fractures, whereas vertebral morphometry has been used to demonstrate both incident vertebral fractures and vertebral body reshaping after fractures. Radiometry offers measurement of cortical changes at the second metacarpal, providing insight into the mechanisms of diseases and their responses to treatment.

Quantitative Computed Tomography

Apart from bone size–related limitations, DXA is unable to distinguish between cortical and trabecular bone. QCT captures a tri-dimensional image, providing an estimation of true density in mass per volume. In addition, cortical and trabecular compartments can be measured separately, along with muscle-bone geometry and muscle density. Both central (also called axial) and peripheral QCT scanners are available; however, radiation exposure is lower for dedicated peripheral QCT scans, registering similar to, or even less than, DXA.[6] The precision from the 3 types of scanners (full-sized/whole-body QCT, peripheral QCT [pQCT], and high-resolution [HR]-pQCT), their radiation exposures relative to DXA and to radiography, and the available reference data for each have been reviewed in detail elsewhere.[7,8]

Full-sized QCT scanners can measure both axial and appendicular sites. Older machines had high radiation and were limited by a large voxel size that exceeded that of the trabeculae, causing volume averaging errors. Newer scanners have addressed this problem and have lower radiation exposure. This technique does not require special positioning, a major advantage for children with motor disabilities.

pQCT measurements are acquired at the radius or tibia, non-dominant side, at different sites along the length of the bone. Examples of measurements acquired in the authors' clinic by tibia pQCT include (according to their proximity to the distal long bone epiphysis) the following: 3% site for trabecular density and bone mineral content (BMC); 38% site for cortical BMC, vBMD, thickness and cross-sectional area, and for periosteal and endosteal circumferences; and 66% site for muscle and fat cross-sectional area and muscle density (**Fig. 3**). Other reported tibial sites of measurement include 4%, 14%, and 20%. At the radius, the 4%, 20%, and 66% sites are most often reported. From these measures, biomechanical indices can be derived (eg, cross-sectional moment of inertia) to estimate skeletal strength. pQCT can also capture bone marrow fat.[9] This novel development reflects interest in bone marrow fat as an endocrine-active tissue that is linked to skeletal strength in adults.[10]

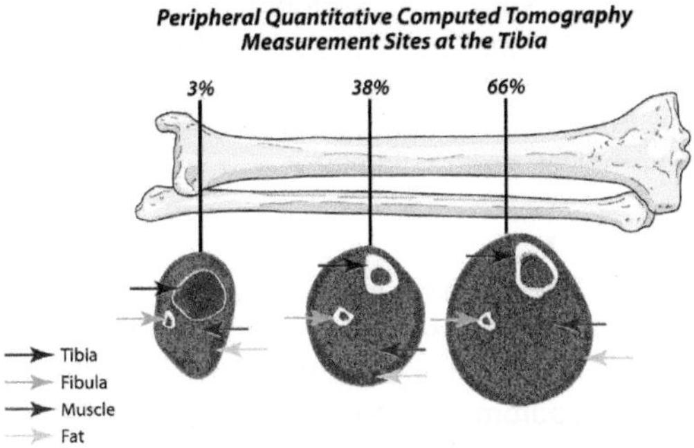

Peripheral Quantitative Computed Tomography Measurement Sites at the Tibia

Fig. 3. Peripheral QCT measurement sites at the tibia. Tibia pQCT scans in a 15-year old boy with chronic recurrent multifocal osteomyelitis, at sites 3%, 38%, and 66% from the growth plate.

The most recent QCT development is HR scanners targeting the peripheral skeleton. HR-pQCT has adequate spatial resolution to enable quantification of not only bone geometry and volumetric trabecular and cortical BMD but also individual trabeculae including trabecular number, thickness, and separation. Only trabecular number is measured directly, with bone volume/total volume, trabecular thickness, and trabecular spacing all derived from a combination of trabecular number and trabecular vBMD.

Although these methods represent precise and sophisticated bone assessment tools, several limitations persist in children. Apart from the need to sit still for an adequate period of time when multiple slices are being obtained (usually possible in children six years of age or older), children must be able to extend their arm or leg comfortably and safely into the gantry of peripheral scanners, which can be challenging to impossible for those with spasticity or contractures. Large calf size has also been a limitation in children with extreme obesity. In addition, central and peripheral QCT scanners are less user-friendly compared with DXA, axial (but not peripheral) QCT has relatively high radiation, and all 3 types of CT scanners are still largely research techniques that are restricted to a small number of pediatric centers around the world.

Magnetic Resonance Imaging

MRI is based on the detection of hydrogen proton excitation that is induced by high magnetic fields. MRI has the unique capacity to simultaneously detect tissue composition changes in the bone and marrow, which have low and high proton densities, respectively. These diametric characteristics are shown as white images for marrow and black for bone. Initially, MRI was used to detect fractures (eg, at the spine) that were indeterminant on standard radiography. Over time, special MRI protocols were developed to measure (apparent) trabecular bone volume per total tissue volume (appBV/TV), characteristics of the trabeculae (number, thickness, and separation), and cortical volume. Bending strength indices can also be derived. The main advantage of MRI is that it provides a volumetric measure without any ionizing radiation. Furthermore, scanning in multiple planes is permissible without repositioning; simultaneous scanning of different limbs is also feasible. However, scans require a long time, take place in a confined ("claustrophobic") environment, are disturbingly noisy for some children, and are expensive.

MRI is currently a research tool, except when used to determine the acuity of a vertebral injury that manifests as edema, if the injury occurred recently (within about 2 months). In children with suspected vertebral fracture but equivocal vertebral radiography/DXA-based VFA (see later discussion), MRI can be a useful diagnostic tool. In addition, MRI is used in children to distinguish vertebral collapse due to osteoporosis from other conditions such as nonbacterial osteomyelitis, congenital vascular-lymphatic anomalies, and malignancy.

Trans-iliac Histomorphometry

Although QCT and MRI techniques have led to major advances in our ability to understand tri-dimensional BMD, bone geometry, and skeletal architecture, only serum bone turnover markers (BTM) and trans-iliac biopsies provide information about bone metabolism. Although serum BTM are used as surrogates for bone metabolism, they are influenced by numerous clinical factors that result in high intra- and inter-individual variability, including gender, age, puberty timing and tempo, serum 25-hydroxyvitamin D status, assay methods, and sample processing. Time of procurement relative to meals, exercise, and recent fractures can also influence results. One of the main factors that has limited their use in children is that serum BTM also reflect linear growth and not just bone turnover per se. In children, the sole technique available to reliably determine bone turnover is trans-iliac bone biopsy.

Trans-iliac biopsies with dual-tetracycline labeling have been around for decades and continue to provide unique information about static and dynamic bone properties that cannot be obtained by any other means. To prepare for a trans-iliac biopsy, tetracycline is taken orally for 2 days, followed by a 10-day free interval, followed by another 2 days of oral prescription. The biopsy is then taken on the fourth or fifth day following the second tetracycline labeling. Full-thickness trans-iliac biopsies are obtained at a standardized site located 2 cm below the anterior superior iliac spine in the supine position. The instrument used for the procedure is a Bordier-Trephine needle, 5 to 7 mm internal diameter depending on the size of the child. Pediatric normative data are available for children, which increases the utility of this technique in clinical practice and in research studies.[11] In addition to quantification of static histomorphometric indices using a Goldner stain, the lamellar pattern can be viewed qualitatively under polarized (birefringent) light. Fluorescent light allows visualization of the pattern of dual tetracycline uptake, and also quantification of dynamic indices such as the bone formation rate (to document bone turnover on trabecular surfaces) and the mineralization lag time (which helps understand, for example, whether increases in osteoid are due to exuberant bone formation, or a mineralization defect).

Trans-iliac bone biopsies gave clues about novel forms of osteogenesis imperfecta (OI) before elucidation about the genetic basis in the past,[12,13] which provided the impetus for gene discovery efforts. Trans-iliac biopsies were also instrumental in teaching us about the unique mechanistic effects of antiresorptive (bisphosphonate) therapy on bone tissue during growth. As an example, large increases in cortical width during growth occurred with intravenous pamidronate in children with OI, due to loss of bone resorption on the endocortical surface at the same time that bone formation continued on the exocortical surface via periosteal apposition.[14] Another important observation in the same clinical context was that retained calcified growth plate carti-lage in horizontally layered trabeculae were responsible for the characteristic meta-physeal "zebra lines" seen on plain radiography.[15]

A recent study documented that among children presenting to a specialized bone clinic with bone fragility, lack of extraskeletal signs of OI, and absence of a family history, 72% had negative state-of-the-art genetic studies.[16] This study suggested there are

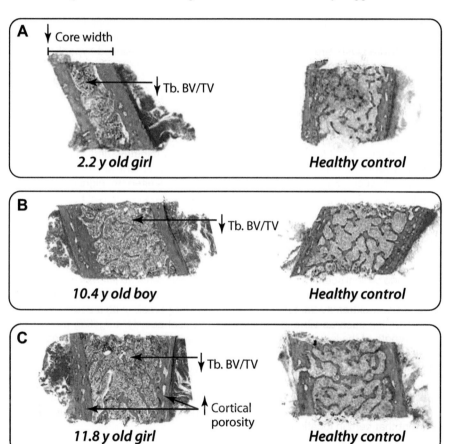

Fig. 4. Trans-iliac histomorphometry in children presenting with bone fragility, lack of extra-skeletal manifestations of OI, lack of family history of osteoporosis, and absence of muta-tions in the known bone fragility genes. On quantitative bone histomorphometry, all 3 children had low trabecular bone volume/tissue volume (Tb. BV/TV), the gold-standard defi-nition of osteoporosis. (A) A 2.2-year-old girl with a small core width, markedly reduced trabecular bone volume, and hyperosteocytosis (the latter, not visible at the magnification shown) consistent with OI or an OI-like condition. (B) A 10.4-year-old boy with low trabec-ular bone volume, reduced bone formation, normal cortical thickness, and lack of hyperos-teocytosis, consistent with juvenile osteoporosis. (C) A 11.8-year-old girl with increased cortical porosity, high osteoblast surface/bone surface, and hyperosteocytosis (the latter, not visible at the magnification shown), consistent with OI or an OI-like condition.

likely as-yet unidentified genetic variants responsible for low bone mass, and bone fragility, in children who otherwise appear healthy. According to the authors' experience, trans-iliac biopsies continue to be useful in definitively diagnosing osteoporosis in such children. For example, hyperosteocytosis and high bone turnover are hallmarks of OI and OI-like conditions, both of which are identifiable on trans-iliac histomorphometry. In juvenile osteoporosis, low bone turnover, thin osteoid seams, and absence of hyperosteocytosis are characteristic signatures. **Fig. 4** provides examples of the trans-iliac histomorphometric findings in 3 children with bone fragility, normal stature, sclerae, and teeth, lack of family history, and normal testing of all the known bone fragility genes. In all 3 cases, biopsy findings were consistent with either an OI-like condition, or juvenile osteoporosis, and provided justification for osteoporosis therapy.

In addition to identifying children with primary osteoporosis, trans-iliac biopsies are also uniquely useful in quantifying changes in osteomalacia, the bone tissue corollary of rickets. This may be particularly helpful when seeking signs of "deep tissue remission" in children with rare mineralization disorders such as X-linked hypophosphatemia and hypophosphatasia who are on specialized drug therapies. The undecalcified samples can also be used to measure BMD distribution, which quantifies the heterogeneity in calcium concentration within bone. Bone matrix mineralization density is high in classic and recessive OI,[17] and in children with low bone turnover due to systemic inflammation.[18]

The main limitations of trans-iliac biopsies, of course, are that they require general anesthesia in children (procedure duration = 15 minutes) and that dedicated training is required for their accurate and safe procurement at the standardized location. As such, this technique continues to be limited to highly specialized clinics.

BONE IMAGING METHODS BY SKELETAL SITE AND THEIR CLINICAL APPLICABILITY

Although the spine has traditionally been the most commonly assessed site, other skeletal sites may be useful depending on the clinical situation. The following examples provide clinical scenarios that benefit from assessments at different skeletal sites: (1) a patient with a peripheral neuropathy, such as Charcot-Marie-Tooth disease and frequent lower extremity fractures (ie, "regional osteoporosis"); (2) a patient receiving an intervention such as vibration therapy or physical activity, targeting muscle and bone strength of the lower extremities; (3) a child with a physical limitation that poses challenges for proper supine positioning, such as a boy with Duchenne muscular dystrophy and lower extremity contractures; or (4) a child with orthopedic hardware that precludes imaging at the spine (scoliosis surgery) or long bones (intramedullary rodding). Having different options for imaging allows the clinician to choose logical sites depending on the underlying problem or intervention, and to have "back-up" sites in the event that certain locations are inaccessible.

SPINE
Radiography

As in adults, vertebral fractures are one of the signatures of osteoporosis in children; however, they are frequently asymptomatic, and go undetected in the absence of routine monitoring.[2] Because one trigger for osteoporosis therapy in children is the presence of vertebral fractures without potential for spontaneous recovery from osteoporosis, vertebral fracture detection is essential in the bone health evaluation. As a result of their clinical significance, standardized reporting using a validated method is critical. To date, radiography has been the gold standard for vertebral fracture detection in children.

The Canadian STeroid-induced Osteoporosis in the Pediatric Population (STOPP) Consortium demonstrated both the clinical significance of vertebral fractures in children with osteoporosis, and the validity in using the Genant semiquantitative method for their detection.[19] By showing that vertebral fractures are linked to biologically-relevant factors including back pain, lower lumbar spine BMD Z-scores, and lower second metacarpal percent cortical area Z-scores,[2,3,20,21] the STOPP Consortium validated that greater than 20% loss of vertebral height ratio according to the modified Genant semiquantitative method[19,22] is an appropriate definition of vertebral fractures in the young. Validity was also affirmed in a study of children with leukemia, in whom Genant-defined vertebral fractures at diagnosis were the strongest predictor of new vertebral *and* long bone fractures over the next 5 years.[3]

In both children and adults, the most common vertebral fracture morphology is anterior wedge deformity, there is a bimodal distribution of all fracture morphologies from T4 to L4, and the peak frequency of vertebral fractures occurs in the midthoracic region. These highly consistent observations in children have been demonstrated in different diseases and at different points in the disease course.[2,20,21,23] The bimodal distributions of fractures in children are slightly more rostral and caudal compared with adults,[24] a finding that is attributed to the less marked curvatures of the developing spine.

Vertebral bodies are scored as grade 0 (normal), grade 1 (mild fracture), grade 2 (moderate), and grade 3 (severe). The grading corresponds to the reduction in height ratios when the anterior height is compared with the posterior height (defined as a wedge fracture), the middle height to the posterior height (uniconcave or biconcave fracture), and the posterior height to the posterior height of the adjacent vertebral bodies (crush fracture). The scores correspond to reductions in height ratios, as follows: Grade 0: less than or equal to 20%; Grade 1: greater than 20% to 25%; Grade 2: greater than 25% to 40%; Grade 3: greater than 40%. **Fig. 5A** shows the visual approach to determining vertebral height ratios, and **Fig. 5B** (images A, B, and C) provides in vivo, pediatric examples. An incident fracture is defined as an increase in the Genant grade by at least 1 compared with a prior image, as previously described.[25] In cases where physiologic anterior rounding of the vertebral body in the mid-thoracic region is difficult to distinguish from a vertebral fracture, the decision can be facilitated by qualitative signs, including loss of endplate parallelism, endplate interruption, and anterior cortical buckling[2] (see **Fig. 5B**, images A, D, and E). Anterior cortical buckling is an uncommon manifestation in children, because the anterior cortex of the vertebral body is not fully formed until the second decade of life. Vertebral fractures can mimic normal variants beyond the physiologic wedging of young children, as described in an atlas compiled from children with glucocorticoid-treated disorders containing both vertebral fractures, and normal variants.[26] This underscores the importance of expertise in adjudicating vertebral fractures in the clinical and research settings.

Children have tremendous potential for recovery from osteoporosis through growth-mediated skeletal modeling, which includes vertebral body reshaping, provided risk factors have abated, and there is sufficient residual linear growth potential. Naturally, the more severe the vertebral collapse, the longer it takes to undergo vertebral body reshaping. To understand the vertebral body reshaping phenomenon in children, the Canadian STOPP Consortium studied factors linked to complete versus incomplete reshaping in bisphosphonate-naïve children with leukemia and vertebral fractures.[3] The "spinal deformity index" (SDI) was used as part of the methodology,[27] which is the simple sum of the Genant grades in a given child. For example, 3 Grade 2 vertebral fractures in a child is equivalent to an SDI of 6, and 2 Grade 1 vertebral fractures in a child equals an SDI of 2. Therefore, the SDI is a barometer of total spine fracture

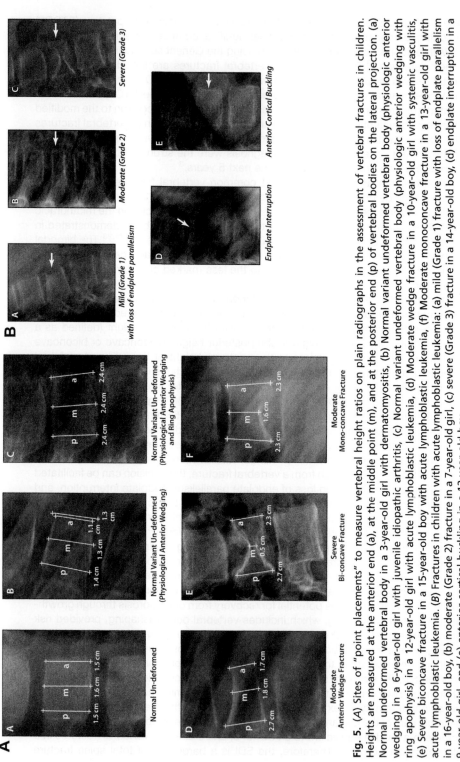

Fig. 5. (A) Sites of "point placements" to measure vertebral height ratios on plain radiographs in the assessment of vertebral fractures in children. Heights are measured at the anterior end (a), at the middle point (m), and at the posterior end (p) of vertebral bodies on the lateral projection. (a) Normal undeformed vertebral body in a 3-year-old girl with dermatomyositis, (b) Normal variant undeformed vertebral body (physiologic anterior wedging) in a 6-year-old girl with juvenile idiopathic arthritis, (c) Normal variant undeformed vertebral body (physiologic anterior wedging with ring apophysis) in a 12-year-old girl with acute lymphoblastic leukemia, (d) Moderate wedge fracture in a 10-year-old girl with systemic vasculitis, (e) Severe biconcave fracture in a 15-year-old boy with acute lymphoblastic leukemia, (f) Moderate monoconcave fracture in a 13-year-old girl with acute lymphoblastic leukemia. (B) Fractures in children with acute lymphoblastic leukemia: (a) mild (Grade 1) fracture with loss of endplate parallelism in a 16-year-old boy, (b) moderate (Grade 2) fracture in a 7-year-old girl, (c) severe (Grade 3) fracture in a 14-year-old boy, (d) endplate interruption in a 9-year-old girl, and (e) anterior cortical buckling in a 12-year-old boy.

burden, one that can be tracked over time to quantify incident VF and vertebral body reshaping. In leukemia, vertebral body reshaping was defined according to the degree of decline in the SDI from baseline to the final follow-up, as follows[3]: (1) complete vertebral body reshaping: a decline in the SDI by 100% (ie, the last available radiograph showed the SDI was 0); (2) incomplete vertebral body reshaping: a decline in the SDI by less than 100% (ie, 0< last SDI < maximum SDI at previous time points); and (3) absence of vertebral body reshaping: no change in the SDI (ie, the last SDI was the same as the maximum SDI at previous time points). An example of complete vertebral body reshaping is provided in **Fig. 6**.

Using this strategy, the Canadian STOPP Consortium showed that more than three-quarters of children with leukemia and vertebral fractures had complete reshaping by their last follow-up, almost 20% had incomplete reshaping, whereas 5% had no improvement in the SDI over 5 years.[3] Those with incomplete or absent vertebral body reshaping were more frequently older (peripubertal at the time of diagnosis) and more often had moderate or severe collapse at the time of the maximum SDI (which occurred between 1 and 2 years following diagnosis). In practical terms, these data revealed that younger children, and those with less severe collapse, are more capable of reshaping vertebral bodies, provided risk factors for bone fragility have resolved. These data further suggested that the peri-pubertal period (ie, 8 years of age in a girl and 9 years of age in a boy) was a critical point in determining whether a child had adequate remaining growth potential to undergo complete restoration of normal vertebral dimensions.

Radiometry

The SDI is particularly useful in situations where the changes in vertebral height ratios are being observed over a longer period of time, given that ranges of vertebral height ratio loss are used to define the fracture severity grades. In situations where smaller changes are being sought, such as differences between 2 groups in a clinical trial, or differences pre-post osteoporosis therapy in short-term, longitudinal observational studies, quantitative vertebral morphometry is useful. With this technique, vertebral heights are directly measured using "six-point vertebral morphometry" (see **Fig. 5A**), to derive the precise vertebral height ratios that were outlined in the prior section on vertebral radiography. This technique has been used in both primary osteoporosis,[28] and in secondary osteoporosis among boys with glucocorticoid-treated Duchenne muscular dystrophy.[29] Determining the morphometrist's intra-rater reliability is important, so that loss of vertebral height, stable vertebral dimensions, and reshaping of vertebral fractures can be defined according to the extent to which height ratio changes exceed, or are within, the precision of the measurement at each vertebral level. For example, if the precision of the measurement is 3% at the T7 vertebral body, and the increase in height ratio is subsequently 6%, this would represent vertebral body reshaping. On the other hand, if the increase in height ratio is 2%, this would indicate no change. These concepts are shown in an observational, pre-post study of intravenous bisphosphonate therapy in boys with glucocorticoid-treated Duchenne muscular dystrophy,[29] in whom 27 vertebral fractures were tracked over 2 years, and vertebral bodies were classified as reshaping, stable, or showing signs of vertebral height ratio loss.

Dual Energy X-Ray Absorptiometry

Newer DXA machines have the capacity to measure not only bone mineral content (BMC), BMD, and bone area on the anterior-posterior projection but also trabecular bone score (TBS) and VFA.

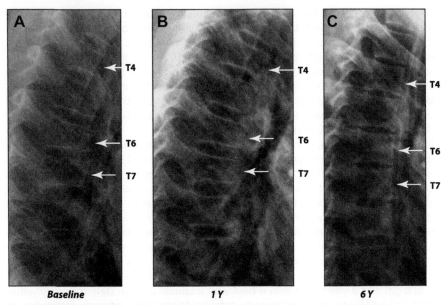

Fig. 6. Lateral spine radiograph showing spontaneous vertebral body reshaping in a 6-year-old, glucocorticoid-treated girl with acute lymphoblastic leukemia. (*A*) Fractures at diagnosis, (*B*) early signs of vertebral body reshaping after 12 months of leukemia therapy, and (*C*) complete vertebral body reshaping after 6 years.

The spine is a highly relevant DXA site, given the predilection of genetic mutations in OI, and glucocorticoid therapy in children with chronic illnesses, to target the trabecular-rich spine. The long-standing challenge, of course, is that children with both primary and secondary osteoporosis are often short, or delayed in their linear growth velocity, relative to healthy peers. For this reason, DXA is well recognized to underestimate BMD in shorter children because of its 2-dimensional quantification. Perhaps less integrated in clinical practice is the reverse, that is, that aBMD in a tall child (as in children with fractures due to Marfan syndrome or familial tall stature) may be overestimated by DXA, giving false reassurances. Fortunately, recommendations to focus on the child's fracture history, the fracture characteristics, and the clinical context when making a diagnosis of osteoporosis take the pressure off DXA as a single diagnostic tool.

To overcome the DXA and bone size issue at the spine, there are two approaches that are frequently used in routine clinical care, and in research studies. Bone mineral apparent density (BMAD) is a term that refers to the fact that the BMD is initially acquired in mass/area (g/cm^2) from the two-dimensional projection, and then converted into a three-dimensional structure (mass/volume, g/cm^3) according to certain assumptions. Using the Kröger technique[30], the vertebrae are considered to be a stack of cylinders. In the Carter technique[31], the spine is considered to be a stack of cuboid volumes. With either method, bone volume is calculated using the projected bone area from the DXA scan, and an estimate of bone depth. With the Kröger method, the projected bone width is used to estimate vertebral body depth (the third dimension), while the Carter approach uses the square root of the projected bone area to estimate the depth of the vertebral body. From these bone volume estimates, an approximate volumetric BMD, referred to in the literature as vBMD or BMAD, is then calculated.

The clinical relevance of these techniques is that both BMAD and aBMD for age associate with fracture risk in healthy children.[32] BMC for height is the simplest method for size adjustment, because it does not require assumptions about bone shape. However, Crabtree and colleagues[33] demonstrated that lumbar spine BMAD gave the highest odds for a vertebral fracture in children with chronic illnesses, compared with lumbar spine aBMD, BMC for height, and bone area for height. Zemel and colleagues[34] developed a height-based size adjustment that uses height-for-age Z scores to predict lumbar spine (and whole body) BMC and aBMD. Deviations from the predicted results represent "height-for-age" BMD Z-scores, abbreviated as "HAZ." In a cohort of children with leukemia at diagnosis, height-adjusted spine aBMD Z-scores associated with vertebral fractures.[35] BMAD reference data are now also available for youth 5 to 19 years of age.[36]

One important technical point relevant to children in the use of lumbar spine BMD is that the cortical processes contribute a significant proportion to the BMD measurement in the anterior-posterior view, whereas the trabecular-rich vertebral body is the true target of osteoporosis assessments. This principle was demonstrated nicely by Dubner and colleagues,[37] who showed lower width-adjusted BMD Z-scores (which exclude the posterior spinous processes) on a lateral spine DXA compared with anterior-posterior aBMD Z-scores in children with juvenile idiopathic arthritis, and that the difference between the 2 measures was greater in younger children.

In routine clinical care, practitioners follow DXA-based BMD Z-score trajectories for signs of decline that signal a child in need of closer monitoring, or signs of recovery in a child whose bone health threats are resolving. In a child showing BMD Z-score declines, size adjustments are important to avoid confounding by poor linear growth. In cases of recovery, concomitant catch-up linear growth is often present, because recuperated BMD usually reflects improved control of the underlying disease, plus or minus progression through puberty (depending on the child's age). Declines in aBMD Z-scores greater than or equal to 0.4 to 0.5 are usually considered significant, a practice that has been informed by natural history studies. For example, a greater decline in lumbar spine BMD Z-score in the first 6 months of glucocorticoid therapy, by a difference of 0.4, was observed in children with glucocorticoid-treated rheumatic disorders who had incident vertebral fractures at 12 months compared to those without fractures.[20] Bone mineral accrual Z-score equations have recently been published, which will be interesting to explore in research studies for their ability to predict future vertebral fractures, or to predict vertebral body reshaping as a measure of recovery from vertebral fractures.[38]

TBS is an indirect index of bone microarchitecture that is determined from lumbar spine (and hip) DXA scans by commercially available software, without any additional scanning procedures.[39,40] Low TBS values are associated with increased risk of both prevalent and incident vertebral and hip fractures in adults,[39,41–46] and the International Society for Clinical Densitometry has endorsed the use of TBS in assessing osteoporotic fracture risk in postmenopausal women.[47] Despite its clinical value, and excellent precision (coefficients of variation of 1.5%), reference data across the lifespan[48] and experience in children are both lacking.

Given the importance of vertebral fracture screening in high-risk populations, there is tremendous interest in the utility of VFA by DXA. Image quality varies significantly depending on the densitometer, as recently reviewed in detail, with newer DXA machines showing high-quality spine images.[4] VFA is indeed attractive in children because of the extremely low radiation.[49–52] The main target population is high-risk children for whom periodic vertebral fracture surveillance is recommended to identify asymptomatic vertebral collapse, such as those with glucocorticoid-treated illnesses and OI. In addition, the test can be done at the same time as routine DXA scanning for BMD, making it a convenient "add-on" for children undergoing routine bone health monitoring. When compared with conventional spine radiographs, the technique shows 95% to 98% agreement in vertebral fracture identification (yes or no), and 87% to 95% agreement in fracture severity in children.[53–55]

Beyond these benefits, the fan-beam technology allows capture of the entire spine on a single image, obviating discrepancies in reporting due to challenges in reading from a spine image that is split into 2 cassettes. The fan-beam technology also avoids divergent beam issues (parallax), making identifying fractures easier. Newer DXA machines have a rotating "c-arm" that obviates the need to reposition the patient from the supine to the lateral position during VFA. Recent guidelines have been published on the use of VFA as an initial screen in children requiring periodic spine imaging for vertebral fracture detection.[4] Because vertebral fracture detection in children involves distinguishing normal variants from pathologic fractures, and because nonfracture pathology can also be seen on a VFA image, pediatric radiologists should still be involved in the assessment of vertebral fractures captured by DXA. Overall, discriminating vertebral fractures from normal vertebral bodies is more challenging than identifying a non-fracture deformity.[26,56] The software also permits automated vertebral morphometry, but human expertise shows better precision in vertebral fracture identification by DXA[4]; therefore, automated vertebral morphometry is best used as a secondary analysis. In such cases, a technician should verify the accuracy of the automatized vertebral height measurements before any results are finalized. Therefore, at the moment automated VFA does not supplant human expertise in the evaluation of pediatric vertebral fractures.

Axial Quantitative Computed Tomography

Spine QCT has not been used widely in children, in large part due to higher radiation exposure compared with both DXA and pQCT, but it does overcome the size limitations of DXA when assessing the small bones of the vertebrae. This technique was used in a study of low-magnitude mechanical loading in children with motor disabilities who stood on vertical oscillating plates for 10 minutes per day, 5 days per week, for over 6 months.[57] In this study, QCT at the proximal tibia and the second lumbar vertebra were assessed. Although proximal tibia vBMD increased significantly by QCT in children who received vibration therapy compared with placebo, no significant differences in spine vBMD were identified. The lack of effect at the spine was hypothesized to result from the abnormal stance in these children with physical disabilities, or the fact that the anabolic effect of the vibrations was only possible at sites with low pre-treatment BMD. The amount of radiation from the QCT tests over the course of the trial (about the equivalent of 4 chest radiographs) makes this technique challenging in a routine clinical care setting where the goal is to undertake serial BMD assessments to assess responses to a treatment.

LONG BONES
Dual Energy X-Ray Absorptiometry

Specific guidance around the use of DXA at the radius, and at the proximal and distal femur, has recently been summarized in an International Society for Clinical Densitometry Pediatric Position Statement.[4] The 33% radius (also referred to as the one-third distal radius) has been a target in children because the forearm is a site of frequent fractures during the growing years, and patient positioning is relatively facile. On the other hand, increases in BMD at this site may not be as relevant to children at risk of spine and lower extremity fractures. Forearm DXA is most useful in children for whom other skeletal sites cannot be measured due to hardware or positioning challenges, or to assess effects of targeted exercise on upper extremity bone mass and density. Recently, reference data for ultra-distal radius BMD by DXA have been published for children.[58]

Proximal femur DXA refers to total hip, largely comprised of cortical bone, and femoral neck, a trabecular-rich site. Historically, the proximal femur was not signaled to be an optimal DXA site because of variability in the structural maturation of the hip. However, pediatric normative data are now available for children older than 5 years,[4] and clinicians have come to appreciate that the hip is a clinically sensitive site. Proximal femur DXA is most useful in patients with neuromuscular disorders, rodding due to scoliosis, or compromised mobility (eg, autism, hypotonia, or reduced walking due to acute or chronic illness). Larger deficits in proximal femur BMD compared with other skeletal sites have been reported in children with OI, Duchenne muscular dystrophy, and leukemia.[59–61] However, numerous aspects of its practical use are still to be resolved, including the relative merit of total hip versus femoral neck regions of interest, the effect of size-adjustment techniques on fracture risks, the optimal age range for high-quality images, and the added value of a proximal femur DXA in different clinical settings.

The distal femur is a frequent site of fracture in children with physical disabilities, making this largely cortical site highly relevant to clinical care. To quantify distal femur BMD, patients lie on their side and the LDF is scanned in a lateromedial direction. In addition to its clinical relevance, side positioning can be more comfortable for children with physical disabilities than the supine positioning required for spine, hip, and total body scans. BMD is determined for 3 regions of interest, corresponding to the metaphysis, metaphyseal-diaphyseal junction and diaphysis[62] (**Fig. 7**). In a large study of children with neuromuscular disorders (cerebral palsy and Duchenne muscular

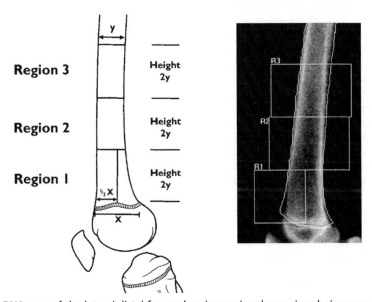

Fig. 7. DXA scan of the lateral distal femur showing regional mapping during scan acquisition. Region 1: anterior distal metaphysis, this is essentially trabecular bone. Region 2: metadiaphysis, composed of both trabecular and cortical bone. Region 3: diaphysis, composed primarily of cortical bone. (*Adapted from* Zemel et al 2009, *J Clinical Densitometry. Assessment of Skeletal Health*, vol. 12, no. 2, 207e218, 2009.)

dystrophy), almost half of the children with very low distal femur BMD Z-scores (less than −5.0) sustained a fragility fracture, while only 15% with Z-scores greater than −1.0 had fractures.[63] Children with neuromuscular disorders also have gracile (thin) bones, which confers an increased risk of bone fragility irrespective of BMD; not surprisingly, a small number of children with LDF BMD Z-scores closer to the mean still had fragile bones. Nevertheless, this study provided proof of principle that LDF BMD was an appropriate measurement for children at risk of long bone fractures due to mobility disorders.

Peripheral Quantitative Computed Tomography

pQCT and HR-pQCT (radius and tibia) have been highly informative in understanding mechanisms of disease and the biology of bone development in the young. In children with Crohn disease assessed by pQCT at the tibia, low metaphyseal trabecular BMD has been a consistent finding, along with reduced diaphyseal cortical bone strength due to expansion of the marrow cavity combined with low periosteal (outer) circumference.[64,65] Calf muscle sarcopenia, measured as muscle cross-sectional area at the 66% tibia site, is also a consistent finding in this population.[64,65] These structural changes were hypothesized to result from a combination of reduced mechanical loading and inflammatory cytokines. Importantly, bone geometry (such as cortical and muscle cross-sectional area, and periosteal and endosteal circumferences) all scale to tibial length, necessitating that Z-scores are generated relative to age, gender, and race, and also to tibial length. These studies provide examples of specific structural changes that together alter bone strength in a serious pediatric chronic illness. A visual of the bone density and structural differences that can be seen by QCT in 3 diseases with bone morbidity is provided in **Fig. 8**.

Another important observation arising from tibia pQCT is that the low trabecular vBMD that is characteristic of glucocorticoid-treated diseases can be overshadowed by high cortical vBMD when using a technique such as DXA, since DXA does not distinguish between the two. For example, cortical vBMD increased in the first 6 months of glucocorticoid therapy in children with Crohn disease, whereas lack of glucocorticoid exposure between 6 and 12 months was associated with cortical vBMD declines.[64] Increasing cortical vBMD during glucocorticoid therapy is hypothesized to result from low bone turnover on trabecular surfaces,[66] resulting in reduced intra-cortical porosity and greater secondary mineralization. This may explain why children on glucocorticoids can have significant bone fragility despite normal DXA-based BMD values, because thinner, denser, cortical bones may be more fragile.[67]

Recently, bone marrow fat, referred to as bone marrow adipose tissue (BMAT), has been of interest to the bone health community as an endocrine-active tissue, with higher BMAT linked to lower bone strength.[10] Esche and colleagues[9] used pQCT at the 65% radius to measure bone marrow density as an inverse surrogate for BMAT. After adjusting for confounders including age, energy intake, and forearm muscle area, an inverse relationship between elevated daily glucocorticoid secretion and higher fat mass index in healthy children and teenagers was found. Similarly, Gao and colleagues[68] showed that BMAT was inversely related to bone area in children.

Most of the HR-pQCT studies to date have been in adults, most often in the healthy population showing associations with fracture risks, but also in adults with OI, as recently reviewed.[69] Anorexia nervosa is one of the most studied clinical populations by QCT methods. A recent cross-sectional report of adolescents with anorexia nervosa compared HR-pQCT at the tibia with healthy controls, with measurements including individual trabecula separation, finite element analysis–derived

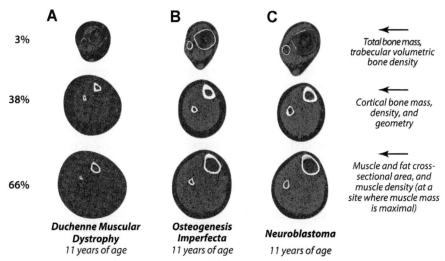

Fig. 8. Peripheral quantitative computed tomography scans of the tibia and fibula (3% site, first row; 38% site, middle row; 66% site, bottom row) in 3 boys, all 11 years of age, with different underlying diseases. Note the differences in bone geometry, in relationship to the nature and duration of their underlying diseases, with Figures (*A*) and (*B*) showing examples of congenital disorders and Figure (*C*) demonstrating an acquired condition. (*A*) Boy with glucocorticoid-treated Duchenne muscular dystrophy, after 3 years of intravenous bisphosphonate therapy for painful vertebral fractures. (*B*) Boy with mild osteogenesis imperfecta, after 3 years of intravenous bisphosphonate therapy for recurrent, low trauma fractures. (*C*) Boy with neuroblastoma on cancer therapy, 1 year following diagnosis.

strength indices, and BMAT at the L4 vertebra (the latter, by magnetic resonance spectroscopy).[70] Girls with anorexia nervosa had numerous bone abnormalities, including higher cortical porosity, and reduced cortical vBMD, thickness and area, lower trabecular number, and lower strength estimates. In addition, BMAT was higher in the anorexia nervosa group, with higher BMAT associated with lower strength estimates. This HR-pQCT study is among the most comprehensive in a pediatric clinical population to date and highlights the breadth of bone density, geometry, and strength indices that are available through combination DXA, HR-pQCT, and MRI.

HAND

Hand radiography is often requested in children to assess the tempo of epiphyseal maturation in relationship to a child's linear growth and bone mineral accrual (aka bone age), providing a ready opportunity to carry out radiometry at this site. Although radiometry to determine second metacarpal morphometry is not new, it is a reminder of the extent to which important information can be derived from fundamental imaging techniques that are readily available in routine clinical care.

Radiometry

Hand radiographs provide the opportunity to assess "hand morphometry" via specific bone measurements on the radiograph ("radiometry"). Second metacarpal length, mid-shaft periosteal diameter, and inner diameter can be measured on a hand radiograph that doubles for bone age, in order to derive combined cortical thickness, cortical area, percent cortical area, and inner diameter area. These indices are then converted to age- and gender-matched Z-scores[71] and provide some insight into changes in skeletal structure at a readily measurable, cortical site. This technique shed light on the mechanisms of bone fragility in children with leukemia, by showing normal length and outer diameter in those with vertebral fractures, but a reduction in the percent cortical area due to increased endosteal resorption (as opposed to loss of periosteal apposition).[2] This finding supported the theory that osteoclast-activating factors are liberated by the leukemic cells, which then act on endocortical surfaces adjacent to the pathological bone marrow. The significance of this finding was further underscored by the association of reductions in second metacarpal percent cortical area Z-scores with an increased risk of vertebral fractures at leukemia diagnosis.[2]

TOTAL BODY
Dual Energy X-Ray Absorptiometry

There is a wealth of information available from a total body (g/cm^2) DXA scan, which is expressed "less head" in children, given the relatively large, but clinically insignificant, contribution of the skull to the total body BMD in young patients. Although total body BMD is typically overshadowed by more clinically relevant, skeletal site-specific BMD measurements (ie, at the lumbar spine or long bones), total body composition is a useful measure if the goal is to evaluate muscle or fat mass, or muscle mass relative to BMD. Specific measures include total body (less head) BMD, BMC (g), fat mass (g), and lean mass (g), from which the following derivatives can be calculated: fat mass index (FMI) = fat mass/[height]^2; lean mass index (LMI) = lean mass/[height]^2, and appendicular LMI = appendicular lean mass/[height]^2. Fat mass distribution can further be assessed as percent fat mass of the trunk/fat mass of the limbs (arms plus legs).[72] Where body size corrections for bone mass are concerned, BMC for height is the simplest method for size adjustment, because it does not require assumptions about bone shape. Total body BMC/height correlates with estimates of bone strength by pQCT,[73] and total body less head for lean mass (adjusted for height) has a high diagnostic odds ratio for a long bone fracture in children with low-trauma fractures.

Total body DXA scans have been used to better understand the *reasons* for reductions in BMC in children with different skeletal phenotypes. The "Mølgaard" model,[74] referring to the Danish doctor who developed this method for children, provides a 3-phase evaluation to explain reductions in total body BMC for a given child. The approach assesses height for age, bone area for height, and BMC for bone area. These 3 phases are then related to 3 different causes of reduced bone mass: short bones, narrow bones, and light bones. It is useful to think about children's bones in this way, because bone density is not the only determinant of bone strength. Indeed, gracile (thinner) tibiae have reduced bone strength independent of cortical density in children with cerebral palsy.[75]

In another approach that considers muscle mass as a key determinant of bone mass, the "mechanostat model" of bone development[76–78] applies a 2-stage algorithm that assumes BMC is a surrogate for bone strength, and lean mass is a surrogate for muscle strength. The 2-stage assessment involves determining whether a child has adequate total body lean mass for height and adequate total body BMC for lean mass. If the child has appropriate lean mass for height, and appropriate BMC for lean mass, the child does not have a muscle-bone problem. If the child has adequate lean mass for height but inadequate BMC for lean mass, the child has a primary bone defect. If the child has reduced lean mass for height but adequate BMC for lean mass, the child has a primary muscle defect. If both are reduced, the child has a mixed muscle-bone defect. This strategy for classifying children holds validity, because children with OI will have a primary bone defect according to this model,[79] whereas children with Crohn disease, who have an "inflammatory cachexia" including sarcopenia, demonstrate a primary muscle defect.[65,80] Excellent examples of how these models are used in clinical practice are provided in a recent review article by Di Iorgi and colleagues.[8]

SUMMARY AND FUTURE DIRECTIONS

The last 2 decades have seen tremendous growth in understanding the clinical characteristics of various childhood bone disorders, their mechanisms and natural histories, and their responses to treatment. This new knowledge would not have been possible without advances in the available bone assessment techniques, particularly bone imaging. New approaches to older techniques including DXA, radiography, and radiometry continue to improve the understanding of pediatric osteoporosis phenotypes. Bone histomorphometry, a now decades-old technique, remains unique in quantifying bone cellular metabolism and mineralization defects.

Going forward, bone marrow fat seems to be an exciting tissue with relevance to skeletal integrity, and DXA-based VFA holds promise for more widespread, low-radiation screening of high-risk children to detect vertebral fractures. Combining muscle and bone outcomes from DXA, or from QCT, have helped understand whether a child's bone fragility is largely due to a primary bone disorder or driven by sarcopenia. Furthermore, the range of sites that can now be assessed by different imaging modalities allows the clinician to select a logical part of the skeleton to monitor in response to bone health threats and bone-active interventions.

Although independent predictors of fractures have been identified in different contexts, formal fracture prediction models are still lacking in children. Future models, if they succeed in overcoming the formidable challenge of adequate sample sizes, should explore newer determinants of bone strength such as DXA-based bone mineral accrual velocity Z-scores, volumetric cortical and trabecular BMD available through quantitative tri-dimensional techniques, metrics of bone geometry and skeletal architecture, and estimates of bone strength.

Whatever bone assessment methods are used or newly developed, their implementation should be based on a standardized approach with acceptable precision, radiation safety, appropriate reference data if required by the questions being asked, acquisition by an operator who is familiar with the challenges of positioning a child for imaging tests, and interpretation that is sensitive to the unique biology of the growing child.

ACKNOWLEDGMENTS

Drs L.M. Ward and V.N. Konji thank the research staff and scientists affiliated with the Ottawa Pediatric Bone Health Research Group who have been dedicated to the care and study of children with bone diseases over many years: Marika Pagé, Maya Scharke, Elizabeth Sykes, Lynn MacLeay, Scott Walker, Colleen Hartigan, and Drs Frank Rauch, Nazih Shenouda, Mary-Ann Matzinger, Jacob Jaremko, Khaldoun Koujok, Brian Lentle, Jinhui Ma, Stefan Jackowski, Nasrin Khan, and Kerry Siminoski.

DISCLOSURE

L.M. Ward has participated in clinical trials with ReveraGen BioPharma, PTC Therapeutics, Catabasis Pharmaceuticals, Novartis, Ultragenyx, and Amgen. Dr L.M.

Ward has also received unrestricted educational grants from Alexion and Ultragenyx, and consulting fees from Ipsen, Ultragenyx, PTC Therapeutics, Novartis, and Amgen, with funds to Dr L.M. Ward's institution. V.N. Konji has no conflict of interest to disclose.

REFERENCES

1. Kalkwarf HJ, Laor T, Bean JA. Fracture risk in children with a forearm injury is associated with volumetric bone density and cortical area (by peripheral QCT) and areal bone density (by DXA). Osteoporos Int 2011;22(2):607–16.

2. Halton J, Gaboury I, Grant R, et al. Advanced vertebral fracture among newly diagnosed children with acute lymphoblastic leukemia: results of the Canadian Steroid-Associated Osteoporosis in the Pediatric Population (STOPP) research program. J Bone Miner Res 2009;24(7):1326–34.

3. Ward LM, Ma J, Lang B, et al. Bone Morbidity and Recovery in Children With Acute Lymphoblastic Leukemia: Results of a Six-Year Prospective Cohort Study. J Bone Miner Res 2018;33(8):1435–43.

4. Weber DR, Boyce A, Gordon C, et al. The Utility of DXA assessment at the forearm, proximal femur, and lateral distal femur, and vertebral fracture assessment in the pediatric population: the 2019 Official Pediatric Positions of the ISCD. J Clin Densitom 2019;22(4):567–89.

5. Ward LM, Weber DR, Munns CF, et al. A contemporary view of the definition and diagnosis of osteoporosis in children and adolescents. J Clin Endocrinol Metab 2020;105(5):e2088–97.

6. Damilakis J, Adams JE, Guglielmi G, et al. Radiation exposure in X-ray-based imaging techniques used in osteoporosis. Eur Radiol 2010;20(11):2707–14.

7. Adams JE, Engelke K, Zemel BS, et al. Quantitative computer tomography in children and adolescents: the 2013 ISCD Pediatric Official Positions. J Clin Densitom 2014;17(2):258–74.

8. Di Iorgi N, Maruca K, Patti G, et al. Update on bone density measurements and their interpretation in children and adolescents. Best Pract Res Clin Endocrinol Metab 2018;32(4):477–98.

9. Esche J, Shi L, Hartmann MF, et al. Glucocorticoids and Body Fat Inversely Associate With Bone Marrow Density of the Distal Radius in Healthy Youths. J Clin Endocrinol Metab 2019;104(6):2250–6.

10. Patsch JM, Li X, Baum T, et al. Bone marrow fat composition as a novel imaging biomarker in postmenopausal women with prevalent fragility fractures. J Bone Miner Res 2013;28(8):1721–8.

11. Glorieux FH, Travers R, Taylor A, et al. Normative data for iliac bone histomorphometry in growing children. Bone 2000;26(2):103–9.

12. Glorieux FH, Rauch F, Plotkin H, et al. Type V osteogenesis imperfecta: a new form of brittle bone disease. J Bone Miner Res 2000;15(9):1650–8.

13. Ward L, Bardai G, Moffatt P, et al. Osteogenesis Imperfecta Type VI in Individuals from Northern Canada. Calcif Tissue Int 2016;98(6):566–72.

14. Rauch F, Travers R, Plotkin H, et al. The effects of intravenous pamidronate on the bone tissue of children and adolescents with osteogenesis imperfecta. J Clin Invest 2002;110(9):1293–9.

15. Rauch F, Travers R, Munns C, et al. Sclerotic metaphyseal lines in a child treated with pamidronate: histomorphometric analysis. J Bone Miner Res 2004;19(7):1191–3.

16. Bardai G, Ward LM, Trejo P, et al. Molecular diagnosis in children with fractures but no extraskeletal signs of osteogenesis imperfecta. Osteoporos Int 2017; 28(7):2095–101.

17. Roschger P, Fratzl-Zelman N, Misof BM, et al. Evidence that abnormal high bone mineralization in growing children with osteogenesis imperfecta is not associated with specific collagen mutations. Calcif Tissue Int 2008;82(4):263–70.

18. Misof BM, Roschger P, Klaushofer K, et al. Increased bone matrix mineralization in treatment-naive children with inflammatory bowel disease. Bone 2017; 105:50–6.

19. Genant HK, Jergas M, Palermo L, et al. Comparison of semiquantitative visual and quantitative morphometric assessment of prevalent and incident vertebral fractures in osteoporosis The Study of Osteoporotic Fractures Research Group. J Bone Miner Res 1996;11(7):984–96.

20. Rodd C, Lang B, Ramsay T, et al. Incident vertebral fractures among children with rheumatic disorders 12 months after glucocorticoid initiation: a national observational study. Arthritis Care Res 2012;64(1):122–31.

21. LeBlanc CM, Ma J, Taljaard M, et al. Incident vertebral fractures and risk factors in the first three years following glucocorticoid initiation among pediatric patients with rheumatic disorders. J Bone Miner Res 2015;30(9):1667–75.

22. Genant HK, Wu CY, van Kuijk C, et al. Vertebral fracture assessment using a semiquantitative technique. J Bone Miner Res 1993;8(9):1137–48.

23. Ma J, McMillan HJ, Karaguzel G, et al. The time to and determinants of first fractures in boys with Duchenne muscular dystrophy. Osteoporos Int 2017;28(2): 597–608.

24. Siminoski K, Lee KC, Jen H, et al. Anatomical distribution of vertebral fractures: comparison of pediatric and adult spines. Osteoporos Int 2012;23(7):1999–2008.

25. Alos N, Grant RM, Ramsay T, et al. High incidence of vertebral fractures in children with acute lymphoblastic leukemia 12 months after the initiation of therapy. J Clin Oncol 2012;30(22):2760–7.

26. Jaremko JL, Siminoski K, Firth GB, et al. Common normal variants of pediatric vertebral development that mimic fractures: a pictorial review from a national longitudinal bone health study. Pediatr Radiol 2015;45(4):593–605.

27. Kerkeni S, Kolta S, Fechtenbaum J, et al. Spinal deformity index (SDI) is a good predictor of incident vertebral fractures. Osteoporos Int 2009;20(9):1547–52.

28. Munns CF, Rauch F, Travers R, et al. Effects of intravenous pamidronate treatment in infants with osteogenesis imperfecta: clinical and histomorphometric outcome. J Bone Miner Res 2005;20(7):1235–43.

29. Sbrocchi AM, Rauch F, Jacob P, et al. The use of intravenous bisphosphonate therapy to treat vertebral fractures due to osteoporosis among boys with Duchenne muscular dystrophy. Osteoporos Int 2012;23(11):2703–11.

30. Krőger H, Kotaniemi A, Vainio P, et al. Bone densitometry of the spine and femur in children by dual-energy X-ray absorptiometry. Bone Miner 1992;17(1):75–85.

31. Carter DR, Bouxsein ML, Marcus R. New approaches for interpreting projected bone densitometry data. J Bone Miner Res 1992;7(2):137–45.

32. Goulding A, Jones IE, Taylor RW, et al. More broken bones: a 4-year double cohort study of young girls with and without distal forearm fractures. J Bone Miner Res 2000;15(10):2011–8.

33. Crabtree NJ, Hogler W, Cooper MS, et al. Diagnostic evaluation of bone densitometric size adjustment techniques in children with and without low trauma fractures. Osteoporos Int 2013;24(7):2015–24.

34. Zemel BS, Leonard MB, Kelly A, et al. Height adjustment in assessing dual energy x-ray absorptiometry measurements of bone mass and density in children. J Clin Endocrinol Metab 2010;95(3):1265–73.

35. Ma J, Siminoski K, Alos N, et al. The choice of normative pediatric reference database changes spine bone mineral density Z-scores but not the relationship between bone mineral density and prevalent vertebral fractures. J Clin Endocrinol Metab 2015;100(3):1018–27.

36. Kindler JM, Lappe JM, Gilsanz V, et al. Lumbar spine bone mineral apparent density in children: results from the bone mineral density in childhood study. J Clin Endocrinol Metab 2019;104(4):1283–92.

37. Dubner SE, Shults J, Leonard MB, et al. Assessment of spine bone mineral density in juvenile idiopathic arthritis: impact of scan projection. J Clin Densitom 2008;11(2):302–8.

38. Kelly A, Shults J, Mostoufi-Moab S, et al. Pediatric bone mineral accrual Z-score calculation equations and their application in childhood disease. J Bone Miner Res 2019;34(1):195–203.

39. Hans D, Goertzen AL, Krieg MA, et al. Bone microarchitecture assessed by TBS predicts osteoporotic fractures independent of bone density: the Manitoba study. J Bone Miner Res 2011;26(11):2762–9.

40. Winzenrieth R, Michelet F, Hans D. Three-dimensional (3D) microarchitecture correlations with 2D projection image gray-level variations assessed by trabecular bone score using high-resolution computed tomographic acquisitions: effects of resolution and noise. J Clin Densitom 2013;16(3):287–96.

41. Briot K, Paternotte S, Kolta S, et al. Added value of trabecular bone score to bone mineral density for prediction of osteoporotic fractures in postmenopausal women: the OPUS study. Bone 2013;57(1):232–6.

42. Leib E, Winzenrieth R, Lamy O, et al. Comparing bone microarchitecture by trabecular bone score (TBS) in Caucasian American women with and without osteoporotic fractures. Calcif Tissue Int 2014;95(3):201–8.

43. Leib E, Winzenrieth R, Aubry-Rozier B, et al. Vertebral microarchitecture and fragility fracture in men: a TBS study. Bone 2014;62:51–5.

44. Leslie WD, Johansson H, Kanis JA, et al. Lumbar spine texture enhances 10-year fracture probability assessment. Osteoporos Int 2014;25(9):2271–7.

45. Leslie WD, Aubry-Rozier B, Lix LM, et al. Spine bone texture assessed by trabecular bone score (TBS) predicts osteoporotic fractures in men: the Manitoba Bone Density Program. Bone 2014;67:10–4.

46. Nassar K, Paternotte S, Kolta S, et al. Added value of trabecular bone score over bone mineral density for identification of vertebral fractures in patients with areal bone mineral density in the non-osteoporotic range. Osteoporos Int 2014;25(1):243–9.

47. Silva BC, Broy SB, Boutroy S, et al. Fracture risk prediction by non-BMD DXA measures: the 2015 ISCD official positions part 2: trabecular bone score. J Clin Densitom 2015;18(3):309–30.

48. Krueger D, Libber J, Binkley N. Spine trabecular bone score precision, a comparison between ge lunar standard and high-resolution densitometers. J Clin Densitom 2015;18(2):226–32.

49. Adiotomre E, Summers L, Allison A, et al. Diagnostic accuracy of DXA compared to conventional spine radiographs for the detection of vertebral fractures in children. Eur Radiol 2017;27(5):2188–99.

50. van Brussel MS, Lems WF. Clinical relevance of diagnosing vertebral fractures by vertebral fracture assessment. Curr Osteoporos Rep 2009;7(3):103–6.

51. Zeytinoglu M, Jain RK, Vokes TJ. Vertebral fracture assessment: Enhancing the diagnosis, prevention, and treatment of osteoporosis. Bone 2017;104:54–65.

52. Jager PL, Jonkman S, Koolhaas W, et al. Combined vertebral fracture assessment and bone mineral density measurement: a new standard in the diagnosis of osteoporosis in academic populations. Osteoporos Int 2011;22(4):1059–68.

53. Crabtree NJ, Chapman S, Hogler W, et al. Vertebral fractures assessment in children: Evaluation of DXA imaging versus conventional spine radiography. Bone 2017;97:168–74.

54. Diacinti D, Pisani D, D'Avanzo M, et al. Reliability of vertebral fractures assessment (VFA) in children with osteogenesis imperfecta. Calcif Tissue Int 2015; 96(4):307–12.

55. Kyriakou A, Shepherd S, Mason A, et al. A critical appraisal of vertebral fracture assessment in paediatrics. Bone 2015;81:255–9.

56. Cosman F. Spine fracture prevalence in a nationally representative sample of US women and men aged >/=40 years: results from the National Health and Nutrition Examination Survey (NHANES) 2013-2014—supplementary presentation. Osteoporos Int 2017;28(8):2319–20.

57. Ward K, Alsop C, Caulton J, et al. Low magnitude mechanical loading is osteogenic in children with disabling conditions. J Bone Miner Res 2004;19(3):360–9.

58. Kindler JM, Kalkwarf HJ, Lappe JM, et al. Pediatric reference ranges for ultradistal radius bone density: results from the bone mineral density in childhood study. J Clin Endocrinol Metab 2020;105(10):dgaa380.

59. Davie MW, Haddaway MJ. Bone mineral content and density in healthy subjects and in osteogenesis imperfecta. Arch Dis Child 1994;70(4):331–4.

60. Larson CM, Henderson RC. Bone mineral density and fractures in boys with Duchenne muscular dystrophy. J Pediatr Orthop 2000;20(1):71–4.

61. Mostoufi-Moab S, Kelly A, Mitchell JA, et al. Changes in pediatric DXA measures of musculoskeletal outcomes and correlation with quantitative CT following treatment of acute lymphoblastic leukemia. Bone 2018;112:128–35.

62. Zemel BS, Stallings VA, Leonard MB, et al. Revised pediatric reference data for the lateral distal femur measured by Hologic Discovery/Delphi dual-energy X-ray absorptiometry. J Clin Densitom 2009;12(2):207–18.

63. Henderson RC, Berglund LM, May R, et al. The relationship between fractures and DXA measures of BMD in the distal femur of children and adolescents with cerebral palsy or muscular dystrophy. J Bone Miner Res 2010;25(3):520–6.

64. Dubner SE, Shults J, Baldassano RN, et al. Longitudinal assessment of bone density and structure in an incident cohort of children with Crohn's disease. Gastroenterology 2009;136(1):123–30.

65. Ward LM, Ma J, Rauch F, et al. Musculoskeletal health in newly diagnosed children with Crohn's disease. Osteoporos Int 2017;28(11):3169–77.

66. Misof BM, Roschger P, McMillan HJ, et al. Histomorphometry and bone matrix mineralization before and after bisphosphonate treatment in boys with duchenne muscular dystrophy: a paired trans-iliac biopsy study. J Bone Miner Res 2016; 31(5):1060–9.

67. Tommasini SM, Nasser P, Schaffler MB, et al. Relationship between bone morphology and bone quality in male tibias: implications for stress fracture risk. J Bone Miner Res 2005;20(8):1372–80.

68. Gao Y, Zong K, Gao Z, et al. Magnetic resonance imaging-measured bone marrow adipose tissue area is inversely related to cortical bone area in children and adolescents aged 5-18 years. J Clin Densitom 2015;18(2):203–8.

69. Mikolajewicz N, Bishop N, Burghardt AJ, et al. HR-pQCT measures of bone microarchitecture predict fracture: systematic review and meta-analysis. J Bone Miner Res 2020;35(3):446–59.
70. Singhal V, Tulsiani S, Campoverde KJ, et al. Impaired bone strength estimates at the distal tibia and its determinants in adolescents with anorexia nervosa. Bone 2018;106:61–8.
71. Garn SM, Poznanski AK, Larson K. Metacarpal lengths, cortical diameters and areas from the 10-state nutrition survey. In: ZFG J, editor. Proceedings of the first workshop on bone morphometry. Ottawa (Canada): University of Ottawa Press; 1976. p. 367–91.
72. Kelly TL, Wilson KE, Heymsfield SB. Dual energy X-Ray absorptiometry body composition reference values from NHANES. PLoS One 2009;4(9):e7038.
73. Leonard MB, Shults J, Elliott DM, et al. Interpretation of whole body dual energy X-ray absorptiometry measures in children: comparison with peripheral quantitative computed tomography. Bone 2004;34(6):1044–52.
74. Molgaard C, Thomsen BL, Prentice A, et al. Whole body bone mineral content in healthy children and adolescents. Arch Dis Child 1997;76(1):9–15.
75. Binkley T, Johnson J, Vogel L, et al. Bone measurements by peripheral quantitative computed tomography (pQCT) in children with cerebral palsy. J Pediatr 2005;147(6):791–6.
76. Frost HM. The mechanostat: a proposed pathogenic mechanism of osteoporoses and the bone mass effects of mechanical and nonmechanical agents. Bone Miner 1987;2(2):73–85.
77. Frost HM, Schonau E. The "muscle-bone unit" in children and adolescents: a 2000 overview. J Pediatr Endocrinol Metab 2000;13(6):571–90.
78. Schoenau E, Frost HM. The "muscle-bone unit" in children and adolescents. Calcif Tissue Int 2002;70(5):405–7.
79. Rauch F, Schoenau E. The developing bone: slave or master of its cells and molecules? Pediatr Res 2001;50(3):309–14.
80. Burnham JM, Shults J, Semeao E, et al. Body-composition alterations consistent with cachexia in children and young adults with Crohn disease. Am J Clin Nutr 2005;82(2):413–20.

Bone Health in Childhood Chronic Disease

David R. Weber, MD, MSCE*

KEYWORDS

- Osteoporosis • Bone density • Fracture • Dual-energy x-ray absorptiometry
- Bone health • Bisphosphonate

KEY POINTS

- Fisk factors for impaired bone health in children with chronic disease include immobility, nutritional deficiency, exposure to bone toxic therapies, hormonal deficiencies, and inflammation.
- Optimizing bone health in children with chronic disease requires a multidisciplinary clinical approach.
- Bisphosphonate therapy should be considered at the first sign of clinically significant skeletal fragility in a child with chronic disease and limited potential for skeletal recovery.

INTRODUCTION

The chronic diseases of childhood that are associated with impaired bone health are numerous and involve nearly all of the pediatric disciplines. These disorders are heterogeneous and the clinical aspects including treatment, course, and prognosis vary widely. Any factor that adversely affects bone mass, quality, or strength may increase the risk of fracture and should be considered a threat to bone health. Common risk factors for impaired bone health include (1) diminished loading of bone due to immobility or muscle weakness, (2) nutritional deficiency, (3) exposure to bone-toxic therapeutics, (4) hormonal deficiencies affecting growth and development, and (5) chronic inflammation (**Fig. 1**). Even a single fracture can dramatically alter the lifecourse of a medically fragile child by limiting mobility or hastening loss of ambulation. With these consequences in mind, there is growing recognition that efforts to optimize bone health in at-risk patients should be undertaken early in the disease course.

Financial Disclosures: The author has nothing to disclose.
Grant Support: National Institutes of Health, K23 DK114477.
Funded by: NIHHYB; *Grant number(s):* DK114477.
Department of Pediatrics - Endocrinology, Golisano Children's Hospital, University of Rochester, Rochester, NY, USA
* Division of Pediatric Endocrinology, University of Rochester Medical Center, Box 690, 601 Elmwood Avenue, Rochester, NY 14642.
E-mail addresses: weberd@email.chop.edu; davidweber118@gmail.com

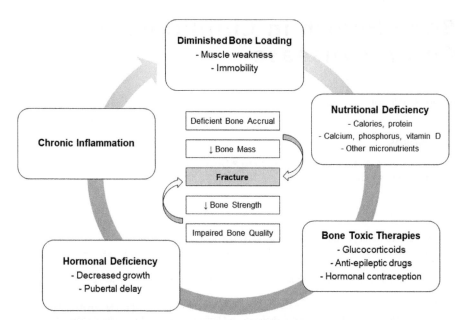

Fig. 1. Risk factors for impaired bone health in childhood chronic disease. Skeletal unloading, inadequate nutrition, exposure to bone toxic medications, hormonal disturbances, and chronic inflammation all may contribute to skeletal fragility by impairing bone accrual and/or negatively affecting bone quality.

The objectives of this review are 2-fold: first, to provide an overview of the chronic diseases of childhood that are most commonly associated with impaired bone health. Key aspects of these conditions relevant to the bone health provider will be summarized, and disease-specific recommendations for clinical management will be discussed when available. Many of these disorders have been the subject of in-depth reviews of bone health, which will be cited. Second, to outline a general approach to the clinical evaluation and treatment of impaired bone health in children with chronic disease.

DISORDERS ASSOCIATED WITH IMPAIRED BONE HEALTH
Neurologic Disorders

Cerebral palsy
Cerebral palsy (CP) is a nonprogressive neuromuscular disorder arising from damage to the developing brain. The clinical severity varies and is commonly classified by degree of motor deficit. Comorbidities including seizures, feeding difficulties, and hypogonadism are common in severely affected individuals.[1] Deficits in bone mineral density (BMD) have been noted in children with CP of all ages and have been shown to be associated with degree of motor deficit, feeding difficulty, and exposure to anti-epileptic drugs (AEDs).[2] Longitudinal studies suggest that children with CP gain bone throughout childhood, albeit at a slower rate than typically developing children.[3] Minimally traumatic fractures are common, especially at the distal femur.[4] Children with CP who suffer a first fracture have been shown to be at high risk of further fracture[5] and should be evaluated.

The evaluation of bone health in children with CP is challenging. Commonly used tools including dual-energy x-ray absorptiometry (DXA) and spine radiograph can be of limited utility in those at highest risk due to contractures, spinal deformities, and in-dwelling hardware. The optimal approach to bone health treatment remains uncertain. Mechanical loading of the skeleton can be achieved in nonambulatory children by use of a stander, but there are minimal data relating standing regimens to bone health outcomes. Physical activity interventions and the use of low-magnitude mechanical stimulation have yielded mixed results.[6,7] Both oral and intravenous (IV) bisphosphonate regimens are widely used to treat osteoporosis in patients with CP[8] and have been associated with gains in BMD and reductions in fracture rate.[9] Guidelines for the management of bone health in childhood CP are available.[10]

Neuromuscular disorders

Duchenne muscular dystrophy (DMD) is the most common heritable neuromuscular disease in childhood. It is a progressive condition that universally results in loss of ambulation by late childhood or early adolescence. Treatment with high-dose glucocorticoids initiated at an early age slows progression of the disease but further weakens the skeleton. The combined risk factors of muscle weakness, immobility, and chronic glucocorticoid exposure contribute to a markedly elevated fracture prevalence (33%–100%, depending on study).[11] Glucocorticoid regimen is a factor in evaluating fracture risk, with daily deflazacort therapy being associated with the greatest risk of fracture.[12]

A notable feature of DMD and other conditions treated with high-dose glucocorticoids is the predilection for vertebral fractures (VF), which can occur even in the absence of low BMD.[13] As a result, routine screening for VF with lateral spine radiography or densitometry is essential.[14] Full considerations for the evaluation and management of bone health in DMD have been extensively reviewed.[15] Other childhood forms of muscular dystrophy are less common. The skeletal effects of these conditions tend to be related to the degree of muscle weakness but have not been systematically studied.

Spinal muscular atrophy is a rare neuromuscular disease of the lower motor neurons. Clinical severity varies from profound weakness with ventilatory dependence from early infancy to mild late-onset disease. Adverse skeletal effects, including scoliosis, low BMD, and atraumatic fracture are common in severely affected children.[16] Treatment advances, including intrathecal injection of nusinersen, improve muscle function and may prolong survival. A small study suggested that IV bisphosphonates were safe and potentially effective in reducing fracture rate.[17]

Epilepsy

A primary concern for children with seizure disorders is that treatments including AEDs and the ketogenic diet may adversely affect the skeleton. The relationships between AEDs and bone mineral metabolism have been extensively reviewed.[18] Many of the classic AEDs induce the CYP-450 enzyme system and thereby lower vitamin D concentration. Direct negative effects of AEDs on skeletal cells have also been reported.[19] Newer generation AEDs seem to have less impact on mineral metabolism but have not been extensively studied.[20] Ketogenic diets are increasingly used to treat refractory epilepsy and may affect the skeleton via acidosis, hypercalciuria, and micronutrient deficiencies.[21] Worsening of BMD deficits in longitudinal studies of children on ketogenic diets have been reported.[22] Current guidelines for patients on a ketogenic diet recommend involvement of a registered dietician (RD), supplementation of calcium and vitamin D as needed, and the consideration of BMD monitoring in children on therapy for 2 or more years.[23]

Neurodevelopment disorders

Children with autism have been shown to have bones that are smaller, weaker, and less dense than typically developing peers.[24] These deficits may be related to inadequate consumption of protein, calcium, and phosphorus and less time spent in physical activity.[25] Girls with Rett Syndrome are also reported to develop skeletal complications including low BMD, fragility fracture, and scoliosis.[26] Guidelines for bone health management in Rett syndrome have been published and include a recommendation for molecular testing in all patients, as specific *MECP2* genotypes seem to confer greater risk of osteoporosis.[27]

Chronic Kidney Disease

The physiologic underpinnings of chronic kidney disease metabolic bone disease (CKD-MBD) include phosphate retention, increased secretion of fibroblast growth factor 23 and parathyroid hormone (PTH), impaired renal 1-α-hydroxylase activity, and hypocalcemia.[28] Skeletal metabolism is affected and can include altered bone turnover, defective mineralization, and skeletal fragility. Fracture rates in children with CKD have been found to be 2 to 3 times greater than the general population.[29] Deficits in BMD, bone structure, and muscle size have been described.[30]

Treatment is directed at controlling phosphate and maintaining normocalcemia.[31] Calcitriol/vitamin D analogues are added for hypocalcemia and to treat secondary hyperparathyroidism. The negative effects of CKD-MBD persist after transplantation. Glucocorticoid sparing immunosuppression is recommended, when possible, and growth hormone should be considered in children who fail to demonstrate catch up growth.[32] The use of bisphosphonates in children with CKD-MBD has not been well studied, and there are concerns it could be detrimental in the setting of low bone turnover.

Inflammatory Disorders

Inflammatory bowel disease (IBD), juvenile idiopathic arthritis, inflammatory arthritis, and systemic lupus erythematosus can all cause skeletal damage.[33] Inflammatory cytokines negatively affect bone by reducing osteoblast mediated formation and promoting osteoclast resorption.[34] Glucocorticoids are frequently used in the initial treatment of inflammatory disease and further weaken bone. Nutritional deficits are possible, especially in IBD in which absorption may be impaired. Inflammatory mediated suppression of pituitary hormone secretion is also a factor. Many of these risk factors are reversible as evidenced by findings that antiinflammatory treatment led to recovery of growth factors, muscle, and bone deficits in children with Crohn disease.[35] Bisphosphonates have been shown to improve BMD in children with IBD[36] and rheumatologic disorders,[37] although indications for use have not been formerly defined.

Liver Disease

Skeletal manifestations of severe liver disease in children include poor growth, low BMD, defects in bone mineralization (including rickets), and fracture.[38] Vitamin D absorption can be profoundly impaired due to fat malabsorption, and very high doses of vitamin D supplementation may be needed. Skeletal recovery is likely after transplant, especially in younger children, as evidenced by findings that long-term survivors of childhood liver transplant had normal BMD and low fracture rate.[39] There are limited data regarding bisphosphonate use in this population. Bisphosphonates should not be administered to patients with active rickets, and care should be taken in those with significant malabsorption, as they may be at increased risk of hypocalcemia following treatment.

Cancer

Glucocorticoids are administered during induction chemotherapy in some forms of childhood cancer. Immobility and deconditioning are also common. Some children require skeletal radiation, which can further damage bone. VF are reported in 25% of children with glucocorticoid-treated acute lymphoblastic leukemia.[40] The prevalence of BMD deficit, fracture, and avascular necrosis may be even higher among patients undergoing hematopoietic stem cell transplantation (HSCT).[41] Many survivors of childhood cancer demonstrate skeletal recovery.[42] Current recommendations suggest annual BMD and VF assessment before and after HSCT, along with attention to calcium and vitamin D repletion as needed. Bisphosphonates can be considered in children with fractures, particularly if symptomatic VF, or if there is a poor prognosis for skeletal recovery based on age, growth potential, or more severe disease.[41]

Diabetes

Impaired bone health is a recognized complication of type 1 diabetes (T1D). In children with T1D, fracture risk was reported to be 14% greater in boys and 35% greater in girls, compared with healthy controls.[43] Deficits in bone density and structure have been described in many[44] but not all studies.[45] When present, the degree of deficit is inadequate to fully explain the fracture risk and suggests impaired bone quality. Hyperglycemia,[46] the coexistence of microvascular disease,[47] and abnormalities in the growth hormone axis[48] have been associated with adverse skeletal outcomes. Vitamin D deficiency and inadequate calcium intake are common.[49] Optimization of calcium and vitamin D intake with dietary modification and supplementation, as needed, is logical and should be incorporated into dietary counseling. Regular weight-bearing physical activity should also be emphasized, noting that children with T1D tend to be less active than peers.[50]

Emerging data in children suggest that cardiometabolic abnormalities associated with type 2 diabetes (T2D) may adversely influence skeletal development.[51] There is growing interest in the use of noninsulin pharmacotherapy to treat childhood T2D. However, some of these agents (sodium-glucose cotransporter 2 inhibitors, for example)[52] may alter bone metabolism and require careful study.

Cystic Fibrosis

Low BMD has been described in some but not all studies of youth with cystic fibrosis (CF).[53] This inconsistency may be due to heterogeneity in CF severity, as studies limited to patients with severe disease have reported significant BMD deficits and fracture risk.[54] Nutritional deficiency leading to low body weight and malabsorption of fat-soluble vitamin D and K, as well as impaired growth and pubertal delay are all risk factors for poor bone accrual.[55] Current guidelines suggest annual assessment of 25-OH vitamin D and a screening DXA scan starting at age 8 years in high-risk children (underweight, poor pulmonary function).[56] Oral alendronate was shown to be safe and effective in improving BMD in youth with CF.[57] However, the indications for initiating bisphosphonates have not been defined.

Congenital Heart Disease

Many children with congenital heart disease (CHD) are critically ill during the early years of skeletal development. Children with single ventricle disease requiring Fontan palliation may be at especially high risk for bone and lean mass deficits that progress with time.[58] Factors shown to impair bone health include diuretics, secondary hyperparathyroidism, and protein losing enteropathy.[59,60] There are few data describing the treatment of bone health in CHD, and specific guidelines have not been published.

Metabolic

Lysosomal storage disorders can result in bony abnormalities and skeletal fragility.[61] Cystinosis in particular can be associated with severe skeletal effects, including rickets, osteoporosis, and CKD-MBD. The cause is multifactorial and related to renal loss of calcium and phosphate, compounded by acidosis and CKD. Treatment is focused on managing rickets and reducing acidosis.[62] Homocystinuria has also been associated with low bone density.[63]

Adolescent Medicine

Gender dysphoria

The treatment of gender dysphoria in youth includes the use of gonadotropin-releasing hormone (GnRH) analogues at the first signs of emotional distress with puberty. Gender-affirming sex steroid therapy typically follows once persistence of gender identify has been established. Concerns about effects of long-term GnRH analogue therapy on skeletal development have been raised. Small studies in adolescents found that GnRH therapy was associated with mild reductions in BMD Z-scores but that catch up bone accrual occurred after initiation of sex steroid therapy.[64] Fracture risk has not been reported in youth but was elevated in adult transwomen.[65] Recent guidelines discuss the issues of bone health in transgender people.[66] A challenge to the evaluation of bone health in this population is that the interpretation of BMD and some bone biomarkers require comparison to sex-matched reference data. DXA reports should therefore include Z-scores referenced to both sex at birth and gender identity.

Eating disorders

Anorexia nervosa, bulimia, and the female athletic triad are associated with impaired bone health.[67] Deficits in BMD and bone structure have been widely described and are the result of energy deficit, low body mass, and hormonal disturbances including hypogonadism.[68] Low body weight is a risk factor for stress fractures in young athletes,[69] and their coexistence should prompt consideration for disordered eating.

Weight restoration therapy is the cornerstone of bone health therapy. Estrogen replacement may be considered in postmenarchal women who fail to resume menses, with or without attaining weight restoration. The decision to institute estrogen replacement should be individualized and must balance skeletal risk against the loss of menses as a biomarker of health. When hormone replacement is desired, evidence supports the use of transdermal estrogen with cyclic progesterone, as this approach has been shown to improve BMD,[70] whereas combined oral contraceptives have not.[71] Studies of bisphosphonates have largely been limited to adults and generally suggest a beneficial effect on BMD.[72] Current opinion states that bisphosphonates should only be used in youth with eating disorders who have clinically significant fractures and poor prognosis for skeletal recovery.[73]

CLINICAL APPROACH

The goals of bone health care in children with chronic disease are to improve health and quality of life by reducing fracture frequency and to promote bone accrual during the critical years for skeletal development. Many children with chronic disease are now living long into adulthood. Maximizing peak bone mass is an important component of mitigating lifelong fracture risk. The accomplishment of these goals requires a multidisciplinary team and close communication with the specialist attending to the child's primary disorder (**Fig. 2**).

The involvement of an RD or other nutrition expert is essential. Risk factors for impaired nutrition are many and include selective eating, gastric- or jejunal-tube dependence, antacids, and malabsorption. Feeding regimens may lead to

Bone Health Evaluation

Medical	Nutrition	Physical Function	Biochemistry	Imaging

Fracture History
• Number
• Location
• Mechanism
 	
Medications
• Glucocorticoids
• Anti-epileptic drugs
• Diuretics
• Contraceptives
 	
Growth
• Height / weight
• Ulnar length if height cannot be assessed
 	
Physical Exam
• Spine for pain, scoliosis
• Long bone deformity
• Joint contracture or laxity
• Pubertal stage
	Dietary Intake
	• Calories, protein
	• Calcium, phosphorus
	• Vitamin D, K, C
	• Other micronutrients
	
	Higher Risk
	• Elemental formula
	• Ketogenic diet
	• Malabsorptive disorder
	  - Cystic fibrosis
	  - Liver disease
	  - IBD
	• Restrictive eating
	  - Anorexia
	  - Autism
	
	Supplements
	• As needed to meet RDA or as dictated by biochemical testing
		Ambulatory
		• Frequency of weight bearing activity
		• Counseling re: fracture avoidance
		
		Non-ambulatory
		• Caregiver education re: safe handling
		• Equipment:
		  - Orthotics
		  - Wheelchair
		  - Transfers
		  - Stander
		• Standing regimen
			Serum
			• CMP
			• Magnesium
			• Phosphorus
			• Intact PTH
			• 25-OH vitamin D
			
			Urine
			• Calcium[a,b]
			• Creatinine
			• Phosphorus[c]
			
			Other[d]
			• TSH, free thyroxine
			• Celiac panel
			• Sex steroids
			• Bone turnover markers
				Lateral spine
				• Patients at high risk of vertebral fracture[e]
				• By radiograph or DXA
				
				DXA
				• Total body less head and lumbar spine are standard
				• Proximal femur, lateral distal femur, distal 1/3 radius in some scenarios[f]
				• Size adjustment in short or tall individuals

Fig. 2. Components of the bone health evaluation. Suggested approach to the initial bone health evaluation. Frequency and extent of follow-up evaluations will depend on initial findings and clinical course. [a] Urine Ca/Cr to assess for hypercalciuria and deficient calcium absorption (see text). [b] Urine Ca/Cr falsely elevated in patients with low muscle mass. Urine Ca/Osmolality or 24-hour quantification should be used instead (see text). [c] Tubular resorption of phosphate [1-(urine phosphorus*serum creatinine)/(serum phosphorus* urine creatinine)] is helpful in determining mechanism of hypophosphatemia and significance of PTH elevations. Values less than 0.9 in presence of hypophosphatemia suggest significant urinary phosphate wasting. [d] Based on clinical suspicion. Thyroid function if growth is impaired. Celiac panel if calcium/vitamin D absorption seems impaired in absence of other cause. Sex steroids (testosterone, estradiol) may be helpful in assessing pubertal status. Bone resorption markers (beta-cross laps, urinary n-telopeptides) may be useful in assessing bisphosphonate dosing. Bone-specific alkaline phosphatase if alkaline phosphatase interpretation is limited by presence of transaminitis. [e] Chronic glucocorticoid use, tenderness over vertebral bodies on examination, low spine bone density by DXA. [f] Choice of site depends on availability of adequate reference data for population and DXA platform. Proximal femur may be appropriate for tracking of BMD through adulthood. Lateral distal femur is used in nonambulatory children at risk of distal femur fracture. Distal one-third radius may be the only option in some patients with significant contractures or indwelling medical hardware. IBD, inflammatory bowel disorder; PTH, parathyroid hormone; RDA, recommended dietary allowance; TSH, thyroid-stimulating hormone.

unexpected complications, as evidenced by reports of hypophosphatemic rickets caused by elemental formula[74] and scurvy due to the ketogenic diet.[75] A dietary history that includes assessment of calcium, phosphorus, vitamin D, as well as macro- and micronutrient intake should be performed at initial evaluation and updated periodically. Many children will require supplementation with cholecalciferol or ergocalciferol. Dosing should be individualized to maintain serum 25-OH-vitamin D levels of 20 to 30 ng/mL (50–75 nmol/L). Routine calcium supplementation is not advised but should be considered if the child is unable to meet the RDA for calcium from dietary sources.

Collaboration with physical therapy (PT) and orthopedic providers is paramount. PT input is essential for the implementation of safe, tolerable weight-bearing regimens. Efforts should be made to optimize bone health before major elective orthopedic procedures such as scoliosis repair or osteotomies for hip dysplasia. This includes the treatment of vitamin D, calcium, and other nutritional deficiencies. In some cases, such as history of fragility fracture, the initiation of bisphosphonate therapy before surgery may be warranted. Deconditioning following surgery or limb immobilization can occur and lead to secondary fractures. PT, under the guidance of the orthopedic surgeon, is a critical component of postimmobilization care.

The assessment of bone health begins with a fracture history. Note should be made of fracture site, timing, and mechanism. Long bone and VF in the absence of trauma are clinically significant and support a diagnosis of osteoporosis in a child with chronic disease. In many cases, biochemical assessment is warranted. Elevations in PTH (in the absence of hypercalcemia) and/or alkaline phosphatase (in the absence of transaminitis) may indicate deficient calcium absorption and can be used to adjust calcium and vitamin D supplementation. Spot urine calcium/creatinine (Uca/Ucr) ratio is helpful in identifying hypercalciuria (>0.2 in children older than 8 years) and deficient calcium absorption (<0.1).[76] Uca/Ucr is not reliable in children with low muscle mass, and spot urine calcium/osmolality[77] or quantification of 24-hour excretion should be performed instead.

Imaging

Imaging is performed to determine BMD and identify VF. DXA provides an estimate of *areal* BMD and is subject to size artifact including underestimation of BMD in short and overestimation of BMD in tall individuals. Techniques for adjusting BMD for size have been developed.[78,79] Size adjustment provides an estimate of the degree of BMD deficit (excess) that may be attributable to short (tall) stature. Delayed (advanced) pubertal development may also affect the assessment of BMD by DXA and should be considered in the clinical interpretation.[80] Total body less head and lumbar spine are the most commonly used DXA sites, although the distal 1/3 radius, proximal hip, and lateral distal femur can be assessed if appropriate reference data are available. The International Society for Clinical Densitometry has sponsored several position development conferences to define best practices for the use of DXA in children. The most recent positions, published in 2019, provide guidance on the use of DXA to assess BMD at the forearm, hip, and lateral distal femur in children. The utility of vertebral fracture assessment by DXA in children was also discussed.[81]

Routine screening for VF should be performed in high-risk patients such as those with back pain, low BMD, or treated with glucocorticoids. Lateral spine radiography or DXA can be used. The Genant semiquantitative method, performed by a provider with pediatric expertise, is recommended for the assessment of VF.[82] Using this approach, VF are graded in severity based on loss of vertebral height as 0 (normal), 1 (mild, <25%), 2 (moderate, 25%–40%), or 3 (severe, >40%). In most cases, the presence of more than or equal to one grade 1 or greater VF, in the absence of trauma, in a child with risk factors for impaired bone health is considered clinically significant and consistent with a diagnosis of osteoporosis. VF assessment is generally repeated annually in children with persistent risk factors and/or being treated with antiosteoporosis agents.

Treatment

The addition of an antiosteoporosis agent to the bone health regimen should be considered when a child with chronic disease suffers a first clinically significant fracture (vertebral, femur) or recurrent low-trauma fractures of other sites when spontaneous recovery of bone health is not anticipated.[83] The decision to initiate therapy must be individualized to balance the benefits and risks. It must incorporate factors including the expected course of underlying disease (limited with possibility of recovery vs progressive), fracture frequency and mechanism (traumatic vs nontraumatic), growth and pubertal status, exposure to bone toxic medications, degree of BMD deficit, and the potential risk and severity of treatment-related adverse events (hypocalcemia, acute phase reaction, renal injury, osteonecrosis of jaw).

The nitrogeneous bisphosphonates are the most widely used agents in children. Bisphosphonates increase BMD and bone strength through the inhibition of osteoclasts. Data from placebo-controlled clinical trials to properly inform indication, dose, or duration of bisphosphonate therapy in children with chronic diseases are lacking. There is, however, growing clinical experience with the use of these drugs in many of the chronic diseases of childhood. Bisphosphonates have generally been shown to be effective in improving bone density, but data for fracture reduction are less conclusive.

Consensus guidelines for the use of bisphosphonates in children have been proposed[84] and protocols for the use of zoledronate[85] and pamidronate[86] have been published. IV formulations are more potent than oral and more widely used. Zoledronate is the most potent, making it the preferred agent in many centers due to its brief infusion time (typically 30 minutes) and dosing duration (typically every 6–12 months). There are a few studies that support the efficacy of oral bisphosphonates to improve BMD in children with chronic disease.[87] A potential role for bisphosphonates in children with low bone density before first fracture requires further study.

SUMMARY

The adverse skeletal effects of childhood chronic disease are now widely recognized. Great strides have been made in defining the pathophysiology underlying impaired bone health in this population. The clinical approach continues to evolve with growing emphasis placed on incorporating bone health care into the multidisciplinary approach to these children. There remains a need for research to more clearly define the optimal indication, dosing, and duration of bisphosphonate therapy. Alternative therapies, including anti-RANKL antibody and anti-sclerostin antibody, are now widely used in adults and should be evaluated in children for whom bisphosphonates are contraindicated or have limited efficacy.

REFERENCES

1. Trinh A, Wong P, Fahey MC, et al. Musculoskeletal and endocrine health in adults with cerebral palsy: new opportunities for intervention. J Clin Endocrinol Metab 2016;101(3):1190–7.

2. Henderson RC, Lark RK, Gurka MJ, et al. Bone density and metabolism in children and adolescents with moderate to severe cerebral palsy. Pediatrics 2002; 110(1 Pt 1):e5.

3. Trinh A, Wong P, Fahey MC, et al. Longitudinal changes in bone density in adolescents and young adults with cerebral palsy: a case for early intervention. Clin Endocrinol (Oxf) 2019;91(4):517–24.

4. Sees JP, Sitoula P, Dabney K, et al. Pamidronate treatment to prevent reoccurring fractures in children with cerebral palsy. J Pediatr Orthop 2016;36(2):193–7.

5. Stevenson RD, Conaway M, Barrington JW, et al. Fracture rate in children with cerebral palsy. Pediatr Rehabil 2006;9(4):396–403.

6. Kim SJ, Kim SN, Yang YN, et al. Effect of weight bearing exercise to improve bone mineral density in children with cerebral palsy: a meta-analysis. J Musculoskelet Neuronal Interact 2017;17(4):334–40.

7. Gusso S, Munns CF, Colle P, et al. Effects of whole-body vibration training on physical function, bone and muscle mass in adolescents and young adults with cerebral palsy. Sci Rep 2016;6:22518.

8. Nasomyont N, Hornung LN, Gordon CM, et al. Outcomes following intravenous bisphosphonate infusion in pediatric patients: A 7-year retrospective chart review. Bone 2019;121:60–7.

9. Kim MJ, Kim SN, Lee IS, et al. Effects of bisphosphonates to treat osteoporosis in children with cerebral palsy: a meta-analysis. J Pediatr Endocrinol Metab 2015; 28(11-12):1343–50.

10. Ozel S, Switzer L, Macintosh A, et al. Informing evidence-based clinical practice guidelines for children with cerebral palsy at risk of osteoporosis: an update. Dev Med Child Neurol 2016;58(9):918–23.

11. Singh A, Schaeffer EK, Reilly CW. Vertebral fractures in duchenne muscular dystrophy patients managed with deflazacort. J Pediatr Orthop 2018;38(6):320–4.

12. Joseph S, Wang C, Bushby K, et al. Fractures and linear growth in a nationwide cohort of boys with Duchenne muscular dystrophy with and without glucocorticoid treatment: results from the UK NorthStar Database. JAMA Neurol 2019; 76(6):701–9.

13. Ma J, McMillan HJ, Karaguzel G, et al. The time to and determinants of first fractures in boys with Duchenne muscular dystrophy. Osteoporos Int 2017;28(2): 597–608.

14. Crabtree NJ, Chapman S, Hogler W, et al. Vertebral fractures assessment in children: evaluation of DXA imaging versus conventional spine radiography. Bone 2017;97:168–74.

15. Ward LM, Hadjiyannakis S, McMillan HJ, et al. Bone health and osteoporosis management of the patient with duchenne muscular dystrophy. Pediatrics 2018;142(Suppl 2):S34–42.

16. Baranello G, Vai S, Broggi F, et al. Evolution of bone mineral density, bone metabolism and fragility fractures in Spinal Muscular Atrophy (SMA) types 2 and 3. Neuromuscul Disord 2019;29(7):525–32.

17. Nasomyont N, Hornung LN, Wasserman H. Intravenous bisphosphonate therapy in children with spinal muscular atrophy. Osteoporos Int 2019.

18. Verrotti A, Coppola G, Parisi P, et al. Bone and calcium metabolism and antiepileptic drugs. Clin Neurol Neurosurg 2010;112(1):1–10.

19. Pitetzis DA, Spilioti MG, Yovos JG, et al. The effect of VPA on bone: From clinical studies to cell cultures-The molecular mechanisms revisited. Seizure 2017;48: 36–43.

20. Fu J, Peng L, Li J, et al. Effects of second-generation antiepileptic drugs compared to first-generation antiepileptic drugs on bone metabolism in patients with epilepsy: a meta-analysis. Horm Metab Res 2019;51(8):511–21.

21. Ruiz Herrero J, Canedo Villarroya E, Garcia Penas JJ, et al. Safety and effectiveness of the prolonged treatment of children with a ketogenic diet. Nutrients 2020;12(2).

22. Simm PJ, Bicknell-Royle J, Lawrie J, et al. The effect of the ketogenic diet on the developing skeleton. Epilepsy Res 2017;136:62–6.

23. Kossoff EH, Zupec-Kania BA, Auvin S, et al. Optimal clinical management of children receiving dietary therapies for epilepsy: updated recommendations of the International Ketogenic Diet Study Group. Epilepsia Open 2018;3(2):175–92.

24. Neumeyer AM, Cano Sokoloff N, McDonnell E, et al. Bone microarchitecture in adolescent boys with autism spectrum disorder. Bone 2017;97:139–46.

25. Neumeyer AM, Cano Sokoloff N, McDonnell EI, et al. Nutrition and bone density in boys with autism spectrum disorder. J Acad Nutr Diet 2018;118(5):865–77.

26. Roende G, Ravn K, Fuglsang K, et al. DXA measurements in Rett syndrome reveal small bones with low bone mass. J Bone Miner Res 2011;26(9):2280–6.

27. Jefferson A, Leonard H, Siafarikas A, et al. Clinical guidelines for management of bone health in Rett syndrome based on expert consensus and available evidence. PLoS One 2016;11(2):e0146824.

28. Hanudel MR, Salusky IB. Treatment of pediatric chronic kidney disease-mineral and bone disorder. Curr Osteoporos Rep 2017;15(3):198–206.

29. Denburg MR, Kumar J, Jemielita T, et al. Fracture burden and risk factors in childhood CKD: results from the CKiD Cohort Study. J Am Soc Nephrol 2016;27(2):543–50.

30. Tsampalieros A, Kalkwarf HJ, Wetzsteon RJ, et al. Changes in bone structure and the muscle-bone unit in children with chronic kidney disease. Kidney Int 2012;3(10):347.

31. Ketteler M, Block GA, Evenepoel P, et al. Executive summary of the 2017 KDIGO Chronic Kidney Disease-Mineral and Bone Disorder (CKD-MBD) Guideline Update: what's changed and why it matters. Kidney Int 2017;92(1):26–36.

32. Haffner D, Leifheit-Nestler M. CKD-MBD post kidney transplantation. Pediatr Nephrol 2019.

33. Huber AM, Ward LM. The impact of underlying disease on fracture risk and bone mineral density in children with rheumatic disorders: A review of current literature. Semin Arthritis Rheum 2016,46(1):49–63.

34. Adamopoulos IE. Inflammation in bone physiology and pathology. Curr Opin Rheumatol 2018;30(1):59–64.

35. DeBoer MD, Lee AM, Herbert K, et al. Increases in IGF-1 After Anti-TNF-alpha therapy are associated with bone and muscle accrual in pediatric Crohn disease. J Clin Endocrinol Metab 2018;103(3):936–45.

36. Sbrocchi AM, Forget S, Laforte D, et al. Zoledronic acid for the treatment of osteopenia in pediatric Crohn's disease. Pediatr Int 2010;52(5):754–61.

37. Rooney M, Bishop N, Davidson J, et al. The prevention and treatment of glucocorticoid-induced osteopaenia in juvenile rheumatic disease: A randomised double-blind controlled trial. EClinicalMedicine 2019;12:79–87.

38. Hogler W, Baumann U, Kelly D. Endocrine and bone metabolic complications in chronic liver disease and after liver transplantation in children. J Pediatr Gastroenterol Nutr 2012;54(3):313–21.

39. Ee LC, Noble C, Fawcett J, et al. Bone mineral density of very long-term survivors after childhood liver transplantation. J Pediatr Gastroenterol Nutr 2018;66(5): 797–801.

40. Cummings EA, Ma J, Fernandez CV, et al. Incident Vertebral Fractures in Children With Leukemia During the Four Years Following Diagnosis. J Clin Endocrinol Metab 2015;100(9):3408–17.

41. Kuhlen M, Kunstreich M, Niinimaki R, et al. Guidance to bone morbidity in children and adolescents undergoing allogeneic hematopoietic stem cell transplantation. Biol Blood Marrow Transplant 2020;26(2):e27–37.

42. Ward LM, Ma J, Lang B, et al. Bone morbidity and recovery in children with acute lymphoblastic leukemia: results of a six-year prospective cohort study. J Bone Miner Res 2018;33(8):1435–43.

43. Weber DR, Haynes K, Leonard MB, et al. Type 1 diabetes is associated with an increased risk of fracture across the life span: a population-based cohort study using The Health Improvement Network (THIN). Diabetes Care 2015;38(10): 1913–20.

44. Chen SC, Shepherd S, McMillan M, et al. Skeletal fragility and its clinical determinants in children with type 1 diabetes. J Clin Endocrinol Metab 2019;104(8): 3585–94.

45. Madsen JOB, Herskin CW, Zerahn B, et al. Unaffected bone mineral density in Danish children and adolescents with type 1 diabetes. J Bone Miner Metab 2020;38(3):328–37.

46. Weber DR, Gordon RJ, Kelley JC, et al. Poor glycemic control is associated with impaired bone accrual in the year following a diagnosis of type 1 diabetes. J Clin Endocrinol Metab 2019;104(10):4511–20.

47. Abdalrahaman N, McComb C, Foster JE, et al. Deficits in trabecular bone microarchitecture in young women with type 1 diabetes mellitus. J Bone Miner Res 2015;30(8):1386–93.

48. Mitchell DM, Caksa S, Joseph T, et al. Elevated HbA1c is associated with altered cortical and trabecular microarchitecture in girls with type 1 diabetes. J Clin Endocrinol Metab 2019.

49. Mayer-Davis EJ, Nichols M, Liese AD, et al. Dietary intake among youth with diabetes: the SEARCH for diabetes in youth study. J Am Diet Assoc 2006;106(5): 689–97.

50. Sundberg F, Forsander G, Fasth A, et al. Children younger than 7 years with type 1 diabetes are less physically active than healthy controls. Acta Paediatr 2012; 101(11):1164–9.

51. Hetherington-Rauth M, Bea JW, Blew RM, et al. Relationship of cardiometabolic risk biomarkers with DXA and pQCT bone health outcomes in young girls. Bone 2019;120:452–8.

52. Cianciolo G, De Pascalis A, Capelli I, et al. Mineral and electrolyte disorders with SGLT2i therapy. JBMR Plus 2019;3(11):e10242.

53. Ubago-Guisado E, Cavero-Redondo I, Alvarez-Bueno C, et al. Bone health in children and youth with cystic fibrosis: a systematic review and meta-analysis of matched cohort studies. J Pediatr 2019;215:178–86.e6.

54. Cairoli E, Eller-Vainicher C, Morlacchi LC, et al. Bone involvement in young adults with cystic fibrosis awaiting lung transplantation for end-stage respiratory failure. Osteoporos Int 2019;30(6):1255–63.

55. Goldsweig B, Kaminski B, Sidhaye A, et al. Puberty in cystic fibrosis. J Cyst Fibros 2019;18(Suppl 2):S88–94.

56. Aris RM, Merkel PA, Bachrach LK, et al. Guide to bone health and disease in cystic fibrosis. J Clin Endocrinol Metab 2005;90(3):1888–96.

57. Bianchi ML, Colombo C, Assael BM, et al. Treatment of low bone density in young people with cystic fibrosis: a multicentre, prospective, open-label observational study of calcium and calcifediol followed by a randomised placebo-controlled trial of alendronate. Lancet Respir Med 2013;1(5):377–85.

58. Diab SG, Godang K, Muller LO, et al. Progressive loss of bone mass in children with Fontan circulation. Congenit Heart Dis 2019;14(6):996–1004.

59. Goldberg DJ, Dodds K, Avitabile CM, et al. Children with protein-losing enteropathy after the Fontan operation are at risk for abnormal bone mineral density. Pediatr Cardiol 2012;33(8):1264–8.

60. Cheng HH, Carmona F, McDavitt E, et al. Fractures related to metabolic bone disease in children with congenital heart disease. Congenit Heart Dis 2016; 11(1):80–6.

61. Langeveld M, Hollak CEM. Bone health in patients with inborn errors of metabolism. Rev Endocr Metab Disord 2018;19(1):81–92.

62. Hohenfellner K, Rauch F, Ariceta G, et al. Management of bone disease in cystinosis: Statement from an international conference. J Inherit Metab Dis 2019;42(5): 1019–29.

63. Weber DR, Coughlin C, Brodsky JL, et al. Low bone mineral density is a common finding in patients with homocystinuria. Mol Genet Metab 2016;117(3):351–4.

64. Stoffers IE, de Vries MC, Hannema SE. Physical changes, laboratory parameters, and bone mineral density during testosterone treatment in adolescents with gender dysphoria. J Sex Med 2019;16(9):1459–68.

65. Wiepjes CM, de Blok CJ, Staphorsius AS, et al. Fracture risk in trans women and trans men using long-term gender-affirming hormonal treatment: a nationwide cohort study. J Bone Miner Res 2020;35(1):64–70.

66. Hembree WC, Cohen-Kettenis PT, Gooren L, et al. Endocrine treatment of gender-dysphoric/gender-incongruent persons: an endocrine society clinical practice guideline. J Clin Endocrinol Metab 2017;102(11):3869–903.

67. Williams NI, Statuta SM, Austin A. Female athlete triad: future directions for energy availability and eating disorder research and practice. Clin Sports Med 2017;36(4):671–86.

68. Robinson L, Aldridge V, Clark EM, et al. A systematic review and meta-analysis of the association between eating disorders and bone density. Osteoporos Int 2016; 27(6):1953–66.

69. Nose-Ogura S, Yoshino O, Dohi M, et al. Risk factors of stress fractures due to the female athlete triad: Differences in teens and twenties. Scand J Med Sci Sports 2019;29(10):1501–10.

70. Misra M, Katzman D, Miller KK, et al. Physiologic estrogen replacement increases bone density in adolescent girls with anorexia nervosa. J Bone Miner Res 2011; 26(10):2430–8.

71. Strokosch GR, Friedman AJ, Wu SC, et al. Effects of an oral contraceptive (norgestimate/ethinyl estradiol) on bone mineral density in adolescent females with anorexia nervosa: a double-blind, placebo-controlled study. J Adolesc Health 2006;39(6):819–27.

72. Robinson L, Aldridge V, Clark EM, et al. Pharmacological treatment options for low bone mineral density and secondary osteoporosis in anorexia nervosa: a systematic review of the literature. J Psychosom Res 2017;98:87–97.

73. Misra M, Klibanski A. Anorexia nervosa and bone. J Endocrinol 2014;221(3): R163–76.

74. Gonzalez Ballesteros LF, Ma NS, Gordon RJ, et al. Unexpected widespread hypophosphatemia and bone disease associated with elemental formula use in infants and children. Bone 2017;97:287–92.

75. Alten ED, Chaturvedi A, Cullimore M, et al. No longer a historical ailment: two cases of childhood scurvy with recommendations for bone health providers. Osteoporos Int 2020;31(5):1001–5.

76. Metz MP. Determining urinary calcium/creatinine cut-offs for the paediatric population using published data. Ann Clin Biochem 2006;43(Pt 5):398–401.

77. Mir S, Serdaroglu E. Quantification of hypercalciuria with the urine calcium osmolality ratio in children. Pediatr Nephrol 2005;20(11):1562–5.

78. Zemel BS, Kalkwarf HJ, Gilsanz V, et al. Revised reference curves for bone mineral content and areal bone mineral density according to age and sex for black and non-black children: results of the bone mineral density in childhood study. J Clin Endocrinol Metab 2011;96(10):3160–9.

79. Crabtree NJ, Shaw NJ, Bishop NJ, et al. Amalgamated reference data for size-adjusted bone densitometry measurements in 3598 children and young adults-the ALPHABET study. J Bone Miner Res 2017;32(1):172–80.

80. Gordon CM, Bachrach LK, Carpenter TO, et al. Dual energy X-ray absorptiometry interpretation and reporting in children and adolescents: the 2007 ISCD pediatric official positions. J Clin Densitom 2008;11(1):43–58.

81. Weber DR, Boyce A, Gordon C, et al. The utility of DXA assessment at the forearm, proximal femur, and lateral distal femur, and vertebral fracture assessment in the pediatric population: 2019 ISCD official position. J Clin Densitom 2019;22(4):567–89.

82. Jaremko JL, Siminoski K, Firth GB, et al. Common normal variants of pediatric vertebral development that mimic fractures: a pictorial review from a national longitudinal bone health study. Pediatr Radiol 2015;45(4):593–605.

83. Ward LM, Weber DR, Munns CF, et al. A contemporary view of the definition and diagnosis of osteoporosis in children and adolescents. J Clin Endocrinol Metab 2019.

84. Simm PJ, Biggin A, Zacharin MR, et al. Consensus guidelines on the use of bisphosphonate therapy in children and adolescents. J Paediatr Child Health 2018;54(3):223–33.

85. George S, Weber DR, Kaplan P, et al. Short-term safety of zoledronic acid in young patients with bone disorders: an extensive institutional experience. J Clin Endocrinol Metab 2015;100(11):4163–71.

86. Palomo T, Andrade MC, Peters BS, et al. Evaluation of a modified pamidronate protocol for the treatment of osteogenesis imperfecta. Calcif Tissue Int 2016;98(1):42–8.

87. Bianchi ML, Cimaz R, Bardare M, et al. Efficacy and safety of alendronate for the treatment of osteoporosis in diffuse connective tissue diseases in children: a prospective multicenter study. Arthritis Rheum 2000;43(9):1960–6.

Inhaled Corticosteroids and Endocrine Effects in Childhood

David B. Allen, MD

KEYWORDS

- Inhaled corticosteroids • Growth • Adrenal suppression

KEY POINTS

- Potential adverse systemic effects of long-term inhaled corticosteroid (ICS) therapy include suppression of adrenal function, growth inhibition, and impaired bone mineralization.
- Dosage, type of inhaler device used, patient technique, and characteristics of the individual drug influence delivery of drug to the systemic circulation and risk for systemic adverse effects.
- Symptomatic hypothalamic-pituitary-adrenal axis suppression, although rare during ICS treatment alone, can occur even in the absence of growth suppression and should be suspected in any ICS-treated child presenting with suspicious signs or symptoms.
- Because detectable slowing in growth rate is not uncommon in prepubertal children treated with continuous ICSs, anticipatory guidance regarding risk-to-benefit perspective and appropriate monitoring should be provided.
- Current evidence indicates that decreased bone mineral acquisition in children is associated only with high doses but not low to medium doses of ICS.

INTRODUCTION

Asthma is the most common chronic inflammatory disease of children, and inhaled corticosteroids (ICSs) are the most effective and commonly used treatment of persistent asthma. ICSs currently approved for and commonly used by children with asthma include beclomethasone dipropionate (BDP), budesonide (BUD), fluticasone propionate (FP), mometasone furoate (MF), ciclesonide (CIC), and triamcinolone acetonide (TA). This article reviews 4 areas critical to understanding potential adverse endocrine outcomes of ICSs and placing them in proper perspective: (1) influence of drug/delivery device properties on systemic steroid burden; (2) adrenal insufficiency during ICS

Division of Pediatric Endocrinology and Diabetes, Department of Pediatrics, University of Wisconsin School of Medicine and Public Health, H4/448 CSC – Pediatrics, 600 Highland Avenue, Madison, WI 53792-4108, USA
E-mail address: dballen@wisc.edu

Endocrinol Metab Clin N Am 49 (2020) 651–665
https://doi.org/10.1016/j.ecl.2020.07.003
0889-8529/20/© 2020 Elsevier Inc. All rights reserved.

treatment; (3) growth effects of ICSs and asthma itself; and (4) bone mineral accretion during ICS therapy. For background information and references, readers are referred to comprehensive reviews.[1,2]

IMPORTANT DIFFERENCES IN INHALED CORTICOSTEROIDS CHARACTERISTICS, DELIVERY, AND ABSORPTION

A challenge in interpreting studies of ICS safety properly is assessing whether clinically equivalent drug/delivery device regimens are being compared. The potency of specific ICS preparations varies widely; judged according to glucocorticoid-receptor binding affinity, the relative topical potencies of ICSs are FP > MF > desisobutyryl (DES)-CIC (DES-CIC is the active metabolite of CIC) > BUD > beclomethasone monopropionate (BMP) (BMP is the active metabolite of BDP) > TA. The amount of systemic absorption depends not only on the actual dose administered but also on the mode of delivery. Although most dry powder inhalers (DPIs) and nebulizers generally deliver only 10% to 30% of the nominal dose to the lung, hydrofluoroalkane (HFA)-propelled metered dose inhalers (MDIs), which have replaced ozone-depleting chlorofluorocarbon (CFC)-propelled MDIs, deliver up to 56% of the nominal dose to airways.[3] The addition of a spacer device to an MDI can further increase the percentage of the nominal dose reaching the lungs by up to 20%. After inhalation, the portion of drug that reaches the lungs exerts therapeutic anti-inflammatory effects prior to essentially complete absorption into the systemic circulation. In contrast, drug swallowed and absorbed exerts systemic effects without substantial organ-specific anti-inflammatory effects.[1]

Although various ICS preparations are thought to have similar clinical efficacy when used at equivalent therapeutic doses, differences in pharmacokinetics affect their safety profiles. The percent of drug systemically available after oral administration varies greatly, estimated to be less than 1% for FP, MF, and CIC but up to 41% for BDP, 23% for TA and 10% for BUD (**Fig. 1**).[3–5] Thus, clinically relevant differences in the ratio of drug absorbed through the lungs to total drug absorbed into the systemic circulation primarily reflects differences in gastrointestinal absorption and first-pass hepatic metabolism. Other important drug attributes (potency and lipophilicity) have important effects on therapeutic microgram-for-microgram comparisons and determination of clinically equivalent doses of various ICS compounds but are less useful than oral bioavailability in predicting differences in the ratio between therapeutic and systemic effects.

Administering an ICS in the form of a prodrug theoretically enhances the ratio of therapeutic to systemic effects. Currently, BDP and CIC are the only ICS prodrugs, inactive in their native forms before metabolism in the lung to BMP and DES-CIC, respectively. These 2 active metabolites of BDP and CIC have 2 of the highest receptor affinities of any corticosteroids (12–13.5 times that of dexamethasone). The 2 prodrugs differ, however, in that BMP is further metabolized to another active drug, beclomethasone, which prolongs systemic exposure following absorption from the lung, whereas DES-CIC, which has no active metabolites, undergoes thorough hepatic first-pass metabolism (>99%) and thus imparts little systemic bioactivity. Optimally, ICSs are engineered to be metabolized rapidly to either inactive products or highly protein bound (and, therefore, inaccessible to the glucocorticoid receptor) once they leave the lung. DES-CIC exhibits both properties because it is highly protein bound and exhibits low lipophilicity (and thus more rapid theoretic clearance), but further study is needed to clarify whether DES-CIC's characteristics target ICS bioactivity to the lungs and minimize adverse systemic effects in a clinically meaningful way.

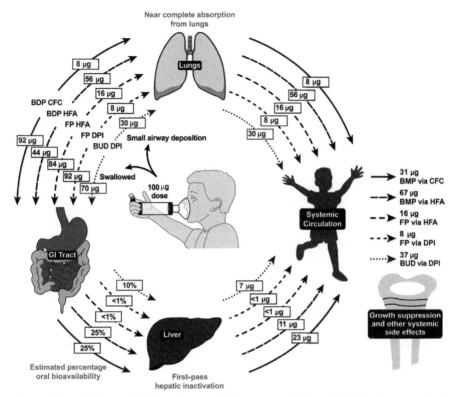

Fig. 1. Effects of drug and device characteristics on systemic bioavailability of a conceptual 100 μg dose of various ICS preparations. GI, gastrointestinal. (*From* Allen DB. Inhaled corticosteroids and growth: still an issue after all these years. J Pediatr. 2015;166(2):466; with permission.)

Studies have demonstrated the importance of drug-specific variations in delivery to the systemic circulation. In particular, The Dose of Inhaled Corticosteroids with Equisystemic Effects study was designed to characterize systemic effects of the ICS to determine equisystemic doses of 6 ICSs using analysis of area under the curve (AUC) for overnight hourly cortisol concentrations.[6] Marked variations in systemic effect were detected that depended not only on the ICS but also the delivery device. For instance, FP, the most potent ICS with regard to receptor binding affinity, was minimally cortisol suppressive, even at high doses, when administered with a DPI but very cortisol suppressive when administered by a CFC-MDI plus valved holding chamber (which increases lung delivery). Furthermore, because lung deposition of FP delivered by HFA-MDI is at least twice that delivered by DPIs (approximately 16% vs approximately 8%), a dose of FP via DPI that has minimal systemic effects could have growth suppressive effects when administered by HFA-MDI (**Fig. 2**).[7] Because FP is absorbed into blood virtually exclusively via the lung, these results show that an equal dose of FP via HFA-MDI resulted in much more drug delivery to the lung than the same dose of FP via DPI. More efficient delivery can also compensate for reduced potency. For instance, equivalent 10% AUC cortisol suppression effect was produced by 268 μg of DPI BUD (approximately 30%–35% delivery of nominal dosage) and 445 μg of DPI FP (approximately 15% delivery of nominal dosage),

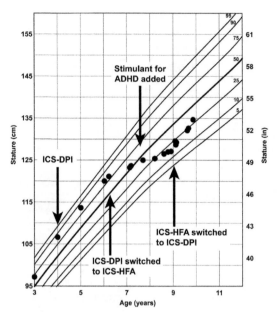

Fig. 2. Growth curve for a boy referred for evaluation of growth failure at age 8.8 years. At age 4 years, asthma was diagnosed and treated with twice-daily dry powder ICS plus a long-acting β-agonist. At age 6.3 years, ICS treatment was changed to twice-daily equal dosages of ICS delivered via an HFA inhaler, which slowed growth rate from 6.5 to ~3 cm/y. At age 7.5 years, stimulant medication for treatment of ADHD was added, and growth rate declined to ~2 cm/y during the ensuing 18 months of combined ICS HFA plus stimulant treatment. Transition of ICS treatment back to equal dosages of dry powder ICS plus a long-acting β-agonist was accompanied by an increase in growth rate. (*From* Allen DB. Inhaled corticosteroids and growth: still an issue after all these years. J Pediatr. 2015;166(2):465; with permission.)

even though the BUD molecule is only one-half as potent as FP in its binding affinity for the glucocorticoid receptor.

Particle size is an important factor in determining delivery of drug to lung versus gut. For example, BDP for use in HFA-propelled MDI was reformulated as a solution (unlike the suspension of the previous CFC-propelled MDI), and the smaller BDP particles of the HFA-propelled solution are delivered more efficiently to the lungs (>50% of the solution's nominal dose reaches the lung vs only 4% to 8% lung delivery with the CFC-propelled suspension). Accordingly, studies show that beclomethasone administered via HFA-MDI produces a clinically equivalent therapeutic response at 35% to 50% of the BDP dose given via CFC-MDI. Furthermore, if equal doses of beclomethasone are given by HFA-MDI and CFC-MDI, the HFA-MDI leads to approximately 70% higher systemic beclomethasone levels than the CFC (see **Fig. 1**).[8,9] Thus, prescribers must consider the potential significance of HFA formulations versus previous CFC formulations because even on the lowest labeled dose of HFA-propelled BDP (40 μg twice daily, which is only 20% of the nominal dose used in previous CFC-propelled BDP inhalers), growth rates were decreased 1.1 cm (compared with placebo) over 44 weeks in 5 year olds to 18 year olds with mild persistent asthma.[10] Importantly, transition to the more environmentally friendly HFA-propelled MDIs did not require changes in the particle size of all corticosteroids, such as was the case with FP, so attention to the characteristics of each ICS is required to tailor therapy.

The phase-out of CFC propellants also accelerated development of multidose DPIs. As discussed previously, the output characteristics of these DPI devices vary markedly; thus, 1 inhaler may generate considerably more fine particles capable of delivery to very small airways (<5 μm) than another. An important study used pharmacokinetics to compare the lung deposition of the 2 most widely prescribed DPI corticosteroids: BUD inhaled from Turbuhaler (AstraZeneca, Lund, Sweden) and FP inhaled from Diskus (GlaxoSmithKline, London, United Kingdom). The mean lung depositions of BUD (via Tubuhaler) and FP (via Diskus) were 30.8% and 8.0%, respectively (see **Fig. 1**). In other words, ICS lung deposition was 4-times higher in children after inhalation from Turbuhaler than after inhalation from Diskus. Given ICS delivered to the lung is almost completely absorbed into the systemic blood stream, the more efficient lung delivery of BUD via DPIs explains why it caused greater suppression of overnight cortisol concentrations than FP via DPIs despite BUD exhibiting a lower glucocorticoid binding affinity.[6] In addition, even if prescribing the same drug delivered by a different inhalation device, awareness of lung delivery is important because a dose of dry powder FP that has poor lung delivery and minimal systemic can have growth suppressive effects when administered by an HFA-MDI (see **Fig. 2**).[7] Thus, to make rational comparisons between various ICS preparations, knowledge of the interaction of drug preparation and delivery device in determining oral and lung drug deposition is essential. It has been proposed that new approach to designing comparative trials of systemic would be to compare the drugs and devices in doses that would be expected to result in significant differences in relative systemic glucocorticoid activity, taking into account relative receptor-binding affinity as well as dosing and bioavailability differences.[11]

ADRENAL INSUFFICIENCY IN INHALED CORTICOSTEROID–TREATED CHILDREN

The presence of exogenous glucocorticoid in the bloodstream will reduce the need for endogenous cortisol production proportionately. Measurements of basal hypothalamic-pituitary-adrenal (HPA) activity, such as AUC cortisol concentrations and urinary-free cortisol excretion, theoretically provide the most sensitive indication of systemic bioavailability of ICS, and these laboratory measures of HPA axis function frequently are used to compare systemic bioavailability of ICS. The mere presence of an exogenous glucocorticoid in circulation, however, does not necessarily indicate risk of adverse consequences. Clinically relevant adverse effects are anticipated only if the exogenous glucocorticoid either approaches or exceeds, in glucocorticoid effect, normal cortisol production or provides a pattern of glucocorticoid exposure that, by differing significantly from normal diurnal fluctuations in cortisol levels, adversely affects other physiologic systems.[12]

Although clinical experience with ICSs over the past 30 years suggests that the risk of adrenal insufficiency due to ICS treatment alone is very low, reports of symptomatic adrenal insufficiency raise appropriate concern about this potential side effect.[13,14] In 1 study from the United Kingdom, 28 children treated with ICS doses within recommended guidelines met diagnostic criteria for adrenal crisis, 23 with overt symptomatic hypoglycemia and 5 with insidious onset of symptoms.[15] The frequency of acute adrenal crisis was greatest in FP-treated children and often precipitated by abrupt termination of high-dose ICS. Close inspection of the reported cases, however, reveals (1) treatment with FP far in excess of recommended dosage for children; (2) lack of follow-up visits to assess disease control and reduce dose of ICS; and (3) provision of care by general practitioners in the absence of subspecialty consultation. Consequently, these cases mirror prior reports of hypoglycemia or laboratory evidence of severe HPA axis suppression, attributable to excessive dosing of ICSs and/or residual effects of prior oral corticosteroid treatment.[16,17] Nevertheless, the potential risks of systemic effects of ICS treatment were highlighted by a report that two-thirds of 143 children attending an allergy specialty clinic had evidence of HPA axis dysfunction correlated with ICS plus nasal corticosteroid daily dose per square meter.[18]

Several tests are available to assess adrenal function. An early morning fasting cortisol level greater than 10 μg/dL (276 nmol/L) still serves as a feasible real-world indicator of intact nocturnal corticotropin stimulation and preservation of diurnal HPA axis rhythmicity. Less invasive tests of adrenal function (eg, early morning salivary cortisol and cortisone) hold promise as screening tests for severe HPA suppression.[19] The low-dose (0.5–1 μg) short Synacthen (synthetic corticotropin) test (SST) is the most widely used dynamic tests of HPA axis function and correlates best with the insulin tolerance test in adults. Although for adults a peak cortisol less than 18 μg/dL (500 nmol/L) is used as a threshold for diagnosing adrenal suppression, literature suggests that for children treated with ICS, a threshold of peak cortisol less than 12.5 μg/dL (350 nmol/L) is more appropriate to identify clinically significant adrenal impairment.[19] Future assessment of risk for HPA axis suppression may include (1) measurement of early morning salivary concentrations[19] or hair cortisol concentrations[20] as noninvasive biomarkers and (2) determining individual susceptibility to ICS-induced adrenal suppression based on genetic variations in the platelet-derived growth factor D (PDGFD) gene locus.[21]

Most long-term studies of ICS effects on the HPA axis are cross-sectional, retrospective, or not controlled by a placebo arm and thus are of limited value. No change in HPA axis function measured by basal cortisol levels was reported in children who received open-label BUD, 400 μg/d, via CFC-MDI after 12 months.[22] Reassuring data subsequently were published, showing no effects of BUD 400 μg/d via CFC-MDI on HPA axis function measured by standard-dose (250-μg) SST and urinary cortisol excretion.[23] On the other hand, a retrospective analysis of adults taking ICS alone found that 20% failed the SST and suppression of adrenal function increased in a dose-dependent fashion. A basal cortisol greater than or equal to 12.6 μg/dL (348 nmol/L) provided 100% specificity for passing the SST whereas a cortisol value less than 1.2 μg/dL (34 nmol/L) had 100% sensitivity for SST failure.[24]

Thus, although the frequency of ICS-induced clinically significant HPA axis suppression remains debatable, there is no debate that children treated with ICSs are at increased risk for this serious and potentially life-threatening adverse effect. Overall, the literature supports these practical recommendations: (1) acute adrenal insufficiency during or after discontinuation of low-to-moderate dose ICS therapy (eg, <176 μg/d FP, BUD, or HFA-BDP) is rare, and these children do not require routine monitoring of the HPA axis unless there is evidence of growth suppression[12]; (2) children receiving chronic ICS treatment at dosages higher than these should have periodic fasting morning cortisol testing and, if results are less than 10 μg/dL (275 nmol/L), consultation with pediatric endocrinology for performance of a low-dose (1 μg) or standard-dose SST; although the precise relationship between abnormal responses to low-dose corticotropin testing and risk for adrenal crisis are unresolved, a reduced adrenal gland responsiveness to low-dose corticotropin suggests that provision of additional hydrocortisone for significant illness or injury and wearing of a cortisol-dependent Medic-Alert bracelet is prudent[25]; and (3) cortisol deficiency should be suspected in any ICS-treated child presenting with lethargy, change in mental status, or other symptoms suggestive of hypoglycemia.[13]

Children who have severe asthma requiring consistent high-dose ICS therapy or who are receiving topical corticosteroids by additional routes (eg, dermal for atopic dermatitis or intranasal for allergic rhinitis) exhibit varying degrees of HPA axis suppression on biochemical testing and are at increased risk for clinically significant HPA axis suppression.[26] Morning plasma cortisol levels should be monitored periodically in these children and, if less than 10 μg/dL, consultation with a pediatric endocrinologist is advised for performance of a low-dose SST and counseling regarding hydrocortisone stress-dosing for illnesses/injuries not treated by an increased ICS dose. Importantly, documentation of HPA axis suppression in ICS-treated children should not prompt prescribing of additional daily hydrocortisone, because the presence of HPA axis suppression indicates that the child already is exposed to supraphysiologic daily glucocorticoid effect. Furthermore, despite these measurable effects of ICSs on the HPA axis, it is critical to recall that effective anti-inflammatory activity is essential for the treatment of severe asthma, that corticosteroids are the most effective anti-inflammatory agents available, and that the suppressive effects of ICSs on the HPA axis are markedly less than clinically equivalent doses of oral corticosteroids.

GROWTH EFFECTS OF INHALED CORTICOSTEROIDS

The potential adverse effect of ICS therapy on growth has attracted the most attention from both those who prescribe ICSs and the parents of children with asthma because (1) normal growth is a sensitive indicator of a child's overall health and well-being and (2) height is a visible and important characteristic to children and parents, and fear of growth suppression promotes treatment nonadherence. Corticosteroids are potent inhibitors of linear growth, exerting suppressive effects at virtually every level of a child's growth axis (**Fig. 3**).[27] Blunting of pulsatile growth hormone release, down-regulation of growth hormone receptor expression, inhibition of insulinlike growth factor-1 bioactivity, and osteoblast activity and suppression of collagen synthesis and adrenal androgen production all are known mechanisms by which corticosteroids can inhibit growth. Glucocorticoids also inhibit intestinal calcium absorption, increase urinary calcium excretion, and disrupt bone formation, all of which can negatively affect linear growth. Even small amounts of exogenous corticosteroid in excess of normal physiologic requirements, if provided consistently over time, are capable of suppressing childhood growth. Such effects can be detected by knemometry, a highly sensitive measurement of lower-leg growth rate and ICS systemic effects (more sensitive than urinary-free cortisol in some studies)[28] over short treatment intervals but unfortunately lack predictive quality for clinically significant systemic adverse effects on annual growth or HPA axis function. Consequently, it is appropriate to still rely on well-designed stadiometer studies to examine potential effects of ICSs on childhood growth.

Earlier, well-designed stadiometer studies conducted in prepubertal children receiving uninterrupted, moderate-dose ICS therapy showed the following: (1) detectable slowing of 1-year growth in prepubertal children can occur with continuous, twice-daily treatment with ICSs (400 μg/d CFC-BDP or BUD or, to a lesser degree, FP 200 μg/d); (2) administration of clinically equivalent doses of ICS with more efficient first-pass hepatic inactivation of swallowed drug reduces risk of growth suppression; (3) the risk for growth suppression is increased when ICS therapy is combined with intranasal or dermal steroid therapy; (4) growth suppression related to asthma itself as a disease occurs only when asthma is persistent and of at least moderate severity; and (5) titration to the lowest effective dose minimizes an already low risk of growth suppression by ICS.[29] A recent Cochrane review offered these conclusions emphasizing both the importance and complexity of drug-device-dosage factor interactions: "FP at an equivalent dose seems to inhibit growth less than BDP and BUD. However,

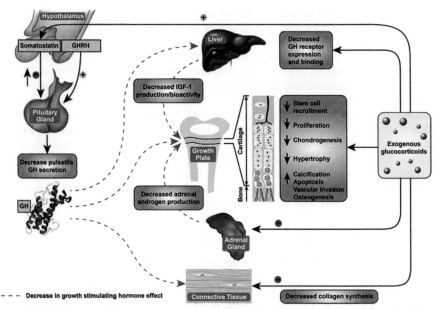

Fig. 3. Mechanisms of growth suppression by glucocorticoids. Glucocorticoids inhibit linear growth by blunting pulsatile growth hormone release through augmentation of hypothalamic somatostatin tone, down-regulating hepatic and growth plate growth hormone receptor expression, inhibiting insulinlike growth factor 1 (IGF-1) bioactivity and osteoblast activity, accelerating chondrocyte apoptosis, and suppressing collagen synthesis and adrenal androgen production. GH, growth hormone; GHRH, growth hormone–releasing hormone. (*From* Allen DB. Inhaled corticosteroids and growth: still an issue after all these years. J Pediatr. 2015;166(2):466; with permission.)

the evidence from this systematic review of head-to-head trials is not certain enough to inform the selection of ICS or inhalation device for the treatment of children with persistent asthma."[30]

Studies also have advanced understanding of the effects of ICS therapy on the growth of very young children, final adult height attainment, and growth in children with concomitant attention-deficit/hyperactivity disorder (ADHD) therapy. It previously was theorized that the faster growth rate of infancy and early childhood would mitigate growth suppressing effects of ICS. A controlled study showed, however, decreased growth (mean −1.6 cm) in toddlers 1 year to 3 years of age during 2 years of treatment with FP, 176 μg/d, via CFC-MDI compared with placebo.[31] Furthermore, this study of toddlers indicated the risk for growth suppression was greatest in the younger (<3 years of age) and lighter (<15 kg) subjects and that growth deficits did not normalize with time or after discontinuation of therapy.

A second prior assumption was that growth deficits sustained during childhood would be subsequently compensated for by later catch-up growth. This has been challenged by a prospective, randomized, controlled trial of 5 year olds to 13 year olds in whom 2 years of therapy with BUD, 400 μg/d, via DPI led to mean adult heights 1.2 cm shorter than if placebo had been given for 2 years (95% CI, 0.5–1.9 cm lower; $P = .001$).[32] The growth attenuation imposed by BUD therapy was greatest in peripubertal subjects, and the relative growth deficit of 1.2 cm incurred during the first 2 years of the study (the 2 years the placebo arm received no ICSs) persisted despite no difference in BUD doses in initial BUD-treatment and placebo arms during the subsequent observational period (mean follow-up, 4.2 years). The finding that subsequent similar BUD doses did not alter the relative growth deficit suggests that growth deficits from ICS therapy are not wholly progressive or cumulative but that exposure of ICSs during peripubertal years may have a sustained, albeit small, effect on adult height attainment. Because the adolescent years of this study were observational with no monitoring of treatment adherence, it also is possible that results did not accurately capture the magnitude of effects of consistent ICS treatment on growth during this period. This concern is supported by 1 recent study focused on pubertal growth during low-to-medium daily-dose ICS treatment, which reported progressive declines in height SDS from prepuberty to final adult height (2.5 cm ± 2.89 cm lower in boys and 2.0 cm ± 2.03 cm lower in girls) in asthmatic patients compared with controls.[33] Thus, further study is needed to determine the effects of ICSs on growth during puberty.

As discussed previously, the risk for ICS-induced growth suppression is greater if additional corticosteroid therapies (intranasal, topical, and so forth) are required for comorbid allergic or dermatologic conditions. Similarly, simultaneous ICS treatment of asthma and stimulant treatment of ADHD is becoming increasingly commonplace, making it important to consider possible growth-inhibiting influences via distinct pathways with additive or synergistic effects (see **Fig. 2**). Studies of growth during continuous treatment with methylphenidate have shown a mean reduction in first year growth rate of 1.25 cm/y (approximately 20% reduction in growth rate for a prepubertal child), with persistence of the effect creating mean differences in height gain compared with control children of between 2 cm and 3 cm after 2 years to 3 years.[34,35] Although often attributed to simultaneous poor weight gain, significant changes in height SD scores in methylphenidate-treated versus control children have been reported in the absence of any change in weight and body mass index values. Although precise mechanisms remain uncertain, increased dopamine and noradrenaline associated with stimulant treatment can inhibit secretion of growth hormone, prolactin, thyroid hormones, sex hormones, and insulin. Decreased growth hormone secretion and slow growth—even during the typically robust growth hormone secreting period of puberty—also have been reported with commonly prescribed selective serotonin reuptake inhibitors (SSRIs), growth effects that normalized when SSRI treatment was discontinued.[36] Thus far, limited analysis of long-term height attainment in stimulant-treated and control children with ADHD has not shown diminished adult height; however, growth slowing as a potential adverse effect during the first years of stimulant treatment appears well established.[37] As a result, when confronted by the increasingly common situation of a child receiving multiple drug therapy—especially involving corticosteroids, stimulants, and perhaps SSRIs—anticipation of and monitoring for medication-induced growth attenuation is prudent as catch-up is not guaranteed.

INHALED CORTICOSTEROIDS AND BONE METABOLISM

Corticosteroid excess affects normal bone metabolism in numerous ways. Calcium homeostasis is disrupted by alteration of osteoblastic and osteoclastic activity, leading to increased bone dissolution and decreased bone formation. Increases in urinary calcium losses coupled with inhibition of vitamin D–mediated intestinal calcium absorption result in total body calcium deficiency and secondary hyperparathyroidism. Particularly in girls, reductions in sex hormone production reduce bone mass further. The rate of bone accretion normally parallels linear growth rate: rapid during the first few years of life, slower during childhood, and with a return to a more rapid rate of accretion during adolescence and early adulthood. Thus, inhibition of bone metabolism by ICSs during early childhood and adolescence could have important consequences.

Cross-sectional studies of children treated with ICSs generally have reported normal bone mass or density and blood markers of bone metabolism.[38,39] Such studies potentially are confounded by effects of underlying asthma itself on bone accretion. As shown by a cross-sectional study of 1041 children, 5 years old to 12 years old (32% ethnic/racial minorities and 40% female), however, even mild-moderate persistent asthma (ie, disease sufficient enough to produce a decrease in baseline lung function) of 4 years' to 7 years' duration has not been found to affect bone mineral density (BMD) adversely.[40]

Few controlled, prospective studies have investigated the effect of ICSs on BMD. Children in the 4-year Childhood Asthma Management Program (CAMP) study showed no effects of BUD treatment on BMD compared with nedocromil sodium (NS) or placebo-treated children.[41] Additionally, a 24-month study of children (ages 6–14 years) with persistent asthma treated with FP, 200 μg/d (if uncontrolled, maximum dose 400 μg/d), or NS is particularly notable. BMD was assessed blindly using dual-energy x-ray absorptiometry measurements of the lumbar spine and femoral neck. In total, 174 children were randomized to treatment (87 received FP and 87 received NS). At month 24, the adjusted mean percentage increase in lumbar spine BMD was 11.6% in the FP group compared with 10.4% in NS-treated children (95% CI for treatment difference, −0.7% to 3.1%). The corresponding increases in femoral neck BMD were 8.9% and 8.5%, respectively. FP was significantly superior for every efficacy parameter investigated and was similarly well tolerated as NS. The investigators concluded that long-term effects of FP and NS on BMD accrual and growth are similar among children with asthma. Although not statistically significant, examination of the data revealed a trend for improved bone mineral accretion with FP treatment. Possible explanations include greater physical activity in the FP-treated children and exposure to fewer oral corticosteroid bursts for treatment of exacerbations.[42]

Given it is well accepted that long-term oral corticosteroid therapy adversely affects BMD, and that systemic glucocorticoid exposure secondary to ICS administration varies, it is not surprising that studies have suggested that as systemic ICS delivery increases, effects on BMD may ensue. Although it is unclear whether a threshold dose exists for any drug and its delivery device, a cross-sectional study of 76 prepubertal children, performed prior to reformulation to HFA-based MDI therapy, indicated bone mass was similar in children treated with 400 μg/d to 800 μg/d of ICS and in children who received no ICS.[43] At higher ICS doses, however, differences in BMD were seen; compared with children treated with 400 μg/d to 800 μg/d, children receiving greater than 800 μg/d of ICS had significantly lower lumbar spine BMD (mean difference −0.05 g/cm^2; 95% CI, −0.02 to −0.09). Thus, current consensus is that decreased BMD acquisition in children is associated with high doses but not low to medium doses of ICSs.[44]

Use of rescue ICS therapy only during asthma exacerbations theoretically would reduce the risk of adverse effects on BMD. A double-blind, randomized study of 136 children (5–10 years old), however, did not support this expectation.[45] In the study, all the subjects received BUD therapy daily for 6 months and then were assigned to BUD, 100 μg twice daily; to BUD as needed for 1 year; or to disodium cromoglycate (DSCG). Compared with the DSCG therapy, subjects on daily BUD had a lower 1-year increase in BMD (0.023 g/cm vs 0.034 g/cm; $P = .023$), whereas no BMD difference was found between DSCG versus as-needed BUD or between as-needed BUD versus daily BUD therapy. As a result, larger and longer studies are needed to establish whether intermittent rescue ICS therapy compared to daily ICS therapy provides BMD benefits.

Besides the use of intermittent bursts of ICS to potentially protect BMD, another modifiable risk factor is treatment of comorbid vitamin D deficiency. In a longitudinal study of 780 children ages 5 years old to 12 years old with mild to moderate asthma, boys with vitamin D insufficiency showed an inverse correlation between the use of oral corticosteroids and bone mineral accretion and (P<.001).[46] There was not a significant interaction (P = .48), however, between the study's prescribed dosing of BUD (400 µg daily via MDI), vitamin D level, and bone mineral accretion during the study (mean length of follow-up 4.3 years). As a result, further study of whether vitamin D levels optimize bone mineral accretion in ICS-treated children is needed. Nevertheless, given that many asthmatic children require oral corticosteroid therapy, supplementation to correct any vitamin D insufficiency appears prudent to optimize bone mineral accretion.

Although BMD and bone mineral accretion function as surrogates for risk of future fractures, a large population-based cohort of children in the United Kingdom estimated incidence rates of fracture among children aged 4 years to 17 years taking ICSs (n = 97,387), those taking bronchodilators only (n = 70,984), and a reference group (n = 345,758). Fracture incidence was increased in children using ICSs as well as in those receiving bronchodilators alone. With an average daily BDP dose of less than 200 µg, the crude fracture risk relative to nonusers was 1.10 (95% CI, 0.96 to 1.26); with dosage of 201 µg to 400 µg, it was 1.23 (95% CI, 1.08–1.39); and with dosages over 400 µg, it was 1.36 (95% CI, 1.11–1.67). This excess risk disappeared, however, after adjustment for indicators of asthma severity. The investigators concluded that increased risk of fracture associated with use of ICSs is likely the result of the underlying illness, rather than directly attributable to ICS therapy.[47] This conclusion is supported by a recent study of more than 19,000 Canadian children; 19,420 children showed that systemic corticosteroids, but not ICSs, were significantly associated with increased odds of fracture in the pediatric asthma population.[48] Similarly, an Australian study found no difference in fracture incidence between children with asthma and healthy controls, and no differences in fracture incidence in the children with asthma subgrouped according to ICS dosage.[49] In summary, risk of impaired bone mineralization appears very low with the use of ICSs alone for the treatment of mild to moderate asthma. This risk is markedly altered by concomitant treatment with oral corticosteroids, which have a well-documented association with osteopenia.[46]

SUMMARY

For children with persistent asthma of any degree, ICS treatment is recommended as first-line therapy. Although topical airway corticosteroid therapy has markedly improved the control of asthma while lessening the risk of corticosteroid side effects, the use of ICSs continues to be accompanied by a fear of potential adverse systemic effects. Unfortunately, these fears result in some children being deprived of appropriate and effective treatment or even exposed to a greater risk of requiring oral corticosteroid treatment. Nevertheless, because these agents may be used for long periods of time in a large number of children, safety issues are paramount.

Some important overall conclusions appear well supported by the literature. First, ICSs used in small doses (eg, <100 µg/d) present no significant risk for systemic side effects. When ICSs are used at higher dosages and continuously for long periods of time, important differences in drug characteristics, in particular the efficiency of inactivation of swallowed drug (which does not exert a therapeutic effect prior to gaining access to the systemic circulation), affect the ratio of therapeutic to systemic effect of individual ICS. From a practical viewpoint, the long-term clinical history of ICS therapy is informative. Clinically significant suppression of the HPA axis due to ICS therapy alone can occur, and, although rare at moderate dosages, should be investigated in children treated with higher ICS dosages or presenting with any symptoms suggesting cortisol deficiency. Detectable suppression of childhood growth likely will occur when ICSs with high percentage of lung deposition and/or relatively poor first-pass inactivation are administered consistently at doses greater than 200 μg/d. Mild ICS-induced growth attenuation during childhood can persist as small decreases in final adult height. Harmful effects of ICSs on bone metabolism, although less studied than growth-related effects, are not expected with the use of an ICS dosage that does not suppress basal HPA axis function or childhood growth, and at higher ICS dosages, effects on BMD can be minimized by increased participation in bone-strengthening physical activity, vitamin D sufficiency, and decreased exposure to oral corticosteroid bursts.

Important caveats include the following: (1) these conclusions are drawn from studies of ICSs used alone and in recommended doses, not in combination with intranasal or other topical corticosteroids or other concomitant growth-suppressing medications[3]; and (2) occurrence of all ICS adverse systemic effects is strongly influenced by strict adherence to prescribed dosage administration, so that high patient/family compliance is a risk factor for potential ICS toxicity that should influence dosage selection and titration.

Differences in safety profiles among the available ICSs exist, but there have been few direct comparative studies attempting to establish rank in benefit-to-risk ratios. Importantly, the safety profiles of all ICS preparations, which focus anti-inflammatory effects on the lung, are markedly better than oral glucocorticoids. Risk of adverse effects is minimized by using the lowest effective dosage, by limiting systemic availability of the drug through careful selection of the inhalation device and proper technique, by the adjunct use of alternative anti-inflammatory agents, and, when higher doses are required, by choice of ICS medication with a higher ratio of therapeutic-to-systemic effects. Monitoring of growth in children is a sensitive method of detecting significant ICS systemic effects and can enhance a family's confidence in the safety of the medication. When long-term, high-dose therapy is required, periodic evaluations of adrenal function and bone density are advisable. For children with persistent asthma, ICSs are highly effective medications that, when prescribed and monitored judiciously, have benefits that clearly exceed potential risks.

DISCLOSURE

The author has nothing to disclose.

REFERENCES

1. Allen DB, Bielory L, Derendorf H, et al. Inhaled corticosteroids: past lessons and future issues. J Allergy Clin Immunol 2003;112(3 Suppl):S1–40.

2. Kelly HW. Comparison of inhaled corticosteroids: an update. Ann Pharmacother 2009;43(3):519–27.

3. Allen DB. Inhaled corticosteroids and growth: still an issue after all these years. J Pediatr 2015;166(2):463–9.

4. Daley-Yates PT, Baker RC. Systemic bioavailability of fluticasone propionate administered as nasal drops and aqueous nasal spray formulations. Br J Clin Pharmacol 2001;51(1):103–5.
5. Derendorf H, Hochhaus G, Rohatagi S, et al. Pharmacokinetics of Triamcinolone Acetonide After Intravenous, Oral, and Inhaled Administration. J Clin Pharmacol 1995;35(3):302–5.
6. Martin RJ, Szefler SJ, Chinchilli VM, et al. Systemic effect comparisons of six inhaled corticosteroid preparations. Am J Respir Crit Care Med 2002;165(10): 1377–83.
7. Leach CL, Kuehl PJ, Chand R, et al. Characterization of respiratory deposition of fluticasone-salmeterol hydrofluoroalkane-134a and hydrofluoroalkane-134a be-clomethasone in asthmatic patients. Ann Allergy Asthma Immunol 2012;108(3): 195–200.
8. Busse WW, Brazinsky S, Jacobson K, et al. Efficacy response of inhaled beclo-methasone dipropionate in asthma is proportional to dose and is improved by formulation with a new propellant. J Allergy Clin Immunol 1999;104(6):1215–22.
9. Harrison LI, Colice GL, Donnell D, et al. Adrenal effects and pharmacokinetics of CFC-free beclomethasone dipropionate: a 14-day dose-response study. J Pharm Pharmacol 1999;51(3):263–9.
10. Martinez FD, Chinchilli VM, Morgan WJ, et al. Use of beclomethasone dipropio-nate as rescue treatment for children with mild persistent asthma (TREXA): a randomised, double-blind, placebo-controlled trial. Lancet 2011;377(9766): 650–7.
11. Kelly HW. Assessing the therapeutic index of inhaled corticosteroids in children: Is knemometry the answer? J Allergy Clin Immunol 2017;140(2):387–8.
12. Allen DB. Sense and sensitivity: assessing inhaled corticosteroid effects on the hypothalamic-pituitary-adrenal axis. Ann Allergy Asthma Immunol 2002;89(6): 537–9.
13. Kapadia CR, Nebesio TD, Myers SE, et al. Endocrine Effects of Inhaled Cortico-steroids in Children. JAMA Pediatr 2016;170(2):163–70.
14. Goldbloom EB, Mokashi A, Cummings EA, et al. Symptomatic adrenal suppres-sion among children in Canada. Arch Dis Child 2017;102(4):338–9.
15. Todd GR, Acerini CL, Ross-Russell R, et al. Survey of adrenal crisis associated with inhaled corticosteroids in the United Kingdom. Arch Dis Child 2002;87(6): 457–61.
16. Hollman GA, Allen DB. Overt glucocorticoid excess due to inhaled corticosteroid therapy. Pediatrics 1988;81(3):452–5.
17. Carrel AL, Somers S, Lemanske RF Jr, et al. Hypoglycemia and cortisol defi-ciency associated with low-dose corticosteroid therapy for asthma. Pediatrics 1996;97(6 Pt 1):921–4.
18. Zöllner EW, Lombard CJ, Galal U, et al. Screening for hypothalamic–pituitary–ad-renal axis suppression in asthmatic children remains problematic: a cross-sectional study. BMJ Open 2013;3(8):e002935.
19. Blair J, Lancaster G, Titman A, et al. Early morning salivary cortisol and cortisone, and adrenal responses to a simplified low-dose short Synacthen test in children with asthma. Clin Endocrinol 2014;80(3):376–83.
20. Smy L, Shaw K, Amstutz U, et al. Assessment of hair cortisol as a potential biomarker for possible adrenal suppression due to inhaled corticosteroid use in children with asthma: A retrospective observational study. Clin Biochem 2018; 56:26–32.

21. Hawcutt DB, Francis B, Carr DF, et al. Susceptibility to corticosteroid-induced adrenal suppression: a genome-wide association study. *The Lancet*. Respir Med 2018;6(6):442–50.

22. Ribeiro LB. Budesonide: safety and efficacy aspects of its long-term use in children. Pediatr Allergy Immunol 1993;4(2):73–8.

23. Bacharier LB, Raissy HH, Wilson L, et al. Long-term effect of budesonide on hypothalamic-pituitary-adrenal axis function in children with mild to moderate asthma. Pediatrics 2004;113(6):1693–9.

24. Woods CP, Argese N, Chapman M, et al. Adrenal suppression in patients taking inhaled glucocorticoids is highly prevalent and management can be guided by morning cortisol. Eur J Endocrinol 2015;173(5):633–42.

25. Kannisto S, Korppi M, Remes K, et al. Adrenal suppression, evaluated by a low dose adrenocorticotropin test, and growth in asthmatic children treated with inhaled steroids. J Clin Endocrinol Metab 2000;85(2):652–7.

26. Zollner EW, Lombard CJ, Galal U, et al. Hypothalamic-pituitary-adrenal axis suppression in asthmatic school children. Pediatrics 2012;130(6):e1512–9.

27. Allen DB. Growth suppression by glucocorticoid therapy. Endocrinol Metab Clin North Am 1996;25(3):699–717.

28. Chawes B, Nilsson E, Nørgaard S, et al. Knemometry is more sensitive to systemic effects of inhaled corticosteroids in children with asthma than 24-hour urine cortisol excretion. J Allergy Clin Immunol 2017;140(2):431–6.

29. Allen DB. Safety of inhaled corticosteroids in children. Pediatr Pulmonol 2002; 33(3):208–20.

30. Axelsson I, Naumburg E, Prietsch SO, et al. Inhaled corticosteroids in children with persistent asthma: effects of different drugs and delivery devices on growth. Cochrane Database Syst Rev 2019;(6):CD010126.

31. Guilbert TW, Morgan WJ, Zeiger RS, et al. Long-term inhaled corticosteroids in preschool children at high risk for asthma. N Engl J Med 2006;354(19):1985–97.

32. Kelly HW, Sternberg AL, Lescher R, et al. Effect of inhaled glucocorticoids in childhood on adult height. N Engl J Med 2012;367(10):904–12.

33. De Leonibus C, Attanasi M, Roze Z, et al. Influence of inhaled corticosteroids on pubertal growth and final height in asthmatic children. Pediatr Allergy Immunol 2016;27(5):499–506.

34. Methylphenidate: growth retardation. Prescrire Int 2011;20(120):238–9.

35. Dura-Trave T, Yoldi-Petri ME, Gallinas-Victoriano F, et al. Effects of osmotic-release methylphenidate on height and weight in children with attention-deficit hyperactivity disorder (ADHD) following up to four years of treatment. J Child Neurol 2012;27(5):604–9.

36. Weintrob N, Cohen D, Klipper-Aurbach Y, et al. Decreased growth during therapy with selective serotonin reuptake inhibitors. Arch Pediatr Adolesc Med 2002; 156(7):696–701.

37. Biederman J, Spencer TJ, Monuteaux MC, et al. A naturalistic 10-year prospective study of height and weight in children with attention-deficit hyperactivity disorder grown up: sex and treatment effects. J Pediatr 2010;157(4):635–40.

38. Konig P, Hillman L, Cervantes C, et al. Bone metabolism in children with asthma treated with inhaled beclomethasone dipropionate. J Pediatr 1993;122(2): 219–26.

39. Griffiths AL, Sim D, Strauss B, et al. Effect of high-dose fluticasone propionate on bone density and metabolism in children with asthma. Pediatr Pulmonol 2004; 37(2):116–21.

40. Kelly HW, Nelson HS. Potential adverse effects of the inhaled corticosteroids. J Allergy Clin Immunol 2003;112(3):469–78 [quiz: 479].
41. The Childhood Asthma Management Program Research Group. Long-term effects of budesonide or nedocromil in children with asthma. N Engl J Med 2000;343(15):1054–63.
42. Roux C, Kolta S, Desfougeres JL, et al. Long-term safety of fluticasone propionate and nedocromil sodium on bone in children with asthma. Pediatrics 2003;111(6 Pt 1):e706–13.
43. Harris M, Hauser S, Nguyen TV, et al. Bone mineral density in prepubertal asthmatics receiving corticosteroid treatment. J Paediatr Child Health 2001;37(1): 67–71.
44. Skoner DP. Inhaled corticosteroids: Effects on growth and bone health. Ann Allergy Asthma Immunol 2016;117(6):595–600.
45. Turpeinen M, Pelkonen AS, Nikander K, et al. Bone mineral density in children treated with daily or periodical inhaled budesonide: the Helsinki Early Intervention Childhood Asthma study. Pediatr Res 2010;68(2):169–73.
46. Tse SM, Kelly HW, Litonjua AA, et al. Corticosteroid use and bone mineral accretion in children with asthma: effect modification by vitamin D. J Allergy Clin Immunol 2012;130(1):53–60.e4.
47. van Staa TP, Bishop N, Leufkens HG, et al. Are inhaled corticosteroids associated with an increased risk of fracture in children? Osteoporos Int 2004;15(10):785–91.
48. Gray N, Howard A, Zhu J, et al. Association Between Inhaled Corticosteroid Use and Bone Fracture in Children With Asthma. JAMA Pediatr 2018;172(1):57–64.
49. Zieck SE, George J, Blakeley BA, et al. Asthma, bones and corticosteroids: Are inhaled corticosteroids associated with fractures in children with asthma? J Paediatr Child Health 2017;53(8):771–7.

New and Emerging Technologies in Type 1 Diabetes

Jordan S. Sherwood, MD, Steven J. Russell, MD, PhD,
Melissa S. Putman, MD, MSc*

KEYWORDS

- Continuous glucose monitoring (CGM) • Automated insulin delivery (AID)
- Artificial pancreas (AP) • Bionic pancreas • Closed-loop • Insulin • Glucagon
- Ultrarapid-acting insulin

KEY POINTS

- Innovative and novel technologies for the management of type 1 diabetes hold promise for improving glycemia, decreasing burden of disease management, and improving long-term outcomes.
- Improvements in the accuracy of real-time continuous glucose monitoring (CGM) have allowed for the development of automated insulin delivery systems that can adjust insulin delivery based on CGM glucose input.
- The development of new drugs, such as ultrarapid-acting insulins that better mimic physiologic insulin secretion, may lead to improved postprandial glycemia. The advent of stable glucagon formulations may allow for development of dual-hormone closed-loop systems that could further improve glycemic regulation.

NEW TECHNOLOGIES IN TYPE 1 DIABETES

Intensive insulin therapy for the management of type 1 diabetes (T1D) was established as the standard of care based on the results of the Diabetes Control and Complication Trial (DCCT), which conclusively demonstrated the benefits of tight glycemic control.[1] However, those who received intensive insulin management were at increased risk for severe hypoglycemia, which can be acutely life threatening and can result in seizures, coma, or death. Based on DCCT and other data, the American Diabetes Association (ADA) recommends glycosylated hemoglobin (HbA1c) less than 7% in adults, and recently also in many children and adolescents, in order to decrease the risk of both macrovascular and microvascular complications.[2] To achieve these recommended glycemic targets, patients must monitor blood glucose multiple times a day, closely

Diabetes Research Center, Massachusetts General Hospital, 50 Staniford Street, Suite 301, Boston, MA 02114, USA
* Corresponding author.
E-mail address: msputman@partners.org

Endocrinol Metab Clin N Am 49 (2020) 667–678
https://doi.org/10.1016/j.ecl.2020.07.006
0889-8529/20/© 2020 Elsevier Inc. All rights reserved.

estimate carbohydrate intake to calculate appropriate meal coverage, and administer multiple doses of insulin, which can have varying effects based on several physiologic factors such as physical activity, illness, or stress. This program results in a significant burden of disease management. Recently published data from the T1D Exchange, which includes more than 22,000 children and adults in the United States, show that less than a quarter of patients with T1D are meeting HbA1c goals.[3] Diabetes technologies are being developed to help decrease disease burden and improve glycemic outcomes. In this article, the authors highlight diabetes technology and therapies including new insulin analogues, continuous glucose monitoring systems (CGM), continuous subcutaneous insulin infusion (insulin pump therapy), as well as automated insulin delivery (AID) systems that integrate CGM and insulin pump technology with mathematical algorithms that automatically adjust insulin delivery (**Box 1**).

GLUCOSE MONITORING

Self-monitoring of blood glucose (SMBG) with finger-stick glucose (FSG) concentrations has become a key component of diabetes care. The ability to obtain a blood glucose measurement and adjust therapy accordingly is a mainstay of treatment to reach glucose targets and prevent hypoglycemia. Glucometer accuracy has increased throughout the years, but not all meters available on the market today meet standards set forth by the Food and Drug Administration (FDA) and International Organization for Standardization.[4] Identifying glucose trends and patterns based on SMBG to make insulin adjustments had been the standard of care set forth by the DCCT, and increased frequency of SMBG is associated with improved glycemic control.[5] Some newer glucometers are Bluetooth enabled and can pair with smartphone applications for patients

---

Box 1
Key definitions

Real-time continuous glucose monitoring (CGM)	Wearable technology that provides real-time continuous glucose measurements with the options of alerts for hyperglycemia, hypoglycemia, or projected glucose out of target ranges
Flash glucose monitoring (FGM)	Glucose monitoring system in which data are stored in a wearable sensor and obtained by scanning the sensor with dedicated receiver or smartphone
Automated insulin delivery, artificial pancreas system, closed-loop system, bionic pancreas	Terms that refer to an insulin delivery system that uses mathematical algorithms that can adjust insulin delivery based on CGM input
Threshold suspend	Automated insulin suspension when glucose level drops less than a specified threshold
Predictive low glucose suspend	Automated insulin suspension when glucose level is predicted to be less than a specified glucose threshold (eg, 70 mg/dL) in a specific period of time (eg, 30 min)
Hybrid-closed loop system	An automated insulin delivery system that modulates insulin delivery but still requires quantitative announcement of carbohydrate intake by the user
Fully closed-loop system	Automated insulin delivery not dependent on user input
Bihormonal (dual hormone) system	An artificial pancreas technology that uses insulin plus an additional hormone (eg, glucagon) intended to achieve better glycemic control than possible with an insulin-only system

to better track and identify patterns.[6] However, FSG has limitations in that they provide only an instantaneous snapshot in time of current glucose and do not provide information on glucose trends or direction of change.

CGM and FGM devices measure interstitial glucose and estimate plasma glucose every 5 to 15 minutes, depending on the system. Real-time CGM systems (Dexcom G6, Senseonics Eversense, Medtronic Guardian) actively transmit glucose information to a dedicated receiver, insulin pump, smartphone/watch, and to a cloud network if desired and can provide real-time information to the user regarding (1) rate of glucose change, (2) hyperglycemia and hypoglycemia based on individualized thresholds, and (3) impending hypoglycemia alarms based on glucose trends. The glucose measurements can also be shared by patients with others, such as family members, in real-time for an added degree of security. In the only currently available FGM system (Abbott Freestyle Libre), data are stored within the sensor and can be obtained by scanning the device with dedicated receiver or smartphone. Of note, the next-generation Freestyle Libre 2 CGM recently approved by the FDA is capable of "pushing" optional real-time threshold alerts to a receiver or smartphone. Both CGM and FGM devices can be used in blinded mode to record glucose data on the device for later analysis of glycemic patterns to assist health care professionals in making therapeutic decisions.

Externally worn CGM (Dexcom G6, Medtronic Guardian) and FGM (Abbott Freestyle Libre) devices measure interstitial glucose via a transcutaneous sensor, a filament placed in the subcutaneous tissue connected to an overlying transmitter. More recently a CGM with an implantable sensor system with an externally worn transmitter, the Senseonics Eversense, has been approved for 3 or 6 months of use before replacement in the United States and Europe, respectively. Some devices require regular calibration, with FSG input required at least twice daily (Medtronic Guardian and Senseonics Eversense), or are factory calibrated with no additional measurements required (Dexcom G6 and Abbott Freestyle Libre).

Data from CGM and FGM devices can be downloaded by clinicians and provide a standardized ambulatory glucose profile with information regarding percentage of time spent in hypo- and hyperglycemic ranges, time in target range, and glucose variability. Mean glucose as determined by CGM can be used to calculate the glucose management indicator, which provides an estimate of HbA1c[7] to help determine if patients are achieving target glucose goals.[8] In fact, because the relationship between HbA1c and average glucose can be modified by the mean red blood cell lifespan, mean CGM glucose may be a better predictor of long-term complications than HbA1c when the measured HbA1c and GMI are not in agreement.[7] Recently the ADA has published consensus guidelines regarding the recommended percentage of time in target range as well as hyper- and hypoglycemic targets for patients with T1D.[9] Time in target range of 70 to 180 mg/dL (TIR) has been shown to correlate with mean glucose and HbA1c. TIR of 70% correlates to an HbA1c of approximately 7%. TIR has been suggested as a new treatment standard based on the argument that TIR is easier for people with diabetes to understand and is more actionable on a day-to-day basis.[2,10] Targets for time below range (TBR) and time above range (TAR) have also been established (**Table 1**).

CGM accuracy has improved significantly since its inception, and many CGM devices have obtained approval for nonadjunctive use (Dexcom G6, Senseonics Eversense, Freestyle Libre), meaning that CGM data can be used as a replacement for FSG when making insulin-dosing decisions.[11] Studies have shown that CGM use is associated with improved HbA1c and a reduction in hypoglycemia.[12,13] More recently,

Table 1
Continuous glucose monitoring recommendations for patients with type 1 diabetes to achieve HbA1c 7%[a]

	Glycemic Target (mg/dL)	% of CGM Readings
Time below range (TBR)	<54	<1%
	<70	<4%
Time in range (TIR)	70–180	>70%
Time above range (TAR)	>180	<25%
	>250	<5%

[a] For a target HbA1c of 7.5% TIR goal is greater than 60%.

Data from Battelino T, Danne T, Bergenstal RM, et al. Clinical targets for continuous glucose monitoring data interpretation: recommendations from the international consensus on time in range. Diabetes Care. 2019;42(8)1593-1603.

the FDA has created an interoperable integrated continuous glucose monitoring system standard, which allows an approved CGM device to be used as part of an integrated system with other compatible medical devices and electronic interfaces, including insulin delivery systems. Approved systems (currently, the Dexcom G6 and the Freestyle Libre 2) meet accuracy and reliability standards set forth by the FDA, securely transmit glucose data to other devices, and may be used interchangeably with AID devices for the purpose of managing glycemia.

INSULIN

One of the major challenges to managing glycemia in patients with diabetes is the inability of currently available insulin formulations to mimic the kinetics and action of endogenous insulin secretion.[14] In individuals without diabetes, incretin-stimulated insulin release and a rapid hepatic exposure to insulin in response to a meal occur and lead to decreased hepatic glucose production.[15] This physiology is no longer intact in patients with T1D. Exogenous insulin administered in the subcutaneous tissue takes time to be absorbed in the systemic circulation. This delayed systemic delivery of exogenous insulin is a major physiologic difference with the immediate entry of endogenous insulin into the hepatic circulation for rapid effects.[16]

Since the discovery of insulin in 1921, insulin therapy has greatly advanced from porcine and bovine insulin derivatives to the development of rapid-acting, and then ultrarapid-acting, insulin analogues. Older insulins such as Neutral Protamine Hagedorn and regular human insulin have a slow action of onset and long duration, which require patients to have rigid food consumption timing and routines to match the kinetics of insulin action. Rapid-acting insulin analogues (aspart, lispro, and glulisine) have a faster onset of action and quicker time to peak insulin action, which help better match postprandial glucose excursion. These rapid-acting insulins permit greater flexibility for patients: doses can be adjusted based on the timing and quantity of carbohydrates consumed rather. However, rapid-acting insulin analogues still require injection 10 to 15 minutes before meal intake for optimal action.[14]

New ultrarapid-acting insulins have even faster on-off kinetics than rapid-acting insulin.[17–21] Faster aspart (also known as Fiasp) is currently FDA approved for adults and children with diabetes and uses nicotinamide as an excipient and L-arginine to increase stability. Ultrarapid lispro (URLi), which has recently completed a phase 3 trial, uses treprostinil to promote vasodilation and citrate as an excipient.[21] BioChaperone lispro, which uses BC222, an oligosaccharide modified with natural molecules and citrate as an excipient, is currently in development. Postprandial glucose were found to be lower with use of faster aspart in both pump and MDI delivery.[19,22] Overall rates of blood glucose–confirmed hypoglycemia and severe hypoglycemia have been reported to be similar between aspart and faster aspart.[19] Faster aspart is labeled for use to be administered up to 20 minutes after meal, which can provide further flexibility to patients. A trial of URLi in patients with T1D showed decreased postprandial glycemic excursions at 1 and 2 hours compared with lispro.[21] A short-term, cross-over trial comparing BioChaperone Lispro with insulin lispro has also shown decreases in early postprandial hyperglycemia.[20] In a head-to-head study, BioChaperone Lispro had slightly faster on-off kinetics than insulin lispro and may more closely mimic normal postprandial insulin secretion.[17] Inhaled insulin (Afrezza) is FDA approved and has much more rapid kinetics than injectable insulin delivered subcutaneously. Limitations in clinical use include lack of dose equivalency with injectable insulin and possible respiratory side effects including lung function decreases that are reversible on discontinuation.[23]

INSULIN DELIVERY MODALITIES
Multiple Daily Injection

Insulin has been traditionally administered via MDI therapy via insulin syringe or insulin pen. *Smart pen* technology pairs the insulin pen with a smartphone to allow patients to more easily calculate and track insulin administration. The InPen (Companion Medical) is currently the only FDA-approved smart pen device, although others are in development. The InPen connects with a smartphone app via Bluetooth allowing patients to track insulin dosing history, calculate insulin doses, keep track of "insulin on board" (an estimate of rapid-acting insulin still in effect) and adjust calculated dosing accordingly, and set dosing reminders.[24] In addition, the phone application can also receive CGM data directly and in real time. Patients can export data collected from the application and share it with their health care team. Smart pen technology may have extra utility in certain patient populations or clinical scenarios, such as those who have difficulty remembering insulin dosing (eg, pediatric patients or those with cognitive or memory impairment) or those with limited health numeracy.[25] Accurate tracking of insulin dose administration is also of use to treatment teams to aid in insulin regimen adjustments. Further research is needed to determine clinical benefits of this technology, and other companies (including major insulin manufacturers) have announced plans to release smart pens in the future.

Insulin Pumps

Insulin pumps deliver a continuous infusion of insulin via a cannula placed in the subcutaneous tissue, sometimes referred to as continuous subcutaneous insulin infusion (CSII). Most of the pumps available use an infusion set with tubing to deliver insulin (in the United States, pumps from Tandem and Medtronic), but some systems known as patch pumps attach directly to the skin without the need for tubing (in the United States, the Insulet Omnipod system). Insulin pumps have programmable basal and bolus settings that can vary based on the time of the day. Insulin pumps track insulin usage and contain bolus calculators to assist in the calculation of meal-time insulin coverage and glucose correction. The pump also keeps track of "insulin on board" and adjusts calculated doses accordingly. The abilities to use different basal rates at different times of the day, to make temporary basal rate adjustments in response to glucose trend or activity level, and to deliver meal-time bolus insulin over extended periods of time based on user input are all unique to insulin pumps.

Patients can achieve target HbA1c goals with either MDI or insulin pump therapy, and extensive research has sought to determine if glycemic control with pump therapy is superior to that of MDI management. A systematic review and meta-analysis showed that both MDI and pump therapy resulted in comparable levels of glycemic control and incidence of severe hypoglycemia in children and adolescents with T1D and that pump therapy may have favorable effects on glycemic control in adults with T1D.[26] Insulin pump therapy is also associated with improved quality of life in both pediatric and adult populations.[27,28] By allowing varied basal rates, insulin pumps permit more flexible and physiologic insulin delivery that can be changed based on time of day and other factors such as exercise, as well as varied delivery of meal-time insulin bolus (eg, dual-wave or square-wave delivery set by the user) based on the type of food consumed. In addition, pump therapy eliminates the need for multiple daily injections of insulin, instead requiring only infusion set be changed every 2 to 3 days. Uptake of CSII has increased over the past decade, and currently nearly half of all patients with T1D in the United States manage their diabetes with pump therapy.[3]

Automated Insulin Delivery

AID systems (also known as closed-loop, artificial pancreas, or bionic pancreas systems) use real-time glucose measurements fed into a control algorithm that automatically adjusts the rate of subcutaneous insulin delivery via an insulin pump (**Table 2**). The earliest approved AID systems used threshold suspend, in which insulin delivery way automatically suspended when blood glucose level dropped less than a certain threshold.[29] Predictive glucose suspend improves on this feature by suspending insulin delivery when a hypoglycemic event is predicted in the future. Predictive low glucose suspend functionality decreases the percentage of time spent in hypoglycemic ranges in both the daytime and overnight.[30] By suspending insulin before a hypoglycemic event, this feature also reduces the duration of hypoglycemic events when they do occur.

Later generation AID systems entail more complex algorithms to not only suspend insulin delivery based on hypoglycemia but continuously adjust insulin delivery in response to glycemic trends. The most advanced AID systems that are commercially available today are referred to as hybrid closed-loop systems. Patient input is still required to count carbohydrates and administer correction boluses, but the system will additionally modulate insulin delivery in the background, and in some systems deliver partial correction boluses, based on glycemic trends. Other systems that have been studied but are not yet available use qualitative meal announcements to estimate carbohydrate content, describing meals as "typical," "more than typical," "less than typical," or "a small bite," rather than requiring quantitative carbohydrate counting.[31]

Table 2
Current Food and Drug Administration–approved automated insulin delivery systems

	MiniMed 530G (Medtronic)	MiniMed 630G Pump (Medtronic)	Basal-IQ System (Tandem)	MiniMed 670G (Medtronic)	Control IQ System (Tandem)
AID system type	Threshold suspend	Predictive low glucose suspend	Predictive low glucose suspend	Hybrid-closed loop	Hybrid-closed loop

Currently available FDA-approved hybrid closed-loop systems include the Medtronic 670G and Tandem t:slim X2 with Control IQ. The first hybrid closed-loop system available in United States, the Medtronic 670G, was approved in 2017 for adult and pediatric patients as young as age 7 years. The approval relied on a nonrandomized study without a control arm.[32] The system can be used as a traditional pump or in "auto mode," in which the pump automatically adjusts basal insulin rates up to every 5 minutes by increasing, decreasing, or suspending delivery of insulin based on CGM trends. Patients are still required to count carbohydrates and enter them into the system, and meal boluses are calculated based on a programmed carbohydrate ratio. As a safety feature, the system may exit auto mode and revert to preprogrammed delivery if insulin delivery approaches maximum or minimum insulin delivery thresholds, if POC and CGM readings are discrepant, or if CGM signal is lost. In a real-world, prospective observational study of 92 youth who started this system, 30% discontinued use of the auto mode within the first 6 months. Another real-world cohort study of 79 pediatric and adult patients reported that 33% discontinued auto mode use within 12 months.[33,34] Reasons cited included the number of alarms, challenges with requiring calibrations, and dissatisfaction with glycemic control.[34]

The second hybrid closed-loop device in the United States, the Tandem t:slim X2 with Control-IQ using the Dexcom G6 as the input CGM, was approved in 2019 for adults and pediatric patients older than or equal to 6 years. In the 6-month, randomized, controlled pivotal trial of this device, participants were randomized to closed-loop control or usual diabetes care with sensor-augmented pump therapy.[35] Patients randomized to closed-loop control had improvements in target range, mean CGM glucose, and HbA1c, as well as reduced rates of hypoglycemia. Unlike the Medtronic 670G, Control-IQ only reverts to preprogrammed insulin delivery when CGM signal is lost and does not require finger-stick calibration to continue AID. Trials are underway evaluating this device in younger children (NCT03844789).

Experimental Automated Insulin Delivery Systems

Several AID systems that rely on different sets of mathematical algorithms, including proportional integral derivative, fuzzy logic, and model predictive control algorithms, are in development. These AID systems have been associated with increased time in target glucose range (typically 70–180 mg/dL) and in some cases with decreased mean glucose, lower HbA1c, and decreased time in the hypoglycemic range. Pivotal trials for several of these AID systems are currently ongoing, including the Omnipod Horizon hybrid closed-loop system (NCT04196140) and the Beta Bionics iLet Bionic Pancreas (NCT04200313).

One class of AID systems, called bihormonal or dual hormone systems, is capable of delivering a second hormone to further improve glycemic control. Given the kinetics of subcutaneous insulin delivery, the reduction and/or suspension of insulin may be insufficient to prevent hypoglycemia, especially in certain scenarios that may result in changes in insulin sensitivity such as exercise. Several bihormonal systems use microdosing of glucagon to prevent and treat hypoglycemia when suspension of insulin delivery is not sufficient. Glucagon has rapid on and off kinetics, and the addition of glucagon can allow for more aggressive glucose targets compared with insulin-only systems by reducing the potential for hypoglycemia. In short-term studies of bihormonal systems, subjects achieved increased time in target range, lower mean glucose, and decreased rates of hypoglycemia compared with sensor-augmented pump therapy.[31,36] Additional studies comparing bihormonal with insulin-only closed-loop systems suggest that bihormonal systems may further improve mean glucose, time in range, as well as reduce the time spent in hypoglycemic ranges.[37]

Other classes of dual hormone systems that have been studied administer pramlintide (an amylin analogue) or glucagon-like peptide-1 (GLP-1) receptor agonist in combination with insulin.[38,39] Amylin is cosecreted with insulin from pancreatic beta cells and helps moderate postprandial glucose excursions by slowing gastric emptying, inhibiting glucagon secretion, and promoting satiety. A recent study examining an automated system delivering fixed dose ratio of insulin and pramlintide found increase in time in range compared with the insulin-only system.[38] Long-term studies of bihormonal systems are needed to establish their potential benefits.

A recent meta-analysis[37] reviewed published studies of artificial pancreas systems including insulin-only and dual hormone systems delivering glucagon in more than 500 adult and pediatric subjects with T1D. Most of these trials were small and for a short duration, but the analyses showed that AID systems achieved higher TIR compared with conventional pump therapy and that dual hormone systems resulted in greater improvements in TIR than insulin-only systems. Both classes of AID systems deliver improved glycemia overnight, which is a substantial benefit to patients, as fear of nocturnal hypoglycemia is a primary concern for patients and families.[37,40]

Challenges to Fully Automated Insulin Delivery

One the main challenges to achieving fully automated closed-loop insulin delivery is overcoming the kinetics of nonphysiologic subcutaneous insulin administration related to postprandial glucose excursions. Given the kinetics of subcutaneous insulin delivery, increased insulin dosing that occurs only after the glucose excursion has begun may lead to prolonged hyperglycemia. Furthermore, because of variations in physiologic insulin needs and the kinetics of current insulin formulations, increased insulin delivery can result in late hypoglycemia. Exercise can compound these challenges by altering insulin sensitivity and increasing insulin-independent glucose uptake into muscles. Several approaches have been studied to ameliorate this issue. Adjunctive therapies including pramlintide (an amylin analogue), GLP-1 receptor agonists, dipeptidyl peptidase-4 inhibitors, and sodium–glucose cotransporter 2 inhibitors have all been studied in patients with T1D with the goal of decreasing postprandial glycemic excursions and reducing the need for aggressive insulin dosing.[41] Alternate approaches to insulin delivery, such as delivery of insulin directly to intraperitoneal space, enable faster pharmacokinetics/pharmacodynamics than subcutaneous insulin delivery.[42] Studies examining the utility of new ultrarapid-acting insulins in AID systems have suggested decreased glycemic variability with these newer insulin analogues.[43]

DATA MANAGEMENT AND TELEHEALTH

Technology including CGM, smartphones, smartwatches, and activity trackers generate large amounts of high-density data that can be difficult for clinicians to synthesize in the limited time available during visits. At present, SMBG, CGM, and pump data can be downloaded to review for patterns and make adjustments in treatment. Currently available software allows patients to download their pump and CGM at home and then share these data via cloud-based services with the patient's clinical team to review, potentially allowing for more frequent patient contact between in-person visits. With advancement of artificial intelligence and machine learning, these data could be analyzed for automated generation of recommendations for therapy adjustment. Software systems have been developed to automatically generate insulin dose decision support recommendations.[44]

The prevalence of technology at home and in clinics has led to great interest in tele-health—a broad term used to describe health care delivery with the aid of technology, which includes video visits, web-based portals, or text messaging. Telehealth has been applied across multiple specialties and conditions and can be used to conduct remote patient visits and patient education and behavioral management sessions. Tel-ehealth strategies can help increase access to health care and reduce barriers to reaching providers, especially in resource limited settings or for those living far from treatment facilities. A recent meta-analysis found that telehealth intervention in pa-tients with diabetes led to HbA1c improvements.[45] Concerns about spread of SARS-CoV-2 have dramatically increased use of telehealth visits for diabetic patients over a very short period of time in the first quarter of 2020 and will likely accelerate the movement of diabetes management visits to virtual formats.

Availability of data in the cloud has allowed companies to publish "real world" studies describing glycemic control in patients using their technologies.[46] The devel-opment of virtual diabetes clinics is likely on the horizon, as patient data are obtained from wearable devices including CGM and insulin pumps and then transmitted into the electronic health record for analysis with machine learning and decision support.[47]

SUMMARY

Diabetes technology holds promise for improving glycemic outcomes and decreasing burden of disease for patients and families with T1D. Rapid advancement of diabetes therapeutics and technologies have enhanced diabetes monitoring and insulin deliv-ery capabilities. Devices that partially automate insulin delivery improve glycemic con-trol, and more capable automated closed-loop systems will likely be available in the near future. Further research should determine the long-term benefits of these devices on glycemic control and quality of life in T1D.

DISCLOSURE

J.S. Sherwood has nothing to disclose. S.J. Russell has patents and patents pending on aspects of the bionic pancreas that are assigned to Massachusetts General Hos-pital and are licensed to Beta Bionics, has received honoraria and/or travel expenses for lectures from Novo Nordisk, Roche, and Ascensia, serves on the scientific advisory boards of Unomedical and Companion Medical, has received consulting fees from Beta Bionics, Novo Nordisk, Senseonics, and Flexion Therapeutics, has received grant support from Zealand Pharma, Novo Nordisk, and Beta Bionics, and has received in-kind support in the form of technical support and/or donation of materials from Zealand Pharma, Ascencia, Senseonics, Adocia, and Tandem Diabetes. M.S. Putman has nothing to disclose.

REFERENCES

1. Effect of intensive diabetes treatment on the development and progression of long-term complications in adolescents with insulin-dependent diabetes mellitus: Diabetes Control and Complications Trial. Diabetes Control and Complications Trial Research Group. J Pediatr 1994;125(2):177–88.

2. American Diabetes Association. 6. Glycemic targets: standards of medical care in diabetes-2020. Diabetes care 2020;43(Suppl 1):S66–76.

3. Foster NC, Beck RW, Miller KM, et al. State of type 1 diabetes management and outcomes from the T1D Exchange in 2016-2018. Diabetes Technol Ther 2019; 21(2):66–72.

4. King F, Ahn D, Hsiao V, et al. A review of blood glucose monitor accuracy. Diabetes Technol Ther 2018;20(12):843–56.

5. Miller KM, Beck RW, Bergenstal RM, et al. Evidence of a strong association between frequency of self-monitoring of blood glucose and hemoglobin A1c levels in T1D exchange clinic registry participants. Diabetes care 2013;36(7):2009–14.

6. Bailey TS, Wallace JF, Pardo S, et al. Accuracy and user performance evaluation of a new, wireless-enabled blood glucose monitoring system that links to a smart mobile device. J Diabetes Sci Technol 2017;11(4):736–43.

7. Bergenstal RM, Beck RW, Close KL, et al. Glucose management indicator (GMI): a new term for estimating A1C from continuous glucose monitoring. Diabetes care 2018;41(11):2275–80.

8. Nathan DM, Kuenen J, Borg R, et al. Translating the A1C assay into estimated average glucose values. Diabetes care 2008;31(8):1473–8.

9. Battelino T, Danne T, Bergenstal RM, et al. Clinical targets for continuous glucose monitoring data interpretation: recommendations from the international consensus on time in range. Diabetes care 2019;42(8):1593–603.

10. Beck RW, Bergenstal RM, Cheng P, et al. The relationships between time in range, hyperglycemia metrics, and HbA1c. J Diabetes Sci Technol 2019;13(4): 614–26.

11. Aleppo G, Ruedy KJ, Riddlesworth TD, et al. REPLACE-BG: a randomized trial comparing continuous glucose monitoring with and without routine blood glucose monitoring in adults with well-controlled type 1 diabetes. Diabetes care 2017; 40(4):538–45.

12. Juvenile Diabetes Research Foundation Continuous Glucose Monitoring Study Group, Tamborlane WV, Beck RW, Bode BW, et al. Continuous glucose monitoring and intensive treatment of type 1 diabetes. N Engl J Med 2008;359(14):1464–76.

13. Beck RW, Riddlesworth T, Ruedy K, et al. Effect of continuous glucose monitoring on glycemic control in adults with type 1 diabetes using insulin injections: the DIAMOND randomized clinical trial. JAMA 2017;317(4):371–8.

14. Hirsch IB. Insulin analogues. N Engl J Med 2005;352(2):174–83.

15. Nauck MA, Meier JJ. Incretin hormones: Their role in health and disease. Diabetes Obes Metab 2018;20(Suppl 1):5–21.

16. Sharma AK, Taneja G, Kumar A, et al. Insulin analogs: Glimpse on contemporary facts and future prospective. Life Sci 2019;219:90–9.

17. Heise T, Meiffren G, Alluis B, et al. BioChaperone Lispro versus faster aspart and insulin aspart in patients with type 1 diabetes using continuous subcutaneous insulin infusion: A randomized euglycemic clamp study. Diabetes Obes Metab 2018;21(4):1066–70.

18. Heise T, Pieber TR, Danne T, et al. A pooled analysis of clinical pharmacology trials investigating the pharmacokinetic and pharmacodynamic characteristics of fast-acting insulin aspart in adults with type 1 diabetes. Clin Pharmacokinet 2017;56(5):551–9.

19. Klonoff DC, Evans ML, Lane W, et al. A randomized, multicentre trial evaluating the efficacy and safety of fast-acting insulin aspart in continuous subcutaneous insulin infusion in adults with type 1 diabetes (onset 5). Diabetes Obes Metab 2018;21(4):961–7.

20. Andersen G, Meiffren G, Lamers D, et al. Ultra-rapid BioChaperone Lispro improves postprandial blood glucose excursions vs insulin lispro in a 14-day crossover treatment study in people with type 1 diabetes. Diabetes Obes Metab 2018; 20(11):2627–32.

21. Klaff L. DC, Dellva M.A., et al. . Utra Rapid Lispro (URLi) Improves Postprandial Glucose (PPG) Control vs. Humalog (Lispro) in T1D: PRONTO-T1D Study. Paper presented at: American Diabetes Association's 79th Scientific Sessions; San Francisco, CA, June 7–11, 2019.

22. Mathieu C, Bode BW, Franek E, et al. Efficacy and safety of fast-acting insulin aspart in comparison with insulin aspart in type 1 diabetes (onset 1): A 52-week, randomized, treat-to-target, phase III trial. Diabetes Obes Metab 2018;20(5): 1148–55.

23. Kim ES, Plosker GL. AFREZZA(R) (insulin human) Inhalation Powder: A Review in Diabetes Mellitus. Drugs 2015;75(14):1679–86.

24. Gildon BW. InPen smart insulin pen system: product review and user experience. Diabetes Spectr 2018;31(4):354–8.

25. Klonoff DC, Kerr D. Smart pens will improve insulin therapy. J Diabetes Sci Technol 2018;12(3):551–3.

26. Yeh HC, Brown TT, Maruthur N, et al. Comparative effectiveness and safety of methods of insulin delivery and glucose monitoring for diabetes mellitus: a systematic review and meta-analysis. Ann Intern Med 2012;157(5):336–47.

27. Lukacs A, Kiss-Toth E, Varga B, et al. Benefits of continuous subcutaneous insulin infusion on quality of life. Int J Technol Assess Health Care 2013;29(1):48–52.

28. Roze S, Smith-Palmer J, Valentine WJ, et al. Long-term health economic benefits of sensor-augmented pump therapy vs continuous subcutaneous insulin infusion alone in type 1 diabetes: a U.K. perspective. J Med Econ 2016;19(3):236–42.

29. Bergenstal RM, Klonoff DC, Garg SK, et al. Threshold-based insulin-pump interruption for reduction of hypoglycemia. N Engl J Med 2013;369(3):224–32.

30. Forlenza GP, Li Z, Buckingham BA, et al. Predictive low-glucose suspend reduces hypoglycemia in adults, adolescents, and children with type 1 diabetes in an at-home randomized crossover study: results of the PROLOG trial. Diabetes care 2018;41(10):2155–61.

31. El-Khatib FH, Balliro C, Hillard MA, et al. Home use of a bihormonal bionic pancreas versus insulin pump therapy in adults with type 1 diabetes: a multicentre randomised crossover trial. Lancet 2017;389(10067):369–80.

32. Bergenstal RM, Garg S, Weinzimer SA, et al. Safety of a hybrid closed-loop insulin delivery system in patients with type 1 diabetes. JAMA 2016;316(13):1407–8.

33. Lal RA, Basina M, Maahs DM, et al. One year clinical experience of the first commercial hybrid closed-loop system. Diabetes care 2019;42(12):2190–6.

34. Messer LH, Berget C, Vigers T, et al. Real world hybrid closed-loop discontinuation: Predictors and perceptions of youth discontinuing the 670G system in the first 6 months. Pediatr Diabetes 2020;21(2):319–27.

35. Brown SA, Kovatchev BP, Raghinaru D, et al. Six-month randomized, multicenter trial of closed-loop control in type 1 diabetes. N Engl J Med 2019;381(18): 1707–17.

36. Haidar A, Legault L, Matteau-Pelletier L, et al. Outpatient overnight glucose control with dual-hormone artificial pancreas, single-hormone artificial pancreas, or conventional insulin pump therapy in children and adolescents with type 1 diabetes: an open-label, randomised controlled trial. Lancet Diabetes Endocrinol 2015;3(8):595–604.

37. Weisman A, Bai JW, Cardinez M, et al. Effect of artificial pancreas systems on glycaemic control in patients with type 1 diabetes: a systematic review and meta-analysis of outpatient randomised controlled trials. Lancet Diabetes Endocrinol 2017;5(7):501–12.

38. Haidar A, Tsoukas MA, Bernier-Twardy S, et al. A novel dual-hormone insulin-and-pramlintide artificial pancreas for type 1 diabetes: a randomized controlled crossover trial. Diabetes care 2020;43(3):597–606.

39. Sherr JL, Patel NS, Michaud CI, et al. Mitigating meal-related glycemic excursions in an insulin-sparing manner during closed-loop insulin delivery: the beneficial effects of adjunctive pramlintide and liraglutide. Diabetes care 2016;39(7):1127–34.

40. Van Name MA, Hilliard ME, Boyle CT, et al. Nighttime is the worst time: Parental fear of hypoglycemia in young children with type 1 diabetes. Pediatr Diabetes 2018;19(1):114–20.

41. Harris K, Boland C, Meade L, et al. Adjunctive therapy for glucose control in patients with type 1 diabetes. Diabetes Metab Syndr Obes 2018;11:159–73.

42. Pasquini S, Da Prato G, Tonolo G, et al. Continuous intraperitoneal insulin infusion: an alternative route for insulin delivery in type 1 diabetes. Acta Diabetol 2020;57(1):101–4.

43. Ruan Y, Thabit H, Leelarathna L, et al. Faster insulin action is associated with improved glycaemic outcomes during closed-loop insulin delivery and sensor-augmented pump therapy in adults with type 1 diabetes. Diabetes Obes Metab 2017;19(10):1485–9.

44. Nimri R, Dassau E, Segall T, et al. Adjusting insulin doses in patients with type 1 diabetes who use insulin pump and continuous glucose monitoring: Variations among countries and physicians. Diabetes Obes Metab 2018;20(10):2458–66.

45. Faruque LI, Wiebe N, Ehteshami-Afshar A, et al. Effect of telemedicine on glycated hemoglobin in diabetes: a systematic review and meta-analysis of randomized trials. CMAJ 2017;189(9):E341–64.

46. Muller L, Habif S, Leas S, et al. Reducing Hypoglycemia in the Real World: A Retrospective Analysis of Predictive Low-Glucose Suspend Technology in an Ambulatory Insulin-Dependent Cohort. Diabetes Technol Ther 2019;21(9):478–84.

47. Cahn A, Akirov A, Raz I. Digital health technology and diabetes management. J Diabetes 2018;10(1):10–7.

Pediatric Type 2 Diabetes: Not a Mini Version of Adult Type 2 Diabetes

Talia Alyssa Savic Hitt, MD, MPH*, Lorraine E. Levitt Katz, MD

KEYWORDS

- Type 2 diabetes • Pediatrics • Diabetes • Obesity • Metabolic syndrome
- Beta-cell failure

KEY POINTS

- Major risk factors for the development of pediatric type 2 diabetes mellitus (T2DM) include obesity, puberty, and T2DM in a first-degree or second-degree relative.
- The incidence of pediatric T2DM has been increasing with the increase in pediatric obesity, disproportionately affecting minorities and children of lower socioeconomic status.
- Recommended screening for T2DM includes hemoglobin A1c for children who are 10 years of age or older, pubertal, and overweight with at least 1 risk factor for T2DM.
- Current treatment options for pediatric T2DM include lifestyle changes (weight reduction, physical activity, and improved sleep), metformin, insulin, and liraglutide.
- Pediatric T2DM has faster beta-cell decline and early progression to complications compared with adult T2DM.

INTRODUCTION

Over the past several decades, it has become clear that type 2 diabetes mellitus (T2DM) is no longer limited to adults. T2DM in pediatrics poses a major challenge to population health, with an increasing incidence (highest in patients of racial minorities and of lower socioeconomic status) and a high rate of complications.[1–5] Childhood-onset T2DM also shows more rapid progression to beta-cell failure, with high treatment failure rates as shown by the TODAY (Treatment Options for Type 2 Diabetes in Adolescents and Youth) trial, the largest multicenter randomized controlled trial on treatment options in pediatric T2DM, in which children with T2DM were randomized to 1 of 3 treatment arms (metformin monotherapy, metformin plus lifestyle

Division of Endocrinology & Diabetes, Department of Pediatrics, Children's Hospital of Philadelphia, 3500 Civic Center Boulevard, Buerger Building -12th Floor, Philadelphia, PA 19104, USA
* Corresponding author.
E-mail address: hittt@email.chop.edu

Endocrinol Metab Clin N Am 49 (2020) 679–693
https://doi.org/10.1016/j.ecl.2020.08.003
0889-8529/20/© 2020 Elsevier Inc. All rights reserved.

endo.theclinics.com

intervention, and metformin plus rosiglitazone) and the primary outcome was treatment failure, defined by persistently increased hemoglobin A1c (HbA1c) level (>8%) over a 6-month period or inability to wean from temporary insulin therapy within 3 months.[6–8] Thus, recognizing and treating T2DM early in its course is imperative. However, few pharmacologic therapies are US Food and Drug Administration (FDA) approved for pediatric T2DM.

PATHOPHYSIOLOGY AND GENETICS OF PEDIATRIC TYPE 2 DIABETES

The pathophysiology of T2DM starts with declines in skeletal muscle, adipose tissue, and hepatic insulin sensitivity, which necessitates increased pancreatic beta-cell insulin secretion to maintain glucose homeostasis.[9,10] Hyperglycemia develops when compensatory insulin secretion fails to counter worsening insulin sensitivity and manifests as prediabetes and, ultimately, T2DM.[9–11] Hyperglycemic clamp testing has shown that, compared with obese controls without T2DM, youth who develop pediatric T2DM have 50% reduced insulin sensitivity, increased fasting hepatic glucose production, and an 86% lower disposition index (a composite measure describing the relationship between insulin sensitivity and beta-cell function).[12] In addition, insulin secretion can be sufficiently deficient to precipitate diabetes ketoacidosis (DKA), which occurs in ~6% of cases of pediatric T2DM but is an uncommon presentation in adult T2DM.[6,13] Similar to adult T2DM, pediatric T2DM can present with hyperosmolar hyperglycemic nonketoacidosis (HHNK), a condition that should be considered if blood glucose level is greater than or equal to 600 mg/dL.[14]

Obesity is a primary risk factor for reduced insulin sensitivity in children and adults.[13] The metabolic syndrome comprises the clustering of disorders related to central obesity, including insulin resistance, hypertension, and dyslipidemia.[15,16] Other risk factors in adults and children include conditions associated with insulin resistance (such as polycystic ovary syndrome [PCOS]), first-degree relative with T2DM, and high-risk racial minority groups (ie, African American, Latino, Native American, Asian American, Pacific Islander) (**Fig. 1**).[13] A first-degree or second-degree relative with T2DM is present in 74% to 100% of youth with T2DM.[17] Moreover, Magge and colleagues[17] showed that siblings of adolescents with T2DM had 4-times greater odds of abnormal glucose tolerance compared with overweight controls. Several adult

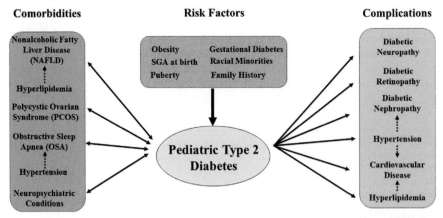

Fig. 1. Common comorbidities, risk factors, and complications in pediatric T2DM.[13] SGA, small for gestational age.

T2DM-related genetic variants, such as the *TCF7L2* locus, have also been identified in African American youth with T2DM and *HNF1A G319S* in Oji-Cree Native Canadian youth.[9,10]

For youth with genetic or other risk factors, obesity and the onset of puberty can precipitate the development of T2DM. Puberty in adolescents leads to an approximately 30% reduction in insulin sensitivity, and most new pediatric T2DM diagnoses occur during puberty.[18,19] Among perinatal risk factors, infants born to mothers with gestational diabetes and children born small-for-gestational-age are at a higher risk for development of metabolic syndrome, insulin resistance, and T2DM in childhood[16,20] (see **Fig. 1**).

PREVALENCE, INCIDENCE, AND DEMOGRAPHICS OF PEDIATRIC TYPE 2 DIABETES

The incidence of pediatric T2DM has been increasing since it was first described in the 1980s and corresponds with the increasing childhood obesity rates.[1–3,21] The SEARCH for Diabetes in Youth database, a population-based registry of diabetes with surveillance of 69,457,475 youths aged less than 20 years, has shown that the prevalence of T2DM in youth in the United States was 0.34 per 1000 in 2001 and increased by ~30% to 0.46 per 1000 (0.046%) in 2009.[2] SEARCH also found that, from 2002 to 2015, the pediatric T2DM incidence in the United States increased by 4.8% annually (from 9.0 cases per 100,000 youths per year in 2002–2003 to 13.8 cases per 100,000 youths per year in 2014–2015).[1,3] In comparison, the US Centers for Disease Control and Prevention estimated that 8.6% of all US adults, about 21 million individuals, were diagnosed with T2DM in 2016.[22]

In 2003, about half or more of new diabetes diagnoses in minority children aged 10 to 19 years were T2DM compared with 15% in non-Hispanic white patients.[23] In addition, the highest annual percentage increase in T2DM incidence in the SEARCH database from 2002 to 2015 was among Asians and Pacific Islanders (7.7% per year), followed by Hispanic patients (6.5% per year), non-Hispanic African Americans (6.0% per year), and Native Americans (3.7% per year).[3] In the TODAY study, the baseline characteristics of the 704 participants showed that youth with T2DM are also disproportionately of lower socioeconomic status: 41.5% with household income less than $25,000, 16.8% had parents with highest education level of a bachelor's degree or higher, and 52.1% live in single-parent households.[4,8] Similar demographics are seen in adults, in whom the T2DM prevalence is highest among non-Hispanic African Americans (11.5%), followed by Hispanic (9.1%), non-Hispanic white (8.0%), and non-Hispanic Asian (6.9%) people, and decreases with higher levels of educational attainment.[22]

SCREENING AND DIAGNOSIS OF PEDIATRIC TYPE 2 DIABETES MELLITUS

The American Diabetes Association (ADA) currently recommends screening for T2DM with HbA1c in youth "after the onset of puberty or greater than or equal to 10 years of age, whichever occurs earlier, who are overweight (body mass index [BMI] ≥85th percentile) or obese (BMI ≥ 95th percentile), and who have 1 or more additional risk factors for diabetes."[13] If HbA1c level is normal, the ADA recommends repeat testing at a minimum of 3-year intervals.[13] The ADA recommends testing for T2DM and prediabetes in obese youth more frequently, such as every 2 years, as suggested by an expert committee obesity guidelines, if BMI continues to increase.[13,24] Children identified with prediabetes should have at least annual repeat testing.[13]

At present, the ADA recommends HbA1c testing for pediatric T2DM screening based on limited data on diabetes screening methods in pediatrics, the known association of increased HbA1c level with long-term diabetes outcomes, and ease of use because patients do not need to fast.[13,25] Other measures of average glycemia, such as fructosamine, can be used in diseases such as iron deficiency anemia, sickle cell disease, thalassemia, and other hemoglobinopathies.[13,25] Glycemic screening includes fasting blood glucose test and oral glucose tolerance test (OGTT), although how these methods compare with HbA1c in pediatrics is unclear.[25]

The diagnostic criteria for diabetes and prediabetes are summarized in **Table 1**.

Differentiating among pediatric T2DM, type 1 diabetes mellitus (T1DM), and monogenic diabetes (MODY) can be difficult because overweight, obesity, and acanthosis nigricans can be present in children with T1DM and MODY.[26,27] In addition, T2DM can present with ketosis or DKA.[28] Testing for diabetes-associated pancreatic islet autoantibodies can be useful to distinguish between T1DM and T2DM. However, these autoantibodies can be positive in patients who seem to have a clinical course more consistent with T2DM.[26,28] In the TODAY study, 9.8% (118) of the 1206 youth with T2DM screened had positive pancreatic autoantibodies: 71 (5.9%) were positive for a single antibody (29 anti-GAD-65 antibody, 42 anti-IA-2 antibody), and 47 (3.9%) were positive for both antibodies.[28] The number of positive antibodies can assist in distinguishing between T2DM and T1DM because the risk of developing T1DM is high in children with more than 1 positive pancreatic islet autoantibody.[13,29]

MODY has also been noted in up to 8% of youth with features suggestive of T2DM.[26] Thus, genetic testing should be considered in youth with multiple family members with diabetes without typical features of T1DM or T2DM, such as negative diabetes autoantibodies, nonobese, and lacking other features of metabolic syndrome.[13,26] Markers of beta-cell insulin secretion, including a fasting C peptide and urinary C peptide/creatinine ratio (UCPCR), may be useful in distinguishing among T2DM, T1DM, and MODY.[26] Katz and colleagues[26,27] showed that fasting C-peptide level greater than 0.85 ng/mL at diagnosis can differentiate T1DM from T2DM with a sensitivity of 83% and a specificity of 89%, and UCPCR greater than 0.7 nmol/mmol has been shown by Besser and colleagues[30] to have 100% sensitivity and 81% specificity to distinguish between T1DM and non-T1DM (MODY or T2DM).[26,27]

COMORBIDITIES IN PEDIATRIC TYPE 2 DIABETES MELLITUS

Comorbid conditions associated with obesity and metabolic syndrome can occur concurrently with prediabetes and T2DM in both youth and adults (see **Fig. 1**).[9] Among

Table 1	
Diagnosis of prediabetes and diabetes	
	Diagnosis Definition
Prediabetes	Any of the following: 1. HbA1c: 5.7%–6.4% 2. Fasting plasma glucose: 100–125 mg/dL 3. Impaired glucose tolerance: 75-g OGTT 2-h glucose 140–199 mg/dL
Diabetes	Two of the following: 1. HbA1c ≥ 6.5% 2. Fasting blood glucose ≥126 mg/dL 3. 75-g OGTT 2-h glucose >200 mg/dL 4. Random plasma glucose ≥200 mg/dL in setting of hyperglycemia symptoms

Data from American Diabetes Association. Standards of Medical Care in Diabetes-2019. Diabetes Care. 2019;42:S1–193.

adults with T2DM, the prevalence of concurrent nonalcoholic fatty liver disease (NAFLD) ranges from 40% to 70%.[31] In a cohort study of 675 children with NAFLD, 30% had comorbid T2DM or prediabetes.[32] A case-control study of 150 overweight children with biopsy-proven NAFLD compared with 150 overweight children without NAFLD showed that the risk factors for NAFLD in pediatrics are aspects associated with metabolic syndrome, including central obesity (waist circumference >102 cm in boys and 88 cm in girls), higher triglyceride level (>150 mg/dL), high total cholesterol level (>200 mg/dL), higher low-density lipoprotein (LDL) cholesterol level (>130 mg/ dL), higher systolic (>130 mm Hg) and diastolic (>85 mm Hg) blood pressure, and lower high-density lipoprotein (HDL) cholesterol levels (<40 mg/dL).[32,33] Signs of NAFLD include increased liver enzyme levels or signs of fatty liver on ultrasonography.[34] Children with NAFLD and comorbid pediatric T2DM have 3.1 times higher odds of developing nonalcoholic steatohepatitis (NASH), a progressive form of NAFLD that has a greater risk of progressing to cirrhosis.[32] In adults with NAFLD, T2DM is associated with higher rates of the development of NASH, liver cirrhosis, and hepatocellular carcinoma.[32]

Obstructive sleep apnea (OSA) is also associated with central obesity and insulin resistance and is an additional independent risk factor for cardiovascular complications, including increased blood pressure, in children and adults.[35,36] Pediatric patients with obesity should be screened for symptoms of OSA, including habitual snoring, apneic pauses while sleeping, or excessive daytime sleepiness; however, history and physical examination have low positive predictive value (65%) in identifying OSA in youth.[37] If symptoms are present, patients should be referred for a diagnostic evaluation for OSA with polysomnography.[38] In addition, sleep disruption and OSA are associated with reduced insulin sensitivity in adults with T2DM, and treatment of OSA may improve glycemic control in patients with pediatric T2DM.[39–41]

PCOS characterized by hyperandrogenism and chronic anovulation, has a higher prevalence in youth with obesity, is associated with insulin resistance with or without obesity, and predisposes youth and adults to the development of diabetes.[42,43] Insulin resistance is present in 30% to 40% of adults with PCOS, including both obese and nonobese.[42] In 27 youth with PCOS and BMIs ranging from 20.4 to 54.4 kg/m^2, OGTT identified impaired glucose tolerance (IGT) in 30% and T2DM in 4%.[42] No relationship between BMI and 2-hour OGTT plasma glucose was found, and the patient with the lowest BMI had IGT.[42]

Psychiatric comorbidities are also common with pediatric T2DM. In a retrospective chart review of 237 patients with pediatric T2DM, Katz and colleagues[44] showed neuropsychiatric disease was present in 19% of patients at diabetes presentation; diagnoses included depression, attention-deficit hyperactivity disorder, schizophrenia, bipolar disorder, and neurodevelopmental disorders. In the TODAY trial, 14.8% screened positive for clinical depression and 30% screened positive for binge eating.[45] Some of these psychiatric comorbidities in pediatric T2DM may be secondary to the use of second-generation antipsychotics, which is associated with weight gain and worsened insulin resistance in pediatric cohort studies.[46,47]

TREATMENT OF PEDIATRIC TYPE 2 DIABETES MELLITUS

At this time, although several pharmacologic medication categories are available for treatment of adult T2DM, only 3 pharmacologic medications are currently FDA approved for pediatric patients with T2DM: metformin, insulin, and the glucagon-like peptide 1 (GLP-1) receptor agonist liraglutide.[13,48] ADA guidelines recommend monitoring of HbA1c level every 3 months to inform treatment.[13] The ADA suggests a target

HbA1c in pediatric T2DM of less than 7% but also states that goal HbA1c less than 6.5% could be used.[13] The latter is supported by the TODAY study, in which hypoglycemia was rare even for patients who progressed to insulin therapy and 5-year diabetic complication rates were high[8,45] (**Fig. 2**).

Metformin is recommended as the first-line therapy for T2DM in adults and youth with normal renal function (see **Fig. 2**).[13] The UK Prospective Diabetes Study Group has shown that, in adults, metformin monotherapy can lead to risk reductions in all diabetes-related clinical endpoint, diabetes-related death and all-cause mortality compared with insulin therapy.[49] Metformin also has a weight loss effect: in the pediatric MOCA (Metformin in Obese Children and Adolescents) trial, in which 151 obese children with prediabetes or IGT were randomized to metformin or placebo,

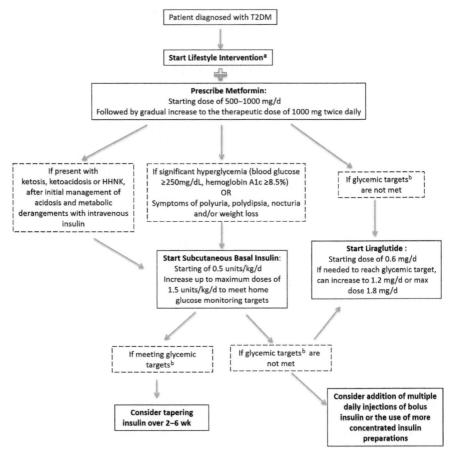

Fig. 2. Treatment algorithm for pediatric T2DM. [a] Lifestyle intervention includes: (1) at least 30 to 60 minutes of moderate to vigorous physical activity at least 5 d/wk and reduction of sedentary behavior; (2) healthy eating patterns and reduction of calorie-dense, nutrition-poor foods, especially sugar-sweetened beverages; (3) sleep 8 to 10 h/night. [b] Glycemic target as recommended by the ADA is hemoglobin A1c less than 7.0% or hemoglobin A1c less than 6.5% for patients with shorter duration of diabetes or lesser degrees of beta-cell dysfunction as long as can be achieved without significant risk factors, including severe hypoglycemia. (*Data from* Refs.[9,13,48])

the metformin group had a statistically significant reduction in BMI (−0.1 standard deviation) and weight (−2.6 kg) after 6 months of treatment.[50]

Basal insulin should be initiated in patients with significant hyperglycemia; ketosis; symptoms of polyuria, polydipsia, nocturia, and/or weight loss; or who are failing to reach glycemic targets on other pharmacologic therapies, but should be tapered once meeting the glycemic target (see **Fig. 2**).[9,13] In the TODAY study, for patients who had treatment failure and progression to add-on insulin therapy in any arm, the response 1-year after insulin initiation was variable, with 33% with HbA1c decrease of greater than or equal to 0.5%, 46% with less than 0.5% change in HbA1c, and 21% with an increase in HbA1c level greater than or equal to 0.5%.[51]

Liraglutide, a daily injectable GLP-1 agonist, was approved for use in pediatric T2DM in spring 2019. Liraglutide is indicated in patients greater than or equal to 10 years of age on metformin plus or minus basal insulin therapy and who have not met glycemic targets (ie, HbA1c<7% or <6.5% based on provider preference) (see **Fig. 2**).[13] In the clinical trial by Tamborlane and colleagues, 134 patients with T2DM on metformin (with or without basal insulin) were randomized to liraglutide or placebo and monitored for 52 weeks: 64% were able to attain HbA1c less than 7% with liraglutide compared with 36% with placebo.[48] In the LEAD (Liraglutide Effect and Action in Diabetes) trial, in which 1091 adults were randomized to liraglutide or placebo added to metformin monotherapy, liraglutide was associated with 1.0% lower HbA1c level compared with a 0.1% HbA1c increase with placebo.[52] Although the adult LEAD trial showed 1.8 to 2.8 kg weight loss in all liraglutide groups, weight and BMI reductions in the pediatric trial were not statistically different in the liraglutide and placebo groups.[48,52] Common side effects of liraglutide include nausea and mild gastrointestinal disturbance that improve over time.[48,52,53] Minor hypoglycemia was more common with liraglutide in youth (0.386 events/patient/y) compared with in adults in LEAD (0.14 events/patient/y).[48,52] Liraglutide is contraindicated in people with personal or family history of medullary thyroid carcinoma or personal history of pancreatitis.[13]

Barriers to use of each of these medications are well recognized. Both insulin and liraglutide are only offered in injectable forms for pediatric T2DM at this time. Metformin has a strong track record of safety, but side effects include abdominal pain and nausea, which can reduce its acceptability.[4,6] Children may also have difficulties with pill swallowing. Although severe insulin resistance in pediatric T2DM makes hypoglycemia less likely, hypoglycemia remains a concern with insulin use.[8] In addition, although liraglutide and metformin contribute to weight loss, if progression to insulin is required, insulin has a weight-positive effect.[13,48,50,52] The TODAY trial also revealed that overall medication adherence (1) declined over time to 56% by 48 months, and (2) was correlated with baseline depressive symptoms.[54]

Because these pharmacologic options currently face barriers to use in pediatric T2DM and adherence is challenging, lifestyle intervention is a therapy mainstay (see **Fig. 2**). Weight loss can improve insulin sensitivity in pediatric T2DM. In a randomized controlled behavioral weight loss trial, an 8% reduction in BMI was associated with improved insulin sensitivity in obese adolescents.[55] In addition, the TODAY trial showed that weight loss was associated with improved cardiometabolic outcomes, including decreases in systolic blood pressure, LDL cholesterol, triglycerides, total cholesterol levels, and increases in HDL cholesterol level over 24 months.[56] Meal replacements in lifestyle modification programs can also be considered because their use has shown short-term weight loss in obese adolescents and improved diet composition in adults.[57,58] However, the 595 participants randomized to the lifestyle intervention combined with metformin therapy arm in the TODAY trial (consisting of a family-based behavioral approach with intensive weekly intervention sessions for the first 6 months followed by biweekly visits alternating with biweekly telephone calls in the second 6 months, followed by monthly visits and telephone calls from months 12–24) had a 5-year treatment failure rate of 46.6%.[8,56] In addition, TODAY study participants who lost weight by month 6 in the weight-management intervention arm did not sustain weight loss in months 12 and 24.[56] Adherence to the lifestyle program was only 60%, and self-monitoring was low for all participants.[59] This low adherence may be partly attributable to the TODAY study design, in which participants with T2DM were randomized to 1 of 3 treatment groups (one-third were in the lifestyle intervention), compared with other successful intensive family-based weight loss trials in pediatrics such as the Bright Bodies program, which directly recruited participants to participate in a weight loss trial, an approach that could contribute to higher baseline patient motivation.[56,60]

For youth with T2DM who fail lifestyle modifications and continue to have morbid obesity, bariatric surgery could be considered as a potential treatment option. Qualifications for bariatric surgery per American Society for Metabolic and Bariatric Surgery guidelines include class III obesity (BMI>140% of the 95th percentile or BMI $\geq$ 40 kg/m^2) or class II obesity (120% of the 95th percentile or BMI $\geq$ 35 to $\leq$39 kg/m^2) with a comorbidity. Of the 30 participants (baseline BMI 54.4 kg/m^2) in the Teen-Longitudinal Assessment of Bariatric Surgery (Teen-LABS) study with baseline T2DM who underwent bariatric surgery, mean HbA1c level decreased from 6.8% to 5.5%.[61]

PROGRESSION OF PEDIATRIC TYPE 2 DIABETES MELLITUS

Pediatric T2DM has been shown to have higher rates of treatment failure compared with adult T2DM. In the TODAY trial, youth with T2DM showed a 45.6% overall treatment failure defined by persistently increased HbA1c level greater than 8% or inability to wean off insulin therapy.[8] Treatment failure at 5 years with metformin monotherapy is higher in pediatric (51.7%) versus adult (21%) T2DM.[8,62] TODAY trial participants on rosiglitazone and metformin combined therapy had a treatment failure rate of 38.6%, higher than seen in an adult retrospective cohort study in which patients on metformin/thiazolidinedione combination therapy had treatment failure of 14.3%.[8,63] These rates of treatment failure in the TODAY trial are particularly striking, with a short mean baseline diabetes duration of only 7.8 months.[8] In addition, youth in the TODAY study on metformin for 3 months with HbA1c level greater than 6.3% or increasing HbA1c level had higher risk for worsening glycemic control.[64]

In addition to high treatment failure rates, pediatric T2DM also has faster progression to beta-cell failure than adult T2DM. Adult patients with T2DM have gradual beta-cell function decline occurring over 10 to 12 years at average rate of 7% per year, whereas youth with T2DM show declines as high as 35% per year.[6,7,10,65,66] Worsening diabetes control on metformin monotherapy occurring as early as 1.5 to 2 years after diagnosis is a manifestation of this rapid beta-cell function decline.[6,10,12,65–67] Higher frequency of DKA in youth with new-onset T2DM also attests to these higher rates of beta-cell failure in pediatric T2DM.[6,13] Baseline predictors of treatment failure and beta-cell decline in pediatric patients are higher fasting glucose level, higher HbA1c level, and DKA.[6,7] These findings suggest earlier diagnosis and treatment may be protective against beta-cell decline.

The Restoring Insulin Secretion (RISE) study compared insulin sensitivity and beta-cell response in 66 youth and 355 adults with IGT or recently diagnosed T2DM and showed that youth with IGT or T2DM have (1) 50% lower insulin sensitivity as measured by hyperglycemic clamp or OGTT, and (2) hyper-responsive beta cells with higher OGTT-stimulated c-peptide and insulin levels.[68] In addition, insulin clearance is lower in pediatric versus adult T2DM, and more insulin is required to achieve the same fasting blood glucose level.[69,70] The RISE trial also attempted to evaluate methods to reduce beta-cell decline in pediatric T2DM and randomized 91 youth with IGT or T2DM to (1) metformin for 1 year, or (2) intensive insulin treatment with insulin glargine for 3 months followed by metformin for 9 months, but did not show any improvement or slowing of beta-cell decline in either arm.[70] Given these findings, early diagnosis and prevention of pediatric T2DM is key before significant beta-cell failure.

COMPLICATIONS OF PEDIATRIC TYPE 2 DIABETES

Diabetes can lead to microvascular complications (ie, nephropathy, retinopathy, and neuropathy) and macrovascular complications (ie, cardiac, cerebrovascular, and peripheral vascular diseases) (see **Fig. 1**).[5] These complications have been described in pediatric T1DM and adult-onset T2DM and generally occur about 15 to 20 years following diagnosis.[5] However, pediatric T2DM is associated with higher risk of complications than pediatric T1DM.[5] By the end of the TODAY trial's 5-year study, increases were found in rates of hypertension from 11.6% to 33.8%, microalbuminuria from 6.3% to 16.6%, and LDL cholesterol from 4.5% to 10.7%.[45] In addition, at the end of the TODAY trial, 14% of participants had retinopathy.[45] The annual albuminuria progression rate in youth based on the TODAY study is 2.6%, similar to the finding in the UK Prospective Diabetes Study (UKPDS) in adults of 2.0%.[45,71,72] From the UKPDS study in adults, diabetic patients without microalbuminuria at diagnosis were predicted to develop nephropathy at a median of 19 years after diagnosis, and those with microalbuminuria at diagnosis were predicted to worsen to macroalbuminuria or worse at a median of 11 years after diagnosis.[71] In a cohort study of 342 youth with T2DM, major diabetic complications (eg, dialysis, blindness, and amputations) were noted in 1.1% at 10 years, 26% at 15 years, and 47.9% at 20 years after diagnosis.[5]

In a retrospective analysis with greater than 20 years of data from 354 patients with T2DM and 470 patients with pediatric T1DM of similar age of onset, pediatric T2DM was also noted to have a significantly higher mortality at shorter disease duration than pediatric T1DM, likely driven by this study's demonstrated higher rate of cardiovascular deaths in T2DM.[73] Cardiovascular changes in pediatric T2DM are prevalent, as shown by echocardiography performed on 455 participants with cardiovascular risk factors (hypertension and obesity) in the TODAY cohort, in which increased mean left ventricular (LV) mass and mean left atrial size and abnormal LV geometry were noted.[74] Carotid intima media thickness, a strong predictor of cardiovascular events in adults, is also high in youth with obesity and T2DM.[75] In addition, cardiac autonomic instability, as measured by heart rate variability, was present in 8% of the TODAY cohort and associated with increased arterial stiffness, as measured by carotid-femoral pulse-wave velocity.[76] Participants with pediatric T2DM in the TODAY trial also had significant dyslipidemia and inflammation, contributors to premature atherosclerosis, with increases in LDL cholesterol level and use of statins (8.6% to 22%) and triglyceride, plasma nonesterified fatty acid, and high-sensitivity C-reactive protein levels.[77] Some studies have also shown higher endothelial dysfunction, measured by lower brachial flow–mediated dilatation, in T2DM youth compared with youth with T1DM who have comparable HbA1c level but longer diabetes duration.[75,78]

Pregnancy complications are also seen in women who have had pediatric-onset T2DM. Pregnancies occurred in 10% of the TODAY study cohort, 26% of whom had loss or stillbirth, and, of the live births, 15.4% were preterm and 20.5% had congenital anomalies (50% cardiac, 50% other).[79] These statistics show the significant complications in pediatric T2DM, particularly compared with pediatric T1DM, and underscore the need for a clear understanding of the cause and progression of pediatric T2DM.

Table 2
Recommendations for monitoring for comorbidities and complications in type 2 diabetes mellitus[a]

	Recommended Monitoring
Comorbidity	
NAFLD	1. Measurement of AST and ALT levels should be done at diagnosis and annually 2. Refer to gastroenterology if persistent increase or worsening of AST and ALT levels
OSA	1. Screen for symptoms of OSA at each visit 2. If symptoms of OSA present, a polysomnogram should be performed and referral to a pediatric sleep specialist if PSG is abnormal
PCOS	1. Female patients with T2DM should be evaluated for symptoms of PCOS. Metformin therapy may improve symptoms of hyperandrogenism
Psychosocial factors	1. Diabetes distress, mental health, and disordered eating behaviors should be assessed regularly 2. Social barriers, including food insecurity, housing instability, and financial barriers, should be assessed and social work consultation should be made if present
Complications	
Nephropathy	1. Blood pressure should be measured at every visit 2. If blood pressure >95th percentile for age, sex, and height, lifestyle management should be initiated. If continued increase, consider antihypertensive therapy (ACE inhibitors or angiotensin receptor blocker) after 6 mo of lifestyle management and referral to nephrology 3. Urine albumin/creatinine ratio should be obtained at diagnosis and annually. If increased (>30 mg/g creatinine), referral to nephrology is indicated
Neuropathy	1. Foot examination should be performed annually with assessment of foot pulses, pinprick, and 10-g monofilament sensation tests; testing of vibration sensation using a 128-Hz tuning fork; and ankle reflexes
Retinopathy	1. Dilated fundoscopy or retinal photography should be done at diagnosis and annually
Cardiovascular	1. Lipid testing at diagnosis and annually 2. Consider therapy with a statin if LDL remains >130 mg/dL after 6 mo of lifestyle intervention 3. Consider therapy with a fibrate if triglyceride levels are increased (fasting level >400 mg/dL) to reduce risk of pancreatitis

Abbreviations: ACE, angiotensin-converting enzyme; ALT, alanine transaminase; AST, aspartate transaminase; PSG, polysomnogram.
[a] Recommendations per American Diabetes Association.[9,13]
Data from Arslanian S, Bacha F, Grey M, et al. Evaluation and management of youth-onset type 2 diabetes: A position statement by the American diabetes association. Diabetes Care. 2018;41(12):2648-2668 and American Diabetes Association. Standards of Medical Care in Diabetes-2019. Diabetes Care. 2019;42:S1–193.

MONITORING FOR COMORBIDITIES AND COMPLICATIONS

The ADA recommendations for monitoring for comorbid conditions and complications are summarized in **Table 2**.

SUMMARY AND FUTURE DIRECTIONS

Pediatric T2DM is an increasing public health concern with an increasing incidence corresponding with the increase in pediatric obesity. Despite a similar pathophysiology to adult T2DM, pediatric T2DM shows faster pancreatic beta-cell decline and increased treatment failure rates compared with adult T2DM. Youth with T2DM will be entering adulthood with significant risks for morbidity and mortality at younger ages than the adult T2DM population. The available treatment options have not been effective in reducing beta-cell decline and are complicated by high nonadherence. Early diagnosis and treatment of pediatric T2DM and development of new pharmacologic therapies; trials of approved adult T2DM therapies, such as the recently approved liraglutide; and effective behavioral interventions are critically needed to stem the continued increase in pediatric T2DM and its sequelae.

DISCLOSURE

The authors have nothing to disclose.

ACKNOWLEDGMENTS

Talia Hitt's work on this chapter was supported, in part, by grant 2T32DK063688-16 (TH) and 2T32DK063688-17 (TH) from the National Institutes of Health (NIH).

REFERENCES

1. Mayer-Davis EJ, Lawrence JM, Dabelea D, et al. Incidence trends of type 1 and type 2 diabetes among youths, 2002-2012. N Engl J Med 2017;376(15):1419–29.

2. Dabelea D, Mayer-Davis EJ, Saydah S, et al. Prevalence of type 1 and type 2 diabetes among children and adolescents from 2001 to 2009. JAMA 2014;311(17): 1778–86.

3. Divers J, Mayer-Davis EJ, Lawrence JM, et al. Trends in incidence of type 1 and type 2 diabetes among youths - selected counties and Indian reservations, United States, 2002-2015. Morb Mortal Wkly Rep 2020;69(6):161–5.

4. Copeland KC, Zeitler P, Geffner M, et al. Characteristics of adolescents and youth with recent-onset type 2 diabetes: the TODAY cohort at baseline. J Clin Endocrinol Metab 2011;96(1):159–67.

5. Dart AB, Martens PJ, Rigatto C, et al. Earlier onset of complications in youth with type 2 diabetes. Diabetes Care 2014;37(2):436–43.

6. Katz LEL, Magge SN, Hernandez ML, et al. Glycemic control in youth with type 2 diabetes declines as early as two years after diagnosis. J Pediatr 2011;158(1): 106–11.

7. Arslanian S, Pyle L, Payan M, et al. Effects of metformin, metformin plus rosiglitazone, and metformin plus lifestyle on insulin sensitivity and -βcell function in TODAY. Diabetes Care 2013;36(6):1749–57.

8. Zeitler P, Hirst K, Pyle L, et al. A clinical trial to maintain glycemic control in youth with type 2 diabetes. N Engl J Med 2012;366(24):2247–56.

9. Arslanian S, Bacha F, Grey M, et al. Evaluation and management of youth-onset type 2 diabetes: a position statement by the American diabetes association. Diabetes Care 2018;41(12):2648–68.

10. Nolan CJ, Damm P, Prentki M. Type 2 diabetes across generations: from pathophysiology to prevention and management. Lancet 2011;378(9786):169–81.

11. Weiss R, Caprio S, Trombetta M, et al. B-cell function across the spectrum of glucose tolerance in obese youth. Diabetes 2005;54(6):1735–43.

12. Gungor N, Bacha F, Saad R, et al. Youth type 2 diabetes. Diabetes Care 2005; 28(3):638–44.

13. American Diabetes Association. Standards of Medical Care in Diabetes-2019. Diabetes Care 2019;42:S1–193.

14. Fourtner SH, Weinzimer SA, Katz LEL. Hyperglycemic hyperosmolar non-ketotic syndrome in children with type 2 diabetes. Pediatr Diabetes 2005;6(3):129–35.

15. Saklayen MG. The global epidemic of the metabolic syndrome. Curr Hypertens Rep 2018;9:1–8.

16. Boney CM, Verma A, Tucker R, et al. Metabolic syndrome in childhood: association with birth weight, maternal obesity, and gestational diabetes mellitus. Pediatrics 2005;115(3):e290–6.

17. Magge SN, Stettler N, Jawad AF, et al. Increased prevalence of abnormal glucose tolerance among obese siblings of children with type 2 diabetes. J Pediatr 2009;154(4):562–6.

18. Caprio S, Plewe G, Diamond MP, et al. Increased insulin secretion in puberty: a compensatory response to reductions in insulin sensitivity. J Pediatr 1989;114(6): 963–7.

19. Goran MI, Gower BA. Longitudinal study on pubertal insulin resistance. Diabetes 2001;50:2444–50.

20. Nam HK, Lee KH. Small for gestational age and obesity: epidemiology and general risks. Ann Pediatr Endocrinol Metab 2018;23(1):9–13.

21. Skinner AC, Ravanbakht SN, Skelton JA, et al. Prevalence of obesity and severe obesity in US children, 1999-2016. Pediatrics 2018;141(3):e20173459.

22. Bullard KM, Cowie CC, Lessem SE, et al. Prevalence of Diagnosed Diabetes in Adults by Diabetes Type — United States, 2016. Morb Mortal Wkly Rep 2018; 67(12):2016–8.

23. Dabelea D, Bell RA, D'Agostino RBJ, et al. Incidence of diabetes in youth in the United States. JAMA 2007;297(24):2716–24.

24. Barlow SE. Expert committee recommendations regarding the prevention , assessment , and treatment of child and adolescent overweight and obesity. Pediatrics 2007;120:S164–92.

25. Kapadia C, Zeitler P. Hemoglobin A1c measurement for the diagnosis of Type 2 diabetes in children. Int J Pediatr Endocrinol 2012;2012(1):2–5.

26. Katz LEL. C-peptide and 24-hour urinary c-peptide as markers to help classify types of childhood diabetes. Horm Res Paediatr 2015;84(1):62–4.

27. Katz LEL, Jawad AF, Ganesh J, et al. Fasting c-peptide and insulin-like growth factor-binding protein-1 levels help to distinguish childhood type 1 and type 2 diabetes at diagnosis. Pediatr Diabetes 2007;8(2):53–9.

28. Klingensmith GJ, Pyle L, Arslanian S, et al. The presence of GAD and IA-2 antibodies in youth with a type 2 diabetes phenotype: results from the TODAY study. Diabetes Care 2010;33(9):1970–5.

29. Ziegler AG, Rewers M, Simell O, et al. Seroconversion to Multiple islet autoantibodies and risk of progression to diabetes in children. JAMA 2013;309(23): 2473–9.

30. Besser RE, Shields BM, Hammersley SE, et al. Home urine C-peptide creatinine ratio (UCPCR) testing can identify type 2 and MODY in pediatric diabetes. Pediatr Diabetes 2013;14(3):181–8.
31. Anstee QM, Mcpherson S, Day CP. How big a problem is non-alcoholic fatty liver disease? BMJ 2011;343:1–5.
32. Newton KP, Hou J, Crimmins NA, et al. Prevalence of prediabetes and type 2 diabetes in children with nonalcoholic fatty liver disease. JAMA Pediatr 2016; 170(10):1–8.
33. Schwimmer JB, Pardee PB, Lavine JE, et al. Cardiovascular risk factors and the metabolic syndrome in pediatric nonalcoholic fatty liver disease. Circulation 2008;118(3):277–83.
34. Middleton JP, Wiener RC, Barnes BH, et al. Clinical features of pediatric nonalcoholic fatty liver disease: a need for increased awareness and a consensus for screening. Clin Pediatr (Phila) 2014;53(14):1318–25.
35. Jean-Louis G, Zizi F, Clark LT, et al. Obstructive sleep apnea and cardiovascular disease: role of the metabolic syndrome and its components. J Clin Sleep Med 2008;4(3):261–72.
36. Kelly A, Dougherty S, Cucchiara A, et al. Catecholamines, Adiponectin, and insulin resistance as measured by homa in children with obstructive sleep apnea. Sleep 2010;33(9):1185–91.
37. Marcus CL, Brooks LJ, Davidson Ward S, et al. Diagnosis and Management of childhood obstructive sleep apnea syndrome. Pediatrics 2012;130(3):e714–35.
38. Bibbins-Domingo K, Grossman DC, Curry SJ, et al. Screening for obstructive sleep apnea in adults us preventive services task force recommendation statement. JAMA 2017;317(4):407–14.
39. Koren D, Katz LEL, Brar PC, et al. Sleep architecture and glucose and insulin homeostasis in obese adolescents. Diabetes Care 2011. https://doi.org/10.2337/dc11-1093.
40. Cappuccio FP, Taggart FM, Kandala NB, et al. Meta-analysis of short sleep duration and obesity in children and adults. Sleep 2008. https://doi.org/10.1093/sleep/31.5.619.
41. Buxton OM, Pavlova M, Reid EW, et al. Sleep restriction for 1 week reduces insulin sensitivity in healthy men. Diabetes 2010. https://doi.org/10.2337/db09-0699.
42. Palmert MR, Gordon CM, Kartashov AI, et al. Screening for abnormal glucose tolerance in adolescents with polycystic ovary syndrome. J Clin Endocrinol Metab 2002;87(3):1017–23.
43. Kelsey MM, Braffett BH, Geffner ME, et al. Menstrual dysfunction in girls from the treatment options for type 2 diabetes in adolescents and youth (TODAY) study. J Clin Endocrinol Metab 2018;103(6):2309–18.
44. Katz LEL, Swami S, Abraham M, et al. Neuropsychiatric disorders at the presentation of type 2 diabetes mellitus in children. Pediatr Diabetes 2005;6(2):84–9.
45. Tryggestad JB, Willi SM. Complications and comorbidities of T2DM in adolescents: findings from the TODAY clinical trial. J Diabet Complications 2015; 29(2):307–12.
46. Coughlin M, Goldie CL, Tregunno D, et al. Enhancing metabolic monitoring for children and adolescents using second-generation antipsychotics. Int J Ment Health Nurs 2018;2009:1188–98.
47. Baeza I, Vigo L, De E, et al. The effects of antipsychotics on weight gain , weight - related hormones and homocysteine in children and adolescents a 1 - year follow - up study. Eur Child Adolesc Psychiatry 2017;26(1):35–46.

48. Tamborlane WV, Barrientos-Pérez M, Fainberg U, et al. Liraglutide in children and adolescents with type 2 diabetes. N Engl J Med 2019;381(7):637–46.

49. Turner R. Effect of intensive blood-glucose control with metformin on complications in overweight patients with type 2 diabetes (UKPDS 34). Lancet 1998; 352(9131):854–65.

50. Kendall D, Vail A, Amin R, et al. Metformin in obese children and adolescents: the MOCA trial. J Clin Endocrinol Metab 2013;98:322–9.

51. Bacha F, El ghormli L, Arslanian S, et al. Predictors of response to insulin therapy in youth with poorly-controlled type 2 diabetes in the TODAY trial. Pediatr Diabetes 2019;20(7):871–9.

52. Nauck M, Frid A, Hermansen K, et al. Efficacy and safety comparison of liraglutide, glimepiride, and placebo, all in combination with metformin, in type 2 diabetes: the LEAD (Liraglutide effect and action in diabetes)-2 study. Diabetes Care 2009;32(1):84–90.

53. Vaag A, Schmitz O, Sethi BK, et al. Liraglutide vs insulin glargine and placebo in combination with metformin and sulfonylurea therapy in type 2 diabetes mellitus (LEAD-5 met + SU): a randomised controlled trial Plasma glucose. Diabetologia 2009;2046–55. https://doi.org/10.1007/s00125-009-1472-y.

54. Katz LEL, Anderson BJ, McKay SV, et al. Correlates of medication adherence in the TODAY cohort of youth with type 2 diabetes. Diabetes Care 2016;39(11): 1956–62.

55. Abrams P, Katz LEL, Moore RH, et al. Threshold for improvement in insulin sensitivity with adolescent weight loss. J Pediatr 2013;163(3):785–90.

56. Marcus MD, Wilfley DE, El ghormli L, et al. Weight change in the management of youth-onset type 2 diabetes: the TODAY clinical trial experience. Pediatr Obes 2017;12(4):337–45.

57. Berkowitz RI, Wadden TA, Gehrman CA, et al. Meal replacements in the treatment of adolescent obesity. Obesity (Silver Spring) 2011;19(6):1193–9.

58. Raynor HA, Anderson AM, Miller GD, et al. Partial meal replacement plan and quality of the diet at 1 year: action for health in diabetes (Look AHEAD) trial. J Acad Nutr Diet 2015;115(5):731–42.

59. Berkowitz RI, Marcus MD, Anderson BJ, et al. Adherence to a lifestyle program for youth with type 2 diabetes and its association with treatment outcome in the TODAY clinical trial. Pediatr Diabetes 2018;19(2):191–8.

60. Savoye M, Shaw M, Dziura J, et al. Effects of a weight management program on body composition and metabolic parameters in overweight. Children 2020; 297(24):2697–704.

61. Inge TH, Laffel LM, Jenkins TM, et al. Comparison of surgical and medical therapy for type 2 diabetes in severely obese adolescents. JAMA Pediatr 2018; 172(5):452–60.

62. Kahn SE, Haffner SM, Heise MA, et al. Glycemic durability of rosiglitazone, metformin, or glyburide monotherapy. N Engl J Med 2006;355(23):2427–43.

63. Rascati K, Richards K, Lopez D, et al. Progression to insulin for patients with diabetes mellitus on dual oral antidiabetic therapy using the US department of defense database. Diabetes Obes Metab 2013;15(10):901–5.

64. Zeitler P, Hirst K, Copeland KC, et al. HbA1c after a short period of monotherapy with metformin identifies durable glycemic control among adolescents with type 2 diabetes. Diabetes Care 2015;38(12):2285–92.

65. Kahn SE. Clinical, review 135: the importance of β-cell failure in the development and progression of type 2 diabetes. J Clin Endocrinol Metab 2001;86(9):4047–58.

66. Gungor N, Arslanian S. Diabetes mellitus of youth. J Pediatr 2004;656–9. https://doi.org/10.1016/j.jpeds.2003.12.045.
67. Bacha F, Gungor N, Lee S, et al. In vivo insulin sensitivity and secretion in obese youth: what are the differences between normal glucose tolerance, impaired glucose tolerance, and type 2 diabetes? Diabetes Care 2009;32(1):100–5.
68. Edelstein SL, Kahn SE, Arslanian SA, et al. Metabolic contrasts between youth and adults with impaired glucose tolerance or recently diagnosed type 2 diabetes: I. Observations using the hyperglycemic Clamp. Diabetes Care 2018;41(8):1696–706.
69. Edelstein SL. Restoring insulin secretion (RISE): design of studies of β-cell preservation in prediabetes and early Type 2 diabetes across the life span. Diabetes Care 2014;37(3):780–8.
70. Nadeau KJ, Hannon TS, Edelstein SL, et al. Impact of insulin and metformin versus metformin alone on β-cell function in youth with impaired glucose tolerance or recently diagnosed type 2 diabetes. Diabetes Care 2018;41(8):1717–25.
71. Adler AI, Stevens RJ, Manley SE, et al. Development and progression of nephropathy in type 2 diabetes: United Kingdom Prospective Diabetes Study. Kidney Int 2003;63:225–32.
72. Chiang JL, Boer IH De, Goldstein-fuchs J. Diabetic kidney disease: a report from an ADA consensus conference. Am J Kidney Dis 2014;64(4):510–33.
73. Constantino MI, Molyneaux L, Limacher-Gisler F, et al. Long-term complications and mortality in young-onset diabetes: Type 2 diabetes is more hazardous and lethal than type 1 diabetes. Diabetes Care 2013;36(12):3863–9.
74. Katz LEL, Gidding SS, Bacha F, et al. Alterations in left ventricular, left atrial, and right ventricular structure and function to cardiovascular risk factors in adolescents with type 2 diabetes participating in the TODAY clinical trial. Pediatr Diabetes 2015. https://doi.org/10.1111/pedi.12119.
75. Shah AS, Urbina EM. Vascular and endothelial function in youth with type 2 diabetes mellitus. Curr Diab Rep 2017;17(6):1–7.
76. Shah AS, El Ghormli L, Vajravelu ME, et al. Heart rate variability and cardiac autonomic dysfunction: prevalence, risk factors, and relationship to arterial stiffness in the treatment options for type 2 diabetes in adolescents and youth (TODAY) study. Diabetes Care 2019;42(11):2143–50.
77. Katz LEL, Bacha F, Gidding SS, et al. Lipid Profiles, inflammatory markers, and insulin therapy in youth with type 2 diabetes. J Pediatr 2018. https://doi.org/10.1016/j.jpeds.2017.12.052.
78. Ohsugi K, Sugawara H, Ebina K, et al. Comparison of brachial artery flow-mediated dilation in youth with type 1 and type 2 diabetes mellitus. J Diabetes Investig 2014;5(5):615–20.
79. Klingensmith GJ, Pyle L, Nadeau KJ, et al. Pregnancy outcomes in youth with type 2 diabetes: the TODAY study experience. Diabetes Care 2016;39(1):122–9.

Overview of Atypical Diabetes

Jaclyn Tamaroff, MD*, Marissa Kilberg, MD, MSEd, Sara E. Pinney, MD, MTR,
Shana McCormack, MD, MTR

KEYWORDS

- Atypical diabetes • Monogenic diabetes
- Maturity-onset diabetes of the young (MODY) • Neonatal diabetes
- Mitochondrial diabetes • Cystic fibrosis–related diabetes (CFRD)

KEY POINTS

- Diagnosis of atypical diabetes requires attention to clinical presentation, specific testing, and personalized treatment based on genetic etiology and comorbidities.
- Atypical diabetes should be considered in patients with disorders associated with diabetes (eg, cystic fibrosis or mitochondrial disease) or age less than 25 years old with non-autoimmune diabetes and lacking typical type 2 diabetes mellitus characteristics.
- Comorbidities, such as deafness, history of hyperinsulinism, renal disease, and liver disease, in a patient with new-onset diabetes should prompt consideration of atypical diabetes.

INTRODUCTION

Although a majority of children and adults with diabetes mellitus (DM) are diagnosed with type 1 diabetes mellitus (T1D) or type 2 diabetes mellitus (T2D), a significant number of patients with DM do not meet T1D or T2D diagnostic criteria or have atypical manifestations of their DM.[1] Monogenic diabetes is estimated to comprise up to 6.5% of the pediatric diabetes population,[1,2] mostly among those classified as T1D but without evidence of pancreatic islet autoimmunity. In 1 study, however, 8% of patients clinically diagnosed with T2D carry mutations in genes associated with monogenic diabetes.[3] Other rare forms of diabetes related to mitochondrial defects, severe insulin resistance syndromes, and lipodystrophy also contribute to the population of patients with atypical forms of diabetes.[4] Collectively, patients who do not have

Funding sources: M. Kilberg receives grant funding from the Cystic Fibrosis Foundation: KIL-BER19D0. J. Tamaroff receives grant funding from T32DK063688-16.
Division of Endocrinology and Diabetes, Children's Hospital of Philadelphia, 3500 Civic Center Boulevard, 12th Floor, Philadelphia, PA 19104, USA
* Corresponding author.
E-mail address: tamaroffj@email.chop.edu

Endocrinol Metab Clin N Am 49 (2020) 695–723
https://doi.org/10.1016/j.ecl.2020.07.004
0889-8529/20/© 2020 Elsevier Inc. All rights reserved.

clear presentations of either T1D or T2D may represent a unique population enriched in both known and as yet undefined monogenic causes of diabetes.

Diagnostic criteria set by the American Diabetes Association remain the same for all forms of DM: hemoglobin (Hb)A$_{1C}$ greater than or equal to 6.5%, fasting blood glucose greater than or equal to 126 mg/dL, oral glucose tolerance test (OGTT) 2-hour glucose greater than or equal to 200 mg/dL, or a random glucose greater than or equal to 200 mg/dL in a patient with classic symptoms of hyperglycemia.[5] Special consideration is needed, however, to select appropriate testing to establish the etiology when atypical diabetes is suspected.

The objective of this article is to provide a brief overview of subtypes, mechanisms, diagnostic considerations, and management approaches in the various forms of atypical diabetes. **Fig. 1** provides an algorithm for considerations in testing for atypical forms of diabetes.

MONOGENIC DIABETES

Monogenic diabetes, including maturity-onset diabetes of the young (MODY) and neonatal DM (NDM), refers to diabetes caused by a single gene mutation.

Neonatal Diabetes Mellitus

NDM, a rare disorder, with incidence of 1 in 90,000 to 1 in 400,000,[6,7] is characterized by onset of persistent hyperglycemia within the first 6 months to 12 months of life.[8] NDM arises from a single-gene mutation that affects pancreatic β-cell development and function.[9] Approximately 25% of cases are transient and resolve by ages 6 months to 18 months, whereas 75% are permanent.[9]

Transient neonatal diabetes mellitus

A majority of transient NDM (TNDM) cases are due to an activating heterozygous mutation in a gene encoding a subunit of the pancreatic β-cell K$_{ATP}$ channel (KCNJ11 and ABCC8) or linked to genetic or epigenetic changes at chromosome 6q24. In 6q24

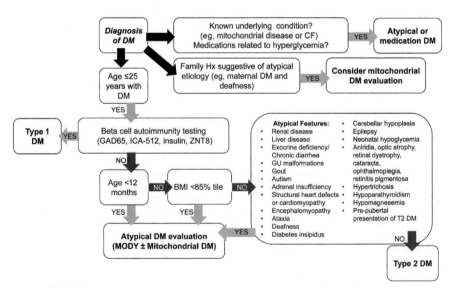

Fig. 1. Diagnostic algorithm for atypical diabetes. GU, genitourinary; Hx, History.

TNDM, hyperglycemia often is followed by a hypoglycemic phase with hyperglycemia re-presenting in adulthood in approximately 50% of individuals.[10]

Permanent neonatal diabetes mellitus

More than 20 mutations, both dominant and recessive, have been reported to cause permanent NDM (PNDM) by altering β-cell function, causing β-cell destruction, or disrupting normal pancreatic development. These mutations result in decreased insulin production and/or secretion and may have associated syndromic comorbidities (**Table 1**). Dominant mutations in KCNJ11 and ABCC8 account for approximately 50% of PNDM cases. Although mutations involving the K_{ATP} channel subunits most commonly present with congenital hyperinsulinism or PNDM, mutations in *ABCC8* and *KCNJ11* also can present with diabetes later in life.

Diagnostic considerations

Patients with NDM may have a history of intrauterine growth restriction or low birth weight due to insulin deficiency in utero.[11] Similar to children with other forms of diabetes, infants often present with polyuria and poor weight gain. Affected infants are at high risk of diabetic ketoacidosis (DKA) at diagnosis, but symptoms (polyuria, tachypnea, irritability, lethargy, and hypovolemia) often are nonspecific and difficult to recognize.[12] Infants with PNMD due to pancreatic aplasia or hypoplasia may present with malabsorptive diarrhea due to pancreatic exocrine insufficiency.[13]

Diagnostic work-up of the neonate with hyperglycemia should include evaluation for alternative etiologies, including sepsis, high glucose infusion rate in parenteral nutrition, or medications (eg, corticosteroids and β-adrenergic agonists). Insulin secretory capacity should be evaluated through measurement of C peptide and insulin, and ketoacidosis should be assessed. HbA_{1C} greater than 6.5% is consistent with a diagnosis of DM, but normal HbA_{1C} in this population is not reassuring and reflects high percent of fetal hemoglobin. Islet cell autoantibodies (insulin, IA-2, GAD65, and Znt8) should be measured to exclude T1D in patients age greater than 6 months. Abdominal ultrasound can assess for pancreatic agenesis, and fecal elastase can evaluate for pancreatic exocrine deficiency.

Genetic diagnosis may focus treatment options, enable counseling regarding associated manifestations, and provide insight regarding the likelihood of permanency. Clinically significant hyperglycemia requires treatment with insulin. Given that a majority of NDM mutations (KCNJ11 and ABCC8) respond to sulfonylureas, however, empiric trial of sulfonylurea therapy under the direction of a pediatric endocrinologist while awaiting genetic testing may be considered.[14]

Maturity-Onset Diabetes of the Young

MODY includes forms of DM that are caused by a single-gene mutation presenting after infancy. Many, but not all, genes linked to MODY also are associated with NDM. Significant variability in the presentation and treatment exists (see **Table 3**). **Fig. 1** provides an algorithm for specific features that may prompt MODY evaluation. **Fig. 2** provides a schematic of the mechanisms of monogenic diabetes.

Diagnostic considerations and mechanisms

The most common genes affected in MODY are *GCK*, *HNF4A*, and *HNF1A*. Each displays unique clinical features.[15] MODY 2 arises from dominant mutations in *GCK*, which increase the glucose threshold required for pancreatic β-cell insulin release. Patients with *GCK* mutations present with mild fasting hyperglycemia that typically does not progress with age, benefit from medical therapy, or result in end organ damage.[15]

Table 1
Overview of causes of monogenic diabetes

MODY Type/Syndrome	Gene	Protein Encoded by Gene	Percent Neonatal Diabetes Mellitus, Nonconsanguineous (%)[9]	Associated Manifestations	Specific Treatments (If Applicable)
Altered β-cell function[a]					
Neonatal Diabetes					
MODY 12	*ABCC8*[16]	K_{ATP} outer subunit SUR1	17%	Developmental delay, epilepsy[9]	Sulfonylureas
DEND MODY 13	*KCNJ11*[17]	K_{ATP} inner subunit Kir6.2	28.9%	Developmental delay and epilepsy (only in severe cases)	Sulfonylureas ± insulin
MODY 10	*INS*[18]	Preproinsulin	10.8%	Typically cause NDM but can lead to DM in older children/adults[18]	Insulin
Fanconi-Bickel syndrome	*SCL2A2 (GLUT2)*	—	0.3%	Hepatic dysfunction Hypergalactosemia Hypoglycemia	—
Rogers syndrome	*SLC19A2*[19]	—	0.3%	Megaloblastic anemia Sensorineural hearing loss	Thiamine
β-cell destruction[b,c]					
Wolcott-Rallison syndrome	*EIFAK3*[22]	Translation initiation factor 2-alpha kinase 3	2.5% (24.3% consanguineous)	Hepatic dysfunction Skeletal dysplasia	Insulin
IPEX	*FOXP3*[23]	Transcription factor	1.4%	Immune dysregulation Polyendocrinopathy Enteropathy	Insulin

	MODY		Percent of all MODY[35]		
MODY 1	HNF4A	Transcription factor	5%[36]	Diazoxide responsive hyperinsulinism / Renal Fanconi syndrome / Liver dysfunction[37]	Sulfonylurea[15]
MODY 2	GCK	Glucokinase	20–50%[36]		None[15]
MODY 3	HNF1A	Transcription factor	20–50%[36]	Diazoxide responsive hyperinsulinism[37]	Sulfonylureas[15]
MODY 4	PDX1	Transcription factor	1%	Pancreatic agenesis (NDM) / Pancreatic exocrine deficiency[38]	Insulin
MODY 5	HNF1B	Transcription factor	<1%	Renal disease (cysts) / Abnormal liver function / Hyperuricemia and gout / Pancreatic exocrine deficiency / Autism spectrum disorder / Genital tract anomalies / Hypomagnesemia[39,40] / Hyperparathyroidism	Insulin
MODY 6	NEUROD1	Transcription factor	<1%	Cerebellar hypoplasia / Vision deficits / Sensorineural hearing loss / Learning difficulties[32]	Insulin
MODY 7	KLF11[41]	Transcription factor	<1%	Present very similarly to "typical" T2D[42]	—
MODY 8	Carboxyl ester lipase		<1%	Defect in bile salt–dependent responsive lipase / Pancreatic exocrine deficiency[43]	—
MODY 9	PAX4	Transcription factor	<1%	Ketosis-prone DM[44] / Identified in groups of patients from West Africa	—
MODY 11	BLK[45]	Tyrosine kinase	<1%	—	—

(continued on next page)

Table 1
(continued)

	MODY		Percent of all MODY[35]		
MODY 14	APPL1	Involved in insulin signaling[46]	<1%	—	Insulin
Pigmented hypertrichotic dermatosis with insulin-dependent DM	SLC29A3[42]	Nucleoside transport hENT3p		Pigmented hypertrichosis Cardiomyopathy Severe chronic inflammation[47]	Insulin

[a] Other mutations leading to altered β-cell function: GCK[20], RFX6[21].

[b] Other mutations leading to β-cell destruction: INS, IER3IPI[24].

[c] Mutations leading to abnormalities in pancreatic development include: PDX1/IPF1,[25] PTF1A (associated with cerebellar agenesis),[26] HNF1B,[27] RFX6,[21] GATA4,[28] GATA6,[29] GLIS3 (associated with hypothyroidism),[30] NEUROD1,[31] NEUROG3,[31] PAX6 (associated with eye anomalies),[33] NKX2-2,[34] MNX1[34]

Abbreviations: DEND, Developmental delay, epilepsy, and neonatal diabetes syndrome; IPEX, Immune dysregulation, polyendocrinopathy, enteropathy, X-linked syndrome.

Data from Refs.[9,15–47]

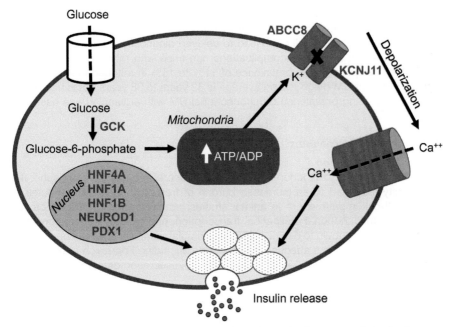

Fig. 2. Mechanisms of monogenic diabetes. In this schematic of a pancreatic β cell, the genes known to cause monogenic diabetes are shown in red. Some mitochondrial disorders also are known to cause diabetes, as reviewed in mitochondrial diabetes section.

Insulin Resistance Syndromes

In contrast to the more common insulin production counterparts, mutations in *INSR* cause Donohue syndrome (severe, neonatal insulin resistance) and Rabson-Mendenhall syndrome (severe insulin resistance that presents in childhood).[48] Lipodystrophies are congenital or acquired conditions that cause severe insulin resistance in the setting of a paucity of subcutaneous fat. They can be generalized or partial (on the basis of extent of deficits) and are associated with multiorgan system involvement.[49] Diagnosis relies on physical examination, including careful survey of subcutaneous adipose depots throughout the body. Individuals with generalized lipodystrophy can receive treatment with recombinant leptin therapy, which reduces the large insulin doses (3–5 times higher than typical total daily insulin dose requirements) required to obtain normoglycemia in these patients.[50] Recombinant leptin also mitigates comorbidities, including fatty liver disease and hypertriglyceridemia.[50]

Treatment

Many treatment considerations for atypical DM are similar to those in typical forms of DM. Management is reviewed in **Table 3**.

MITOCHONDRIAL DIABETES MELLITUS
Background

Mitochondrial diseases are estimated to affect 1 in 5000 individuals and are caused by genetic defects that occur in either the mitochondrial DNA (mtDNA) (de novo or maternal inheritance) or the nuclear DNA (most commonly autosomal recessive) that encode protein constituents of mitochondria or proteins responsible for mitochondrial maintenance.[51] The heterogeneity, variable expressivity, age independence, and multiorgan system involvement all often lead to delayed diagnoses.

Multiple potential endocrine complications can arise with mitochondrial disease. Foremost is DM, which has a prevalence of 11% to 15% in mitochondrial disorders (**Table 2**).[52] Age of DM diagnosis on average is 32 years to 38 years but is highly variable, and increasing prevalence of mitochondrial DM with advancing age has been reported.[52,53]

Brief Overview of Mechanisms

Impaired insulin secretion

In the setting of primary mitochondrial impairment, decreased oxidative phosphorylation capacity may lead to an increased burden of free radicals that contributes to pancreatic β-cell impairment.[54] In animal studies, administration of streptozotocin, which inhibits mitochondrial replication, transcription, and oxidative phosphorylation capacity, has been shown to diminish glucose-stimulated insulin release from islets.[55] In some genetic disorders affecting mitochondria, including Friedreich ataxia (FA),[56] decreased β-cell mass also may contribute to insulin secretion defects.

Insulin resistance

Some studies of mitochondrial DM have demonstrated skeletal muscle insulin resistance even when β-cell function is not yet impaired.[57] The detailed pathophysiology of muscle insulin resistance in mitochondrial disorders is the focus of ongoing investigation. Increased oxidative stress may be one cause of tissue-specific insulin resistance in the setting of decreased mitochondrial oxidative phosphorylation capacity.[54,58] Importantly, in some settings, increased mitochondrial respiration can be protective against diabetes. An animal model of *ANT1* deficiency, a disorder affecting adenosine triphosphate transport, illustrates this phenomenon.[59]

Additional mechanistic considerations, including the role of mitochondria in the development of typical forms of DM[60] and the role of hyperglycemia in mitochondrial dysfunction,[61] are beyond the scope of this overview.

Diagnosis

General and subtype specific expert consensus guidelines regarding screening for mitochondrial DM exist. General guidelines published by Newcastle University in the United Kingdom recommend screening with HbA$_{1C}$ at diagnosis of mitochondrial disease and annually thereafter. Additionally, random glucose and HbA$_{1C}$ should be obtained if patients endorse new or worsening polyuria or polydipsia; an OGTT is recommended for individuals with HbA$_{1C}$ between 6.0% and 6.5%.[95] Some mitochondrial disorders have disease-specific recommendations. For example, FA clinical management guidelines note that HbA$_{1C}$ alone may be an inadequate screening/diagnostic test for FA-related DM and recommend fasting blood glucose measurement annually.[96] Regardless of specific disease, all patients and families should be counseled about DM risk and symptoms that should prompt contacting the care team.

DM can be the presenting feature in mitochondrial diseases. Individuals with Wolfram syndrome (WS) can present first with nonautoimmune, insulin-deficient DM (average age 6 years) and subsequently are diagnosed with WS when optic atrophy manifests.[77] Similarly, in individuals with maternally inherited diabetes and deafness (MIDD), although hearing loss often precedes DM, DM can be the first presenting feature. Approximately 1% of individuals with MIDD initially were misclassified as having T1D or T2D.[97] DM as the first presenting feature of mitochondrial disease has been

Table 2
Overview of diabetes in mitochondrial disorders

Typical Underlying Genetic Mutation(s)	Mitochondrial Disease Clinical Syndrome	Percentage with Diabetes Mellitus (%)	Frequently Encountered Nonendocrine Manifestations	Other Associated Endocrinopathies: In Many of Them, High Prevalence of Risk Factors for Poor Bone Health[62]
mtDNA deletion syndromes				
mtDNA deletion syndrome	Pearson syndrome[63]	Neonatal and/or infantile DM may occur	Macrocytic anemia, neutropenia, thrombocytopenia Renal tubular defects Liver disease Exocrine pancreatic insufficiency	Adrenal insufficiency
mtDNA deletion syndrome	Kearns-Sayre Syndrome (KSS)[64-66]	11–14	Retinitis pigmentosa Progressive external ophthalmoplegia Cardiac conduction abnormalities Cerebellar ataxia Muscle weakness Sensorineural hearing loss Renal tubular acidosis	Short stature (38%) Gonadal dysfunction (20%) Hypoparathyroidism Growth hormone deficiency Hypothyroidism Adrenal insufficiency Hyperaldosteronism Hypomagnesaemia Bone abnormalities
mtDNA sequencing mutations				
MT-TL1 m.3243A>G	Mitochondrial Encephalopathy, Lactic acidosis, and stroke-like episodes (MELAS)[67]	38	Epilepsy, dementia, headaches, ataxia, cognitive deficits Lactic acidosis Stroke-like episodes Cardiomyopathy/cardiac conduction defects Myopathy, neuropathy Pigmentary Retinopathy/optic atrophy	Hypothyroidism (12%) Atypical growth and sexual maturation Dyslipidemia[52]

(continued on next page)

Table 2
(continued)

Typical Underlying Genetic Mutations(s)	Mitochondrial Disease Clinical Syndrome	Percentage with Diabetes Mellitus (%)	Frequently Encountered Nonendocrine Manifestations	Other Associated Endocrinopathies: In Many of Them, High Prevalence of Risk Factors for Poor Bone Health[62]
MT-TL1 m.3243A>G	Maternally Inherited Diabetes and Deafness (MIDD)[67]	38; nearly 100 have IGT by age 70 y[68]	Sensorineural hearing loss Macular retinal dystrophy Myopathy Ptosis Cardiac and renal disease Spectrum of MELAS	Short stature Growth hormone deficiency
MT-TK m.8344A>G (this mutation may cause Leigh syndrome)	Myoclonic epilepsy with ragged red fibers[69]	11	Myoclonus, muscle weakness, ataxia, seizures Sensorineural hearing loss Optic atrophy, ptosis, progressive external ophthalmoplegia Cognitive impairment Cardiomyopathy Recurrent lipomas	Hypothyroidism (2/34 in 1 case series) Hypogonadism (1/34)[69]
MT-TS2 m.12258C>A	MT-TS2–related mitochondrial disease	Approaches 100[70]	Retinitis pigmentosa Sensorineural hearing loss[71]	None reported to date
MT-TE m.14709T>C.[72]	Myoclonic epilepsy with ragged red fibers, MIDD	~60 12/20 reported (and 1 gestational DM)[73]	Congenital encephalomyopathy Retinitis pigmentosa Cardiomyopathy Juvenile or adult-onset myopathy[74]	None reported to date
Nuclear DNA disorders				
WFS1 (primary lesion in endoplasmic reticulum)[75] (AR or AD) CISD2 (WFS2) (AR)[76]	WS: historically considered a mitochondrial disorder[77]	100[78]	Optic nerve atrophy Sensorineural hearing loss (65%) Neurologic disabilities (60%) Urinary tract problems	Diabetes insipidus (70%) Hypogonadism

Gene	Associated disorder	Prevalence of DM	Clinical features	Other manifestations
GAA triplet repeat in frataxin (FXN)[79]	Friedreich's Ataxia (FA)	8-40[56]	Ataxia Cardiomyopathy Visual loss Hearing concerns Cognition spared	Short stature
Polymerase gamma (POLG)[80]	POLG-related mitochondrial disease spectrum (Alpers syndrome, childhood myocerebrohepatopathy spectrum, myoclonic epilepsy myopathy sensory ataxia, sensory ataxic neuropathy with dysarthria and ophthalmoparesis, ataxia neuropathy spectrum, and chronic progressive external ophthalmoplegia)	Case reports of DM, prevalence unknown	Ataxia, seizures, neuropathy Leukodystrophy Optic atrophy, CPEO Cardiac arrhythmias/cardiomyopathy Liver failure, gastrointestinal dysmotility Gastrointestinal dysmotility Myopathy	Adrenal insufficiency Hypothyroidism[81] Hypogonadism[82]
RRM2B	RRM2B-related mtDNA maintenance disorder (rarely can cause childhood KSS and mitochondrial neurogastrointestinal encephalomyopathy)	Case reports of DM, prevalence unknown	Adult-onset ophthalmoparesis Myopathy Neurologic complications Sensorineural hearing loss Renal tubulopathy Gastrointestinal disturbance[83]	Hypothyroidism Hypoparathyroidism Hypogonadism Short stature[83]
MPV17[53,84]	MPV17-related mtDNA maintenance disorder	Case reports of DM, prevalence unknown	Neurohepatopathy Failure to thrive Lactic acidosis Gastrointestinal dysmotility[84]	Hypoglycemia Hypoparathyroidism[85]
TYMP[86]	Mitochondrial neurogastrointestinal encephalomyopathy	~44/102[86]	Leukoencephalopathy Neuropathy Sensorineural hearing loss Weight loss Gastroparesis pseudo-obstruction	Dyslipidemia

(continued on next page)

Table 2
(continued)

Typical Underlying Genetic Mutation(s)	Mitochondrial Disease Clinical Syndrome	Percentage with Diabetes Mellitus (%)	Frequently Encountered Nonendocrine Manifestations	Other Associated Endocrinopathies: In Many of Them, High Prevalence of Risk Factors for Poor Bone Health[62]
ELAC2[87]	Combined oxidative phosphorylation deficiency type 17	Case reports of DM, prevalence unknown	Cognitive deficiencies; Failure to thrive; Hypertrophic cardiomyopathy; Myopathy; Typically, infantile onset	None reported
GFM2[88]	Leigh syndrome; combined oxidative phosphorylation deficiency type 39	Case reports of DM, prevalence unknown	Microcephaly; Axial hypotonia, peripheral hypertonia; Developmental delays/regression; Brain magnetic resonance imaging abnormalities; Seizures; Contractures; Arthrogryposis multiplex congenita	Hypoglycemia
TRIT1[89]	Combined oxidative phosphorylation deficiency 35	Case reports of DM, prevalence unknown	Microcephaly; Abnormal brain magnetic resonance imaging; Myoclonic epilepsy; Developmental delay; Optic disc hypoplasia; Cardiac septal defects	None reported

Additional mitochondrial mutations that cannot yet be clearly linked to diabetes

MT-TK m.8296A>G[90]	Found in 0.9% of 1000 patients with DM but may be a benign polymorphism[91]
MT-ND6 m.14577T>C[92]	Found in 3/253 patients with DM but also has a high frequency in the general population.
OPA1[93]	Diabetes reported but not at rates greater than in typical DM.
RNASEH1	Genetic changes associated with concurrent mitochondrial disorder and autoimmune diabetes.
HNF1B	Reviewed in the MODY section of this article but may be related to mitochondrial dysfunction.[94]

reported even in mitochondrial disorders whose initial manifestation typically is neurologic, such as FA.[98]

Diabetes presentation, although often insidious, can be variable within and across the various mitochondrial disorders. Percentages of individuals with impaired glucose tolerance (IGT) vary among mitochondrial disorders (for example, at least 49% in FA and approaching 100% in MIDD by age 70 years).[56,68] Although not typical, DKA has been reported in FA,[99] mitochondrial encephalopathy, lactic acidosis, and stroke-like episodes (MELAS)[100]; Kearns-Sayre syndrome (KSS)[101]; and WS[102] and hyperosmolar hyperglycemia has been documented in KSS.[64] One of these reports is of a child who died from DKA after oral corticosteroids, which can precipitate or worsen hyperglycemia.[103] Collaborating clinicians should be alert to DM risk and potential need for blood glucose monitoring when prescribing medications associated with hyperglycemia. Mitochondrial-related myopathy also may increase the risk of DKA-related respiratory failure.[104]

Fig. 1 reviews when to consider mitochondrial DM evaluation.

Management

Established clinical guidelines for management of T1D and T2D should be the starting place for management decisions in atypical DM. Some glucose-lowering medications, however, carry risks related to kidney disease and/or heart failure,[105] comorbidities that are common in mitochondrial disorders. Additionally, risks for lactic acidosis, arrhythmias, pancreatitis, and ketoacidosis are important to consider.

The UK Newcastle guidelines emphasize that if ketones are present and/or C peptide is low, then insulin is the starting treatment of choice.[95] The authors recommend measuring serum β-hydroxybutyrate instead of urine acetoacetate in patients with mitochondrial diabetes at risk for ketoacidosis. In individuals with mitochondrial disorders, the accumulation of NADH relative to NAD^+ in the setting of mitochondrial respiratory chain impairment shifts the ratio of acetoacetate to β-hydroxybutyrate in favor of β-hydroxybutyrate.[106,107] Therefore, urinary acetoacetate measurements could falsely underestimate the degree of ketosis in individuals with mitochondrial diabetes.[108]

Case series of mitochondrial DM discuss the requirement for insulin but often do not mention whether other antidiabetic treatments were considered.[66,77] Oral antidiabetic agents have not been tested rigorously in this patient population. At the time of this publication, only insulin, metformin, and liraglutide are approved in populations aged less than 18 years. Ultimately, appropriate medical therapy requires individualized risks and benefits assessment (**Table 3**).

Lifestyle measures are important in management of mitochondrial DM but may be difficult to enact.[109] Current guidance recommends individualizing nutritional interventions and encouraging physical activity in typical DM. Extending these recommendations to individuals with mitochondrial DM appears reasonable, but evidence surrounding their efficacy is limited.[110] Improving nutrition and physical activity also may be more difficult due to gastrointestinal manifestations,[111] nonambulatory status, decreased bone strength,[62] cardiomyopathy,[112] and intellectual disability.[113]

CYSTIC FIBROSIS–RELATED DIABETES
Background

Cystic fibrosis (CF) is an autosomal recessive disorder caused by mutations in the CFTR gene on chromosome 7, resulting in a defective or absent CFTR ion channel, increased airway fluid viscosity, and impaired mucociliary clearance. CFTR

Table 3
Overview of antidiabetic medications in mitochondrial diseases and monogenic diabetes

Treatment	Examples[105,114]	Possible Benefits	Risks to Consider in Mitochondrial Diabetes and Monogenic Diabetes

Insulin		Necessary for use in those with minimal insulin secretion[95]	• Hypoglycemia
			  ○ Risk factors for hypoglycemia (deficits in gluconeogenesis, growth deficiency, and adrenal insufficiency).[63,115]
			  ○ Decreases seizure threshold in those with seizures[116]
			• Dose adjustments needed in chronic kidney disease[117]
			• Weight gain[118]
			• Special considerations due to impairment in dexterity or vision (insulin injection aids or pens recommended)[119]
			• Possible increased risk for insulin edema[120]

Biguanides	Metformin	Frequently used and long-term data in other populations	• Gastrointestinal side effects
			• Risk of lactic acidosis
			  ○ Reports of use in MIDD and FA
			  ○ Risk of lactic acidosis is a concern (although no reported cases in MIDD)[67,68,79,95]
			• Risk of vitamin B_{12} deficiency/neuropathy[121]
			• Inhibits complex I
			  ○ Not clear if this affects use in mitochondrial DM[122]
			• Discontinue in chronic kidney disease stages 3b–5[123]

Sulfonylureas	Glipizide
	Glyburide
	Glimepiride
	Chlorpropamide
	Tolbutamide
		Frequently used and long-term data in other populations
		Prior to the development of other agents, has historically been a first option[95]
		Depolarizes β-cell membrane to stimulate insulin secretion (KCNJ11 and ABCC8 mutations)[14]
			• Hypoglycemia (start on low dose using medicine with short half-life)[53]
			• Discontinue in chronic kidney disease stages 4–5[123]
			• MODY: may require higher doses
			  ○ One algorithm: initial twice-daily dose of 0.1 mg/kg of glyburide with escalation up to 1 mg/kg/d within 5–6 d[14]
			  ○ HNF1A and HNF4A may respond to sulfonylurea at lower doses

Thiazolidinediones	Pioglitazone Rosiglitazone	Possibly improved mitochondrial function[124] Can be used in chronic kidney disease[123]	• Caution in cardiomyopathy/heart failure[125] • Increased risk for bone fractures[126]
GLP-1 agonists	Liraglutide Exenatide Semaglutide Lixisenatide Dulaglutide	Possibly improved mitochondrial function[56] Antidiabetic and possibly improved neuroinflammation (WS)[127] Possibly cardioprotective[128]	• Gastrointestinal side effects • Weight loss (could be benefit or risk) • Risk of acute pancreatitis[129] • Risk of tachycardia[130] • Discontinue in chronic kidney disease stages 4–5[123] • Increased risk of medullary thyroid cancer in at risk individuals
Dipeptidyl-peptidase IV inhibitors	Sitagliptin Saxagliptin Alogliptin Linagliptin	Possibly improved mitochondrial function[131] Linagliptin can be used in chronic kidney disease[123]	• Unclear effect on hospitalizations for heart failure (mixed data)[132] • Risk of acute pancreatitis[133] • Risk of arthralgias[134]

(continued on next page)

Table 3
(continued)

Treatment	Examples[105,114]	Possible Benefits	Risks to Consider in Mitochondrial Diabetes and Monogenic Diabetes

Sodium-glucose cotransport 2 inhibitors	Dapagliflozin Empagliflozin Canagliflozin Ertugliflozin	Benefit in heart failure[135]	• Possible risk of genitourinary infections[136]
			 • Possible risk of urinary tract infections[136]
			 • Euglycemic DKA
			   ○ Consider monitoring β-hydroxybutyrate (illness, poor intake, alcohol consumption, or decreased insulin doses)[137]
			   ○ Measure serum β-hydroxybutyrate because urinalysis may not be as accurate.[106-108]
			 • Discontinue in chronic kidney disease stages 3b-5.[123]

Data from Refs. [14,53,56,63,67,68,79,95,106–108,115–137]

expression in the lung, intestine, and pancreas, among other tissues, explains the wide breadth of disease manifestations. The name *cystic fibrosis*, originated in the 1930s as a description of the fibrotic and cystic pancreas. For many years, therapies targeted mucus viscosity and infections, but the first successful modulator therapy aimed at correcting the CFTR defect has revolutionized advances in the disease.[138] With median age of survival approaching 50 years,[139] later manifestations of the disease are more relevant. CF-related diabetes (CFRD) affects 20% of adolescents and up to 50% of adults aged greater than 30 years[140] and is associated with worse pulmonary function, poorer nutritional status, and overall greater mortality.[141–144]

Brief Overview of Mechanisms

While initially considered solely a product of collateral damage from the fibrotic and inflamed exocrine pancreas, CFRD now is understood to be multifactorial. β-cell defects—including dysfunction and total islet loss,[145,146] impairment in incretin signaling,[147,148] possible α-cell defects,[149] and T2D risk variants[150]—all play important roles in disease development. Whether CFTR is expressed in β cells to contribute directly to insulin secretion defects remains a topic of debate.[145,151,152] Although this disease is wrought with inflammation/infection and corticosteroid exposure, the resulting insulin resistance is observed primarily in times of illness and is not considered a principal mechanism for CFRD.

The earliest clinical presentation of CF-related glucose abnormalities arises from loss of β-cell secretory capacity as manifested by declines in early-phase insulin secretion in response to meals and oral glucose load[153] and elevated plasma glucose at 1 hour (**Fig. 3**). Progressive insulin secretory defects lead to worsening hyperglycemia with fasting hyperglycemia as a late manifestation. Both pulmonary function and nutritional status decline in the years prior to CFRD onset and are associated with subtle glucose abnormalities defined as continuous glucose monitoring (CGM) time above glucose range.[154–156] These findings suggest CF-related glucose abnormalities occur on a clinically relevant continuum prior to CFRD diagnosis.

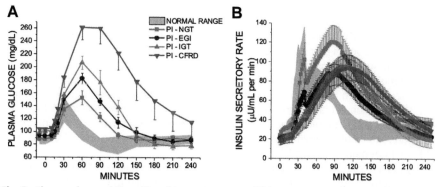

Fig. 3. Plasma glucose (*A*) and insulin secretory rates (*B*) in response to the mixed-meal tolerance test in subjects with pancreatic insufficient (PI) CF. Individuals were categorized based on a preceding OGTT (EGI, early glucose intolerance [plasma glucose at 1 hour greater than or equal to 155 mg/dL and plasma glucose at 2 hours less than or equal to 140 mg/dL]; NGT, normal glucose tolerance). Significant decline in β-cell secretory capacity is evident in PI-EGI. (*From* Nyirjesy SC, Sheikh S, Hadjiliadis D, et al. β-Cell secretory defects are present in pancreatic insufficient cystic fibrosis with 1-hour oral glucose tolerance test glucose ≥155 mg/dL. Pediatr Diabetes. 2018;19(7):1173-1182; with permission.)

The impact of the newest modulator therapies currently is unknown. Promising improvements in insulin secretion in response to ivacaftor give hope that the landscape of CFRD may be changing.[148]

Diagnosis

The Cystic Fibrosis Foundation recommends annual CFRD screening using an OGTT (1.75 g/kg, maximum 75 g) by age 10 years.[144,146] OGTT 1 hour greater than 155 mg/dL has been associated impaired β-cell secretory capacity and inconsistently greater declines in pulmonary function.[153,157] CGM currently is not recommended as a screening or diagnostic tool, given the lack of management recommendations for early derangements.[158]

Other screening opportunities include blood glucose monitoring during the first 48 hours of acute illness/hospitalization and while on overnight enteral feedings. Stress-induced hyperglycemia lasting greater than 48 hours warrants CFRD diagnosis given associated worsened morbidity.[144] Blood glucose greater than 200 mg/dL during or after overnight feeds on 2 separate occurrences is diagnostic of CFRD.[159]

Although HbA$_{1C}$ greater than 6.5% remains diagnostic for CFRD and can be used for monitoring diabetes control; it is not recommended for screening purposes because it fails to capture early glucose abnormalities.[144,146,160] No thresholds for HbA$_{1C}$; fructosamine; 1,5-anhydroglucitol; and glycated albumin were sufficiently sensitive or specific to replace OGTT in identifying CFRD.[161]

Management Considerations

High caloric density and salt and fat consumption are recommended for people with CF, and a diagnosis of CFRD does not change these recommendations. Instead, patients should be instructed in carbohydrate counting and to modulate carbohydrate intake throughout the day.[162] This approach may be relevant particularly in individuals experiencing reactive hypoglycemia after large glycemic loads.[163] Patients on enteral feed supplementation should receive full caloric formula and not low-glycemic dietary supplements.[164] Finally, sensitivity to patients when providing recommendations for nutritional modification is important: adequate weight gain and increased caloric intake are emphasized from a young age in this population and changes to nutritional habits may be overwhelming.

The mainstay of diabetes medical management is subcutaneous insulin, which benefits glycemic control and boasts anabolic properties that can improve nutritional status.[165] The most common regimen in individuals without fasting hyperglycemia includes multiple daily injections with rapid-acting insulin to cover meals.[146,165] Insulin sensitivity tends to be normal (requiring <0.5–0.8 U/kg/d) across the age continuum.[166] Basal insulin is required for individuals with fasting hyperglycemia but also sometimes is administered in the absence of fasting hyperglycemia.[146,165] Continuous subcutaneous insulin administration via an insulin pump for more individualized diabetes management also can be considered.

Early insulin treatment and other medical therapies have been studied in CF. Repaglinide treatment results in similar glycemic control to insulin but without body mass index (BMI) improvement, limiting its widespread application in this population.[140] Currently, the efficacy of glucagon-like peptide-1 (GLP-1) agonists in treating early incretin abnormalities is being evaluated, but potential concerns in CF include gastrointestinal symptoms and weight loss.[164]

Hypoglycemia, in the absence of diabetes and insulin therapy, has been noted after long periods of fasting as well as postprandially.[167] Long-term implications of hypoglycemia remain unclear, with some studies demonstrating early glucose derangements and impaired early-phase insulin secretion concerning for β-cell function decline[163] but others suggesting that these individuals do not progress more rapidly to CFRD.[168]

Microvascular complications are restricted to individuals with fasting hyperglycemia, and patients should be screened for retinopathy, microalbuminuria, and neuropathy starting 5 years after a diagnosis of CFRD.[146] Macrovascular complications have not been appreciated in CF. The contribution of decreased life expectancy and absence of other metabolic derangements, such as dyslipidemia, hypertension, and obesity, to the cardioprotection is unknown but requires further study in the changing landscape of CF.[169,170]

Cystic Fibrosis–Related Diabetes Conclusions

CFRD is viewed as a spectrum of abnormal glucose tolerance with early abnormalities seen in early-phase insulin secretion followed by progressive β-cell decline. The etiology of CFRD development is multifactorial. Early diagnosis and treatment are crucial given implications for morbidity and mortality. At present, insulin therapy is paramount but investigations are geared at further understanding pathogenesis to suggest less burdensome treatment strategies.

SUMMARY

Providers should be suspicious for atypical DM, particularly in youth with a known condition that confers risk and in youth who lack both islet autoantibodies and classic signs of T2D. Strong family history of DM and conditions associated with atypical DM also are features that may prompt additional testing. Although some forms of atypical DM have clear treatment recommendations, many require an empiric evaluation of the patient's presentation, associated conditions, and individualized risks in order to determine the best treatment. More studies are needed in the area of identification of subtypes, screening for detection, and treatment of atypical forms of DM.

ACKNOWLEDGMENTS

The authors would like to thank James Peterson, MS, LCGC.

DISCLOSURE

The authors have nothing to disclose.

REFERENCES

1. Pacaud D, Schwandt A, de Beaufort C, et al. A description of clinician reported diagnosis of type 2 diabetes and other non-type 1 diabetes included in a large international multicentered pediatric diabetes registry (SWEET). Pediatr Diabetes 2016;17(Suppl 23):24–31.
2. Johansson BB, Irgens HU, Molnes J, et al. Targeted next-generation sequencing reveals MODY in up to 6.5% of antibody-negative diabetes cases listed in the Norwegian Childhood Diabetes Registry. Diabetologia 2017;60(4): 625–35.
3. Pihoker C, Gilliam LK, Ellard S, et al. Prevalence, characteristics and clinical diagnosis of maturity onset diabetes of the young due to mutations in HNF1A, HNF4A, and glucokinase: results from the SEARCH for Diabetes in Youth. J Clin Endocrinol Metab 2013;98(10):4055–62.
4. Kadowaki T, Kadowaki H, Mori Y, et al. A subtype of diabetes mellitus associated with a mutation of mitochondrial DNA. N Engl J Med 1994;330(14):962–8.

5. American Diabetes Association. 2. classification and diagnosis of diabetes: standards of medical care in diabetes-2020. Diabetes Care 2020;43(Suppl 1): S14–31.

6. Grulich-Henn J, Wagner V, Thon A, et al. Entities and frequency of neonatal diabetes: data from the diabetes documentation and quality management system (DPV). Diabet Med 2010;27(6):709–12.

7. Polak M, Cavé H. Neonatal diabetes mellitus: a disease linked to multiple mechanisms. Orphanet J Rare Dis 2007;2(1):12.

8. Lemelman MB, Letourneau L, Greeley SAW. Neonatal diabetes mellitus: an update on diagnosis and management. Clin Perinatol 2018;45(1):41–59.

9. De Franco E, Flanagan SE, Houghton JA, et al. The effect of early, comprehensive genomic testing on clinical care in neonatal diabetes: an international cohort study. Lancet 2015;386(9997):957–63.

10. Flanagan SE, Patch A-M, Mackay DJG, et al. Mutations in ATP-Sensitive K$^+$ Channel Genes Cause Transient Neonatal Diabetes and Permanent Diabetes in Childhood or Adulthood. Diabetes. 2007;56(7):1930–7.

11. Rubio-Cabezas O, Ellard S. Diabetes mellitus in neonates and infants: genetic heterogeneity, clinical approach to diagnosis, and therapeutic options. Horm Res Paediatr 2013;80(3):137–46.

12. Letourneau LR, Carmody D, Wroblewski K, et al. Diabetes presentation in infancy: high risk of diabetic ketoacidosis. Diabetes Care 2017;40(10):e147–8.

13. Winter WE, Maclaren NK, Riley WJ, et al. Congenital pancreatic hypoplasia: a syndrome of exocrine and endocrine pancreatic insufficiency. J Pediatr 1986; 109(3):465–8.

14. Carmody D, Bell CD, Hwang JL, et al. Sulfonylurea treatment before genetic testing in neonatal diabetes: pros and cons. J Clin Endocrinol Metab 2014; 99(12):E2709–14.

15. McDonald TJ, Ellard S. Maturity onset diabetes of the young: identification and diagnosis. Ann Clin Biochem 2013;50(Pt 5):403–15.

16. Babenko AP, Polak M, Cave H, et al. Activating mutations in the ABCC8 gene in neonatal diabetes mellitus. N Engl J Med 2006;355(5):456–66.

17. Gloyn AL, Cummings EA, Edghill EL, et al. Permanent neonatal diabetes due to paternal germline mosaicism for an activating mutation of the KCNJ11 Gene encoding the Kir6.2 subunit of the beta-cell potassium adenosine triphosphate channel. J Clin Endocrinol Metab 2004;89(8):3932–5.

18. Edghill EL, Flanagan SE, Patch AM, et al. Insulin mutation screening in 1,044 patients with diabetes: mutations in the INS gene are a common cause of neonatal diabetes but a rare cause of diabetes diagnosed in childhood or adulthood. Diabetes. 2008;57(4):1034–42.

19. Shaw-Smith C, Flanagan SE, Patch AM, et al. Recessive SLC19A2 mutations are a cause of neonatal diabetes mellitus in thiamine-responsive megaloblastic anaemia. Pediatr Diabetes 2012;13(4):314–21.

20. Njolstad PR, Sovik O, Cuesta-Munoz A, et al. Neonatal diabetes mellitus due to complete glucokinase deficiency. N Engl J Med 2001;344(21):1588–92.

21. Smith SB, Qu HQ, Taleb N, et al. Rfx6 directs islet formation and insulin production in mice and humans. Nature 2010;463(7282):775–80.

22. Senee V, Vattem KM, Delepine M, et al. Wolcott-Rallison Syndrome: clinical, genetic, and functional study of EIF2AK3 mutations and suggestion of genetic heterogeneity. Diabetes. 2004;53(7):1876–83.

23. Rubio-Cabezas O, Minton JAL, Caswell R, et al. Clinical heterogeneity in patients with FOXP3 mutations presenting with permanent neonatal diabetes. Diabetes Care 2009;32(1):111–6.

24. Shalev SA, Tenenbaum-Rakover Y, Horovitz Y, et al. Microcephaly, epilepsy, and neonatal diabetes due to compound heterozygous mutations in IER3IP1: insights into the natural history of a rare disorder. Pediatr Diabetes 2014;15(3): 252–6.

25. Stoffers DA, Zinkin NT, Stanojevic V, et al. Pancreatic agenesis attributable to a single nucleotide deletion in the human IPF1 gene coding sequence. Nat Genet 1997;15(1):106–10.

26. Sellick GS, Barker KT, Stolte-Dijkstra I, et al. Mutations in PTF1A cause pancreatic and cerebellar agenesis. Nat Genet 2004;36(12):1301–5.

27. Yorifuji T, Kurokawa K, Mamada M, et al. Neonatal diabetes mellitus and neonatal polycystic, dysplastic kidneys: Phenotypically discordant recurrence of a mutation in the hepatocyte nuclear factor-1beta gene due to germline mosaicism. J Clin Endocrinol Metab 2004;89(6):2905–8.

28. D'Amato E, Giacopelli F, Giannattasio A, et al. Genetic investigation in an Italian child with an unusual association of atrial septal defect, attributable to a new familial GATA4 gene mutation, and neonatal diabetes due to pancreatic agenesis. Diabet Med 2010;27(10):1195–200.

29. De Franco E, Shaw-Smith C, Flanagan SE, et al. GATA6 mutations cause a broad phenotypic spectrum of diabetes from pancreatic agenesis to adult-onset diabetes without exocrine insufficiency. Diabetes. 2013;62(3):993–7.

30. Senee V, Chelala C, Duchatelet S, et al. Mutations in GLIS3 are responsible for a rare syndrome with neonatal diabetes mellitus and congenital hypothyroidism. Nat Genet 2006;38(6):682–7.

31. Pinney SE, Oliver-Krasinski J, Ernst L, et al. Neonatal diabetes and congenital malabsorptive diarrhea attributable to a novel mutation in the human neurogenin-3 gene coding sequence. J Clin Endocrinol Metab 2011;96(7): 1960–5.

32. Rubio-Cabezas O, Minton JA, Kantor I, et al. Homozygous mutations in NEU-ROD1 are responsible for a novel syndrome of permanent neonatal diabetes and neurological abnormalities. Diabetes. 2010;59(9):2326–31.

33. Solomon BD, Pineda-Alvarez DE, Balog JZ, et al. Compound heterozygosity for mutations in PAX6 in a patient with complex brain anomaly, neonatal diabetes mellitus, and microophthalmia. Am J Med Genet A. 2009;149a(11):2543 6.

34. Flanagan SE, De Franco E, Lango Allen H, et al. Analysis of transcription factors key for mouse pancreatic development establishes NKX2-2 and MNX1 mutations as causes of neonatal diabetes in man. Cell Metab 2014;19(1):146–54.

35. Naylor R, Knight Johnson A, del Gaudio D. Maturity-onset diabetes of the young overview. In: Adam MP, Ardinger HH, Pagon RA, et al, editors. GeneReviews((R)). Seattle (WA): University of Washington, Seattle University of Washington, Seattle. GeneReviews is a registered trademark of the University of Washington, Seattle; 1993.

36. Ellard S, Bellanne-Chantelot C, Hattersley AT. Best practice guidelines for the molecular genetic diagnosis of maturity-onset diabetes of the young. Diabetologia 2008;51(4):546–53.

37. Tung JY, Boodhansingh K, Stanley CA, et al. Clinical heterogeneity of hyperinsulinism due to HNF1A and HNF4A mutations. Pediatr Diabetes 2018;19(5):910–6.

38. Caetano LA, Santana LS, Costa-Riquetto AD, et al. PDX1 -MODY and dorsal pancreatic agenesis: New phenotype of a rare disease. Clin Genet 2018; 93(2):382–6.

39. Heidet L, Decramer S, Pawtowski A, et al. Spectrum of HNF1B mutations in a large cohort of patients who harbor renal diseases. Clin J Am Soc Nephrol 2010;5(6):1079–90.

40. Clissold RL, Hamilton AJ, Hattersley AT, et al. HNF1B-associated renal and extra-renal disease-an expanding clinical spectrum. Nat Rev Nephrol 2015; 11(2):102–12.

41. Neve B, Fernandez-Zapico ME, Ashkenazi-Katalan V, et al. Role of transcription factor KLF11 and its diabetes-associated gene variants in pancreatic beta cell function. Proc Natl Acad Sci U S A 2005;102(13):4807–12.

42. Schwitzgebel VM. Many faces of monogenic diabetes. J Diabetes Investig 2014;5(2):121–33.

43. Johansson BB, Torsvik J, Bjorkhaug L, et al. Diabetes and pancreatic exocrine dysfunction due to mutations in the carboxyl ester lipase gene-maturity onset diabetes of the young (CEL-MODY): a protein misfolding disease. J Biol Chem 2011;286(40):34593–605.

44. Mauvais-Jarvis F, Smith SB, Le May C, et al. PAX4 gene variations predispose to ketosis-prone diabetes. Hum Mol Genet 2004;13(24):3151–9.

45. Borowiec M, Liew CW, Thompson R, et al. Mutations at the BLK locus linked to maturity onset diabetes of the young and beta-cell dysfunction. Proc Natl Acad Sci U S A 2009;106(34):14460–5.

46. Prudente S, Jungtrakoon P, Marucci A, et al. Loss-of-function mutations in APPL1 in familial diabetes mellitus. Am J Hum Genet 2015;97(1):177–85.

47. Senniappan S, Hughes M, Shah P, et al. Pigmentary hypertrichosis and non-autoimmune insulin-dependent diabetes mellitus (PHID) syndrome is associated with severe chronic inflammation and cardiomyopathy, and represents a new monogenic autoinflammatory syndrome. J Pediatr Endocrinol Metab 2013;26(9–10):877–82.

48. Ben Harouch S, Klar A, Falik Zaccai TC. INSR-related severe syndromic insulin resistance. In: Adam MP, Ardinger HH, Pagon RA, et al, editors. GeneReviews((R)). Seattle (WA): University of Washington, Seattle, University of Washington, Seattle. GeneReviews is a registered trademark of the University of Washington, Seattle; 1993.

49. Gonzaga-Jauregui C, Ge W, Staples J, et al. Clinical and molecular prevalence of lipodystrophy in an unascertained large clinical care cohort. Diabetes. 2020; 69(2):249–58.

50. Brown RJ, Meehan CA, Cochran E, et al. Effects of metreleptin in pediatric patients with lipodystrophy. J Clin Endocrinol Metab 2017;102(5):1511–9.

51. Chow J, Rahman J, Achermann JC, et al. Mitochondrial disease and endocrine dysfunction. Nat Rev Endocrinol 2016;13(2):92–104.

52. Al-Gadi IS, Haas RH, Falk MJ, et al. Endocrine disorders in primary mitochondrial disease. J Endocr Soc 2018;2(4):361–73.

53. Schaefer AM, Walker M, Turnbull DM, et al. Endocrine disorders in mitochondrial disease. Mol Cell Endocrinol 2013;379(1–2):2–11.

54. Karaa A, Goldstein A. The spectrum of clinical presentation, diagnosis, and management of mitochondrial forms of diabetes. Pediatr Diabetes 2015; 16(1):1–9.

55. Giroix MH, Rasschaert J, Bailbe D, et al. Impairment of glycerol phosphate shuttle in islets from rats with diabetes induced by neonatal streptozocin. Diabetes. 1991;40(2):227–32.

56. Cnop M, Igoillo-Esteve M, Rai M, et al. Central role and mechanisms of beta-cell dysfunction and death in friedreich ataxia-associated diabetes. Ann Neurol 2012;72(6):971–82.

57. Lindroos MM, Majamaa K, Tura A, et al. m.3243A>G mutation in mitochondrial DNA leads to decreased insulin sensitivity in skeletal muscle and to progressive beta-cell dysfunction. Diabetes. 2009;58(3):543–9.

58. Blake R, Trounce IA. Mitochondrial dysfunction and complications associated with diabetes. Biochim Biophys Acta 2014;1840(4):1404–12.

59. Morrow RM, Picard M, Derbeneva O, et al. Mitochondrial energy deficiency leads to hyperproliferation of skeletal muscle mitochondria and enhanced insulin sensitivity. Proc Natl Acad Sci U S A 2017;114(10):2705–10.

60. Lowell BB, Shulman GI. Mitochondrial dysfunction and type 2 diabetes. Science 2005;307(5708):384–7.

61. Cardoso S, Santos MS, Seica R, et al. Cortical and hippocampal mitochondria bioenergetics and oxidative status during hyperglycemia and/or insulin-induced hypoglycemia. Biochim Biophys Acta 2010;1802(11):942–51.

62. Gandhi SS, Muraresku C, McCormick EM, et al. Risk factors for poor bone health in primary mitochondrial disease. J Inherit Metab Dis 2017;40(5):673–83.

63. Williams TB, Daniels M, Puthenveetil G, et al. Pearson syndrome: unique endocrine manifestations including neonatal diabetes and adrenal insufficiency. Mol Genet Metab 2012;106(1):104–7.

64. Ho J, Pacaud D, Rakic M, et al. Diabetes in pediatric patients with Kearns-Sayre syndrome: clinical presentation of 2 cases and a review of pathophysiology. Can J Diabetes 2014;38(4):225–8.

65. Harvey JN, Barnett D. Endocrine dysfunction in Kearns-Sayre syndrome. Clin Endocrinol (Oxf) 1992;37(1):97–103.

66. Khambatta S, Nguyen DL, Beckman TJ, et al. Kearns-Sayre syndrome: a case series of 35 adults and children. Int J Gen Med 2014;7:325–32.

67. Murphy R, Turnbull DM, Walker M, et al. Clinical features, diagnosis and management of maternally inherited diabetes and deafness (MIDD) associated with the 3243A>G mitochondrial point mutation. Diabet Med 2008;25(4):383–99.

68. Maassen JA, Hart LMT, Van Essen E, et al. Mitochondrial diabetes: molecular mechanisms and clinical presentation. Diabetes 2004;53(Suppl 1):S103–9.

69. Mancuso M, Orsucci D, Angelini C, et al. Phenotypic heterogeneity of the 8344A>G mtDNA "MERRF" mutation. Neurology 2013;80(22):2049–54.

70. Whittaker RG, Schaefer AM, McFarland R, et al. Prevalence and progression of diabetes in mitochondrial disease. Diabetologia 2007;50(10):2085–9.

71. Mansergh FC, Millington-Ward S, Kennan A, et al. Retinitis pigmentosa and progressive sensorineural hearing loss caused by a C12258A mutation in the mitochondrial MTTS2 gene. Am J Hum Genet 1999;64(4):971–85.

72. Mezghani N, Mkaouar-Rebai E, Mnif M, et al. The heteroplasmic m.14709T>C mutation in the tRNA(Glu) gene in two Tunisian families with mitochondrial diabetes. J Diabet Complications 2010;24(4):270–7.

73. Ban R, Guo JH, Pu CQ, et al. A novel mutation of mitochondrial T14709C causes myoclonic epilepsy with ragged red fibers syndrome in a chinese patient. Chin Med J 2018;131(13):1569–74.

74. McFarland R, Schaefer AM, Gardner JL, et al. Familial myopathy: new insights into the T14709C mitochondrial tRNA mutation. Ann Neurol 2004;55(4):478–84.

75. Riggs AC, Bernal-Mizrachi E, Ohsugi M, et al. Mice conditionally lacking the Wolfram gene in pancreatic islet beta cells exhibit diabetes as a result of enhanced endoplasmic reticulum stress and apoptosis. Diabetologia 2005; 48(11):2313–21.

76. Chen YF, Kao CH, Chen YT, et al. Cisd2 deficiency drives premature aging and causes mitochondria-mediated defects in mice. Genes Dev 2009;23(10): 1183–94.

77. Urano F. Wolfram syndrome: diagnosis, management, and treatment. Curr Diab Rep 2016;16(1):6.

78. Chaussenot A, Bannwarth S, Rouzier C, et al. Neurologic features and genotype-phenotype correlation in Wolfram syndrome. Ann Neurol 2011;69(3): 501–8.

79. McCormick A, Farmer J, Perlman S, et al. Impact of diabetes in the Friedreich ataxia clinical outcome measures study. Ann Clin Transl Neurol 2017;4(9): 622–31.

80. Scuderi C, Borgione E, Castello F, et al. The in cis T251I and P587L POLG1 base changes: description of a new family and literature review. Neuromuscul Disord 2015;25(4):333–9.

81. Hopkins SE, Somoza A, Gilbert DL. Rare autosomal dominant POLG1 mutation in a family with metabolic strokes, posterior column spinal degeneration, and multi-endocrine disease. J Child Neurol 2010;25(6):752–6.

82. Rahman S, Copeland WC. POLG-related disorders and their neurological manifestations. Nat Rev Neurol 2019;15(1):40–52.

83. Pitceathly RD, Smith C, Fratter C, et al. Adults with RRM2B-related mitochondrial disease have distinct clinical and molecular characteristics. Brain 2012;135(Pt 11):3392–403.

84. Garone C, Rubio JC, Calvo SE, et al. MPV17 mutations causing adult-onset multisystemic disorder with multiple mitochondrial DNA deletions. Arch Neurol 2012;69(12):1648–51.

85. El-Hattab AW, Wang J, Dai H, et al. MPV17-related mitochondrial dna maintenance defect. In: Adam MP, Ardinger HH, Pagon RA, et al, editors. GeneReviews((R)). Seattle (WA): University of Washington, Seattle, University of Washington, Seattle. GeneReviews is a registered trademark of the University of Washington, Seattle; 1993.

86. Garone C, Tadesse S, Hirano M. Clinical and genetic spectrum of mitochondrial neurogastrointestinal encephalomyopathy. Brain 2011;134(Pt 11):3326–32.

87. Paucar M, Pajak A, Freyer C, et al. Chorea, psychosis, acanthocytosis, and prolonged survival associated with ELAC2 mutations. Neurology 2018;91(15): 710–2.

88. Glasgow RIC, Thompson K, Barbosa IA, et al. Novel GFM2 variants associated with early-onset neurological presentations of mitochondrial disease and impaired expression of OXPHOS subunits. Neurogenetics 2017;18(4):227–35.

89. Forde KM, Molloy B, Conroy J, et al. Expansion of the phenotype of biallelic variants in TRIT1. Eur J Med Genet 2020;63:103882.

90. Kameoka K, Isotani H, Tanaka K, et al. Novel mitochondrial DNA mutation in tRNA(Lys) (8296A->G) associated with diabetes. Biochem Biophys Res Commun 1998;245(2):523–7.

91. Ahadi AM, Sadeghizadeh M, Houshmand M, et al. An A8296G mutation in the MT-TK gene of a patient with epilepsy - a disease-causing mutation or rare polymorphism? Neurol Neurochir Pol 2008;42(3):263–6.

92. Tawata M, Hayashi JI, Isobe K, et al. A new mitochondrial DNA mutation at 14577 T/C is probably a major pathogenic mutation for maternally inherited type 2 diabetes. Diabetes. 2000;49(7):1269–72.
93. Yu-Wai-Man P, Griffiths PG, Gorman GS, et al. Multi-system neurological disease is common in patients with OPA1 mutations. Brain 2010;133(Pt 3):771–86.
94. Casemayou A, Fournel A, Bagattin A, et al. Hepatocyte nuclear factor-1beta controls mitochondrial respiration in renal tubular cells. J Am Soc Nephrol 2017;28(11):3205–17.
95. Newcastle Mitochondrial Disease Guidelines. 2013. Available at: https://mitochondrialdisease.nhs.uk/media/diabetic-guideline.pdf.
96. Consensus Clinical Management Guidelines for Friedreich's Ataxis. 2014. Available at: https://curefa.org/clinical-care-guidelines.
97. Majamaa K, Moilanen JS, Uimonen S, et al. Epidemiology of A3243G, the mutation for mitochondrial encephalomyopathy, lactic acidosis, and strokelike episodes: prevalence of the mutation in an adult population. Am J Hum Genet 1998;63(2):447–54.
98. Garg M, Kulkarni SD, Shah KN, et al. Diabetes mellitus as the presenting feature of friedreich's ataxia. J Neurosci Rural Pract 2017;8(Suppl 1):S117–9.
99. Pappa A, Hausler MG, Veigel A, et al. Diabetes mellitus in Friedreich Ataxia: A case series of 19 patients from the German-Austrian diabetes mellitus registry. Diabetes Res Clin Pract 2018;141:229–36.
100. Strachan J, McLellan A, Kirkpatrick M, et al. Ketoacidosis: an unusual presentation of MELAS. J Inherit Metab Dis 2001;24(3):409–10.
101. Isotani H, Fukumoto Y, Kawamura H, et al. Hypoparathyroidism and insulin-dependent diabetes mellitus in a patient with Kearns-Sayre syndrome harbouring a mitochondrial DNA deletion. Clin Endocrinol (Oxf) 1996;45(5):637–41.
102. Kinsley BT, Swift M, Dumont RH, et al. Morbidity and mortality in the Wolfram syndrome. Diabetes Care 1995;18(12):1566–70.
103. Flynn JT, Bachynski BN, Rodrigues MM, et al. Hyperglycemic acidotic coma and death in Kearns-Sayre syndrome. Trans Am Ophthalmol Soc 1985;83:131–61.
104. Konstantinov NK, Rohrscheib M, Agaba EI, et al. Respiratory failure in diabetic ketoacidosis. World J Diabetes 2015;6(8):1009–23.
105. Davies MJ, D'Alessio DA, Fradkin J, et al. Management of Hyperglycemia in Type 2 Diabetes, 2018. A Consensus Report by the American Diabetes Association (ADA) and the European Association for the Study of Diabetes (EASD). Diabetes Care 2018;41(12):2669–701.
106. Yang H, Shan W, Zhu F, et al. Ketone Bodies in Neurological Diseases: Focus on Neuroprotection and Underlying Mechanisms. Front Neurol 2019;10:585.
107. Khan NA, Auranen M, Paetau I, et al. Effective treatment of mitochondrial myopathy by nicotinamide riboside, a vitamin B3. EMBO Mol Med 2014;6(6):721–31.
108. Klocker AA, Phelan H, Twigg SM, et al. Blood beta-hydroxybutyrate vs. urine acetoacetate testing for the prevention and management of ketoacidosis in Type 1 diabetes: a systematic review. Diabet Med 2013;30(7):818–24.
109. Camp KM, Krotoski D, Parisi MA, et al. Nutritional interventions in primary mitochondrial disorders: Developing an evidence base. Mol Genet Metab 2016;119(3):187–206.
110. American Diabetes Association. 5. Facilitating behavior change and well-being to improve health outcomes: standards of medical care in diabetes-2020. Diabetes Care 2020;43(Suppl 1):S48–65.

111. Chapman TP, Hadley G, Fratter C, et al. Unexplained gastrointestinal symptoms: think mitochondrial disease. Dig Liver Dis 2014;46(1):1–8.

112. Meyers DE, Basha HI, Koenig MK. Mitochondrial cardiomyopathy: pathophysiology, diagnosis, and management. Tex Heart Inst J 2013;40(4):385–94.

113. Guevara-Campos J, Gonzalez-Guevara L, Cauli O. Autism and intellectual disability associated with mitochondrial disease and hyperlactacidemia. Int J Mol Sci 2015;16(2):3870–84.

114. Gourgari E, Wilhelm EE, Hassanzadeh H, et al. A comprehensive review of the FDA-approved labels of diabetes drugs: Indications, safety, and emerging cardiovascular safety data. J Diabet Complications 2017;31(12):1719–27.

115. Matsuzaki M, Izumi T, Shishikura K, et al. Hypothalamic growth hormone deficiency and supplementary GH therapy in two patients with mitochondrial myopathy, encephalopathy, lactic acidosis and stroke-like episodes. Neuropediatrics 2002;33(5):271–3.

116. Badawy RA, Vogrin SJ, Lai A, et al. Cortical excitability changes correlate with fluctuations in glucose levels in patients with epilepsy. Epilepsy Behav 2013; 27(3):455–60.

117. Rajput R, Sinha B, Majumdar S, et al. Consensus statement on insulin therapy in chronic kidney disease. Diabetes Res Clin Pract 2017;127:10–20.

118. Russell-Jones D, Khan R. Insulin-associated weight gain in diabetes–causes, effects and coping strategies. Diabetes Obes Metab 2007;9(6):799–812.

119. American Diabetes Association. 7. Diabetes technology: standards of medical care in diabetes-2020. Diabetes Care 2020;43(Suppl 1):S77–88.

120. Suzuki Y, Kadowaki H, Taniyama M, et al. Insulin edema in diabetes mellitus associated with the 3243 mitochondrial tRNA(Leu(UUR)) mutation; case reports. Diabetes Res Clin Pract 1995;29(2):137–42.

121. Luigetti M, Sauchelli D, Primiano G, et al. Peripheral neuropathy is a common manifestation of mitochondrial diseases: a single-centre experience. Eur J Neurol 2016;23(6):1020–7.

122. Cameron AR, Logie L, Patel K, et al. Metformin selectively targets redox control of complex I energy transduction. Redox Biol 2018;14:187–97.

123. Davies M, Chatterjee S, Khunti K. The treatment of type 2 diabetes in the presence of renal impairment: what we should know about newer therapies. Clin Pharmacol 2016;8:61–81.

124. Sauerbeck A, Gao J, Readnower R, et al. Pioglitazone attenuates mitochondrial dysfunction, cognitive impairment, cortical tissue loss, and inflammation following traumatic brain injury. Exp Neurol 2011;227(1):128–35.

125. Erdmann E, Charbonnel B, Wilcox RG, et al. Pioglitazone use and heart failure in patients with type 2 diabetes and preexisting cardiovascular disease: data from the PROactive study (PROactive 08). Diabetes Care 2007;30(11):2773–8.

126. Viscoli CM, Inzucchi SE, Young LH, et al. pioglitazone and risk for bone fracture: safety data from a randomized clinical trial. J Clin Endocrinol Metab 2017; 102(3):914–22.

127. Seppa K, Toots M, Reimets R, et al. GLP-1 receptor agonist liraglutide has a neuroprotective effect on an aged rat model of Wolfram syndrome. Sci Rep 2019;9(1):15742.

128. Marso SP, Bain SC, Consoli A, et al. Semaglutide and cardiovascular outcomes in patients with type 2 diabetes. N Engl J Med 2016;375(19):1834–44.

129. Storgaard H, Cold F, Gluud LL, et al. Glucagon-like peptide-1 receptor agonists and risk of acute pancreatitis in patients with type 2 diabetes. Diabetes Obes Metab 2017;19(6):906–8.

130. Wang T, Wang F, Zhou J, et al. Adverse effects of incretin-based therapies on major cardiovascular and arrhythmia events: meta-analysis of randomized trials. Diabetes Metab Res Rev 2016;32(8):843–57.

131. Pintana H, Apaijai N, Chattipakorn N, et al. DPP-4 inhibitors improve cognition and brain mitochondrial function of insulin-resistant rats. J Endocrinol 2013; 218(1):1–11.

132. Scherntaner G, Cahn A, Raz I. Is the use of DPP-4 inhibitors associated with an increased risk for heart failure? lessons from EXAMINE, SAVOR-TIMI 53, and TECOS. Diabetes Care 2016;39(Suppl 2):S210–8.

133. Zheng SL, Roddick AJ, Aghar-Jaffar R, et al. Association between use of sodium-glucose cotransporter 2 inhibitors, glucagon-like peptide 1 agonists, and dipeptidyl peptidase 4 inhibitors with all-cause mortality in patients with type 2 diabetes: a systematic review and meta-analysis. JAMA 2018;319(15): 1580–91.

134. Men P, He N, Song C, et al. Dipeptidyl peptidase-4 inhibitors and risk of arthralgia: A systematic review and meta-analysis. Diabetes Metab 2017; 43(6):493–500.

135. McMurray JJV, Solomon SD, Inzucchi SE, et al. Dapagliflozin in patients with heart failure and reduced ejection fraction. N Engl J Med 2019;381(21): 1995–2008.

136. Liu J, Li L, Li S, et al. Effects of SGLT2 inhibitors on UTIs and genital infections in type 2 diabetes mellitus: a systematic review and meta-analysis. Sci Rep 2017; 7(1):2824.

137. Rosenstock J, Ferrannini E. Euglycemic diabetic ketoacidosis: a predictable, detectable, and preventable safety concern with SGLT2 inhibitors. Diabetes Care 2015;38(9):1638–42.

138. Boyle MP, De Boeck K. A new era in the treatment of cystic fibrosis: correction of the underlying CFTR defect. Lancet Respir Med 2013;1(2):158–63.

139. Corriveau S, Sykes J, Stephenson AL. Cystic fibrosis survival: the changing epidemiology. Curr Opin Pulm Med 2018;24(6):574–8.

140. Moran A, Dunitz J, Nathan B, et al. Cystic fibrosis-related diabetes: current trends in prevalence, incidence, and mortality. Diabetes Care 2009;32(9): 1626–31.

141. Stephenson AL, Tom M, Berthiaume Y, et al. A contemporary survival analysis of individuals with cystic fibrosis: a cohort study. Eur Respir J 2015;45(3):670–9.

142. Ramos KJ, Quon BS, Heltshe SL, et al. Heterogeneity in survival in adult patients with cystic fibrosis with FEV1 < 30% of predicted in the United States. Chest 2017;151(6):1320–8.

143. Lewis C, Blackman SM, Nelson A, et al. Diabetes-related mortality in adults with cystic fibrosis. Role of genotype and sex. Am J Respir Crit Care Med 2015; 191(2):194–200.

144. Moran A, Brunzell C, Cohen RC, et al. Clinical care guidelines for cystic fibrosis-related diabetes: a position statement of the American Diabetes Association and a clinical practice guideline of the Cystic Fibrosis Foundation, endorsed by the Pediatric Endocrine Society. Diabetes Care 2010;33(12):2697–708.

145. Hart NJ, Aramandla R, Poffenberger G, et al. Cystic fibrosis-related diabetes is caused by islet loss and inflammation. JCI Insight 2018;3(8):e98240.

146. Moran A, Pillay K, Becker D, et al. ISPAD Clinical Practice Consensus Guidelines 2018: Management of cystic fibrosis-related diabetes in children and adolescents. Pediatr Diabetes 2018;19(Suppl 27):64–74.

147. Frost F, Jones GH, Dyce P, et al. Loss of incretin effect contributes to postprandial hyperglycaemia in cystic fibrosis-related diabetes. Diabet Med 2019; 36(11):1367–74.

148. Kelly A, De Leon DD, Sheikh S, et al. Islet hormone and incretin secretion in cystic fibrosis after four months of ivacaftor therapy. Am J Respir Crit Care Med 2019;199(3):342–51.

149. Aitken ML, Szkudlinska MA, Boyko EJ, et al. Impaired counterregulatory responses to hypoglycaemia following oral glucose in adults with cystic fibrosis. Diabetologia 2020;63(5):1055–65.

150. Blackman SM, Commander CW, Watson C, et al. Genetic modifiers of cystic fibrosis-related diabetes. Diabetes. 2013;62(10):3627–35.

151. Sun X, Yi Y, Xie W, et al. CFTR influences beta cell function and insulin secretion through non-cell autonomous exocrine-derived factors. Endocrinology 2017; 158(10):3325–38.

152. Guo JH, Chen H, Ruan YC, et al. Glucose-induced electrical activities and insulin secretion in pancreatic islet beta-cells are modulated by CFTR. Nat Commun 2014;5:4420.

153. Nyirjesy SC, Sheikh S, Hadjiliadis D, et al. beta-Cell secretory defects are present in pancreatic insufficient cystic fibrosis with 1-hour oral glucose tolerance test glucose >/=155 mg/dL. Pediatr Diabetes 2018;19(7):1173–82.

154. Rolon MA, Benali K, Munck A, et al. Cystic fibrosis-related diabetes mellitus: clinical impact of prediabetes and effects of insulin therapy. Acta Paediatr 2001;90(8):860–7.

155. Leclercq A, Gauthier B, Rosner V, et al. Early assessment of glucose abnormalities during continuous glucose monitoring associated with lung function impairment in cystic fibrosis patients. J Cyst Fibros 2014;13(4):478–84.

156. Hameed S, Morton JR, Jaffe A, et al. Early glucose abnormalities in cystic fibrosis are preceded by poor weight gain. Diabetes Care 2010;33(2):221–6.

157. Brodsky J, Dougherty S, Makani R, et al. Elevation of 1-hour plasma glucose during oral glucose tolerance testing is associated with worse pulmonary function in cystic fibrosis. Diabetes Care 2011;34(2):292–5.

158. Chan CL, Ode KL, Granados A, et al. Continuous glucose monitoring in cystic fibrosis - A practical guide. J Cyst Fibros 2019;18(Suppl 2):S25–31.

159. Kelly A, Moran A. Update on cystic fibrosis-related diabetes. J Cyst Fibros 2013; 12(4):318–31.

160. Chan CL, Hope E, Thurston J, et al. Hemoglobin A1c accurately predicts continuous glucose monitoring-derived average glucose in youth and young adults with cystic fibrosis. Diabetes Care 2018;41(7):1406–13.

161. Tommerdahl KL, Brinton JT, Vigers T, et al. Screening for cystic fibrosis-related diabetes and prediabetes: Evaluating 1,5-anhydroglucitol, fructosamine, glycated albumin, and hemoglobin A1c. Pediatr Diabetes 2019;20(8):1080–6.

162. Kaminski BA, Goldsweig BK, Sidhaye A, et al. Cystic fibrosis related diabetes: nutrition and growth considerations. J Cyst Fibros 2019;18(Suppl 2):S32–7.

163. Kilberg MJ, Sheikh S, Stefanovski D, et al. Dysregulated insulin in pancreatic insufficient cystic fibrosis with post-prandial hypoglycemia. J Cyst Fibros 2019;19(2):310–5.

164. Granados A, Chan CL, Ode KL, et al. Cystic fibrosis related diabetes: Pathophysiology, screening and diagnosis. J Cyst Fibros 2019;18(Suppl 2):S3–9.

165. Moran A, Pekow P, Grover P, et al. Insulin therapy to improve BMI in cystic fibrosis-related diabetes without fasting hyperglycemia: results of the cystic fibrosis related diabetes therapy trial. Diabetes Care 2009;32(10):1783–8.

166. Scheuing N, Thon A, Konrad K, et al. Carbohydrate intake and insulin require-ment in children, adolescents and young adults with cystic fibrosis-related dia-betes: A multicenter comparison to type 1 diabetes. Clin Nutr 2015;34(4):732–8.
167. Armaghanian N, Brand-Miller JC, Markovic TP, et al. Hypoglycaemia in cystic fibrosis in the absence of diabetes: A systematic review. J Cyst Fibros 2016; 15(3):274–84.
168. Mannik LA, Chang KA, Annoh PQK, et al. Prevalence of hypoglycemia during oral glucose tolerance testing in adults with cystic fibrosis and risk of developing cystic fibrosis-related diabetes. J Cyst Fibros 2018;17(4):536–41.
169. Costa M, Potvin S, Berthiaume Y, et al. Diabetes: a major co-morbidity of cystic fibrosis. Diabetes Metab 2005;31(3 Pt 1):221–32.
170. Alves Cde A, Aguiar RA, Alves AC, et al. Diabetes mellitus in patients with cystic fibrosis. J Bras Pneumol 2007;33(2):213–21.

Insights into the Genetic Underpinnings of Endocrine Traits from Large-Scale Genome-Wide Association Studies

Diana L. Cousminer, PhD[a,b], Struan F.A. Grant, PhD[a,b],*

KEYWORDS

- Genome-wide association studies • BMI • Height • Puberty • Diabetes
- Bone density • Endocrine traits

KEY POINTS

- Thousands of genetic variants across the genome have been associated with endocrine-related traits and diseases via genome-wide association studies.
- Individuals at the tails of the phenotypic distribution may have a polygenic load of associated risk alleles resulting in a phenotype similar to monogenic syndromes.
- Still, only part of the genetic contribution to these traits (heritability) has been identified.
- Studies of these traits in childhood lag behind large adult studies.
- Understanding the molecular mechanisms tagged by associated variation has been slow because of the need for in-depth functional investigation of each locus.

INTRODUCTION

Genome-wide association studies (GWAS) have rapidly increased in both size and statistical power to detect genetic loci associated with traits and diseases over the past ~15 years. Thousands of genomic variants have been associated with endocrine traits, many of which are related to disease pathogenesis. Although these studies have provided key insights into the genetic architecture of these traits, specific investigation of the genetic contribution to pediatric endocrine-related traits during childhood mostly lags behind advancements in adults. A key issue is to understand how adult-associated loci operate in children. Furthermore, understanding the molecular

[a] Center for Spatial and Functional Genomics, Division of Human Genetics, Department of Pediatrics, Children's Hospital of Philadelphia, 3615 Civic Center Boulevard, Philadelphia, PA 19104, USA; [b] Department of Genetics, Perelman School of Medicine, University of Pennsylvania, Clinical Research Building 500, 415 Curie Boulevard, Philadelphia, PA 19104, USA
* Corresponding author. Children's Hospital of Philadelphia, 3615 Civic Center Boulevard, Room 1102D, Philadelphia, PA 19104.
E-mail address: grants@chop.edu

Endocrinol Metab Clin N Am 49 (2020) 725–739
https://doi.org/10.1016/j.ecl.2020.07.007
0889-8529/20/© 2020 Elsevier Inc. All rights reserved.

endo.theclinics.com

mechanisms that underlie identified loci has been slow, partly because of the need to identify the underlying causal effector genes at these loci through in-depth functional follow-up studies.

Many endocrine-related traits that have been subjected to genetic association studies have principally considered variation in the normal range, such as variability in adult height, but these findings also have clinical or translational implications. For example, studying the genetics of variation in height, body mass index (BMI), and bone mineral density (BMD) is providing insights into the pathologic extremes of these traits, such as idiopathic short stature, extreme obesity, and cases with significant fracture, respectively. In addition, studying normal variation in the pediatric setting can have ramifications for disease risk in adulthood, such as genetic determinants of BMD during childhood influencing later-life risk for bone loss, fracture, and osteoporosis. Other genetic studies have investigated endocrine-related diseases, such as type 2 diabetes (T2D), largely in the adult setting, but which can now be subsequently tested in the pediatric setting given the increasing rates of such diseases in children. Furthermore, genetic studies of immune-related diabetes (type 1 diabetes [T1D], latent autoimmune diabetes in adults [LADA]) can shed light on innate contributions to the pathophysiology of the spectrum of diabetes traits throughout the life course and help distinguish diabetes subtypes.

In this review, the authors provide an update on the latest GWAS efforts for endocrine-related traits, beginning with a discussion of quantifying how much trait variance is due to genetic factors (ie, heritability) and how much of that variance studies have described to date. In addition, the authors contrast the genetic discovery efforts made in adults against pediatric settings and highlight both the challenges and the opportunities in translating such findings into novel diagnostic and therapeutic strategies going forward.

For a summary of recent GWAS of pediatric endocrine traits highlighted in this review, see **Table 1**.

Height

Given its relative ease of measurement and wide availability, adult stature has served as a model polygenic trait at the leading edge of large sample sizes and number of loci discovered. The most recent study included more than 700,000 individuals, revealing 3290 near-independent genome-wide significant signals across the genome. Despite the large number of discovered loci, these variants together explain approximately a quarter of the variation in height attributable to genetic factors (**Fig. 1, Table 2**),[1] a measure known as heritability. Although heritability has traditionally been estimated using twin or family studies, recent methods using directly genotyped/imputed single nucleotide polymorphism (SNP) variants (so-called SNP-heritability) have aided in clarifying the amount of heritability one can expect to characterize in genetic association studies. An understanding of the total genetic contribution to a trait helps estimate how much of this variance has been captured in genetic associations to date, and how much remains to be uncovered in future studies.

With only a quarter of the SNP-heritability of height identified, some of the "missing heritability" may be filled in by lower frequency (1%–5% allele frequency) and rare variants (<1% allele frequency) with relatively large effect sizes, that is, fewer people carry the variant, but for those who do, it is more impactful on the phenotype. Indeed, a recent study identified 83 low-frequency coding variants associated with height (with allele frequencies of 0.1%–4.8%) with effect sizes up to 10 times larger than those found for common variants (with the largest single-variant effects of up to 2 cm per allele).[2] However, these 83 variants explain just 1.7% of the heritability of

Table 1
Recent genome-wide association studies of pediatric endocrine traits highlighted in this review

Trait	Population	Sample Size	Reference
Birth weight	Transethnic	321,223	EGG Consortium et al,[6] 2019
Height standard deviation score at age 10 in girls and 12 in boys	European	13,960	Cousminer et al,[9] 2013
Childhood BMI	European	47,541	Felix et al,[13] 2016
Childhood obesity	Transethnic	Up to 14,893 obese cases and 20,288 lean controls	Bradfield et al,[14] 2019
Infant and early childhood adiposity	European	9286	Helgeland et al,[20] 2019
Six early growth and adiposity traits	European	Up to 22,769	Couto Alves et al,[17] 2019
Age at menarche	European	370,000	Day et al,[40] 2017
Age at voice break	European	55,871	Day et al,[41] 2015
Total body bone mineral density	Transethnic	Up to 66,628	Medina-Gomez et al,[31] 2018
Type 1 diabetes	European	8967 cases and 6076 controls	Aylward et al,[47] 2018

Data from Refs.[6,9,13,14,17,20,31,40,41,47]

height. Similarly, in a Japanese study, 64 rare and low-frequency variants were identified, comprising only 1.7% of the variability in height.[3] Meanwhile, going below the traditional genome-wide significance level of $P<5 \times 10^{-8}$ may yield additional information; a study including ~20,000 SNPs, most of which were below the traditional genome-wide significance threshold, claimed to have predicted closer to the full SNP-heritability for height.[4] Thus, increasing GWAS sample sizes will continue to yield additional common variants of increasingly small effect sizes that explain more of the missing heritability. Notably, heritability is not fixed but depends on the specific population investigated as well as environmental/socioeconomic factors. Most current heritability estimates, and most GWAS efforts, come from cohorts consisting primarily of European ancestry samples. Clearly, additional studies are needed to better understand the heritability of traits in other ethnicities.

Given the extent of the genetic characterization of height, predicting a subject's height based on genetic data becomes a prospect on the horizon. In aggregate, genetic variation associated with a trait can be combined into a polygenic risk score (PRS), calculated as the sum of the associated alleles weighted by their estimated effect sizes (**Fig. 2**). In Yengo and colleagues,[1] the correlation between height predicted by the PRS using genome-wide significant independent SNPs and actual height was 19.7%; this increased to 24.4% when including variants under the traditional GWAS significance threshold (going down to $P<.001$). Clearly, a PRS cannot capture nongenetic contributions to a trait, but it serves as a benchmark of how genetic information may be used to predict clinical outcomes, particularly in combination with other epidemiologic information.

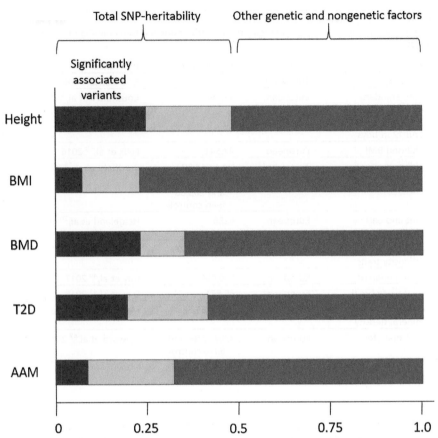

Fig. 1. Heritability of endocrine-related traits. Heritability is the amount of trait variance that is due to genetic factors. SNP-heritability (the sum of the orange plus yellow bar) is the amount of variability that can be captured by directly genotyped and imputed SNPs in GWAS. Currently, a substantial amount of the SNP-heritability can be explained by the hundreds to thousands of common variants associated in large-scale studies of endocrine-related traits. Orange represents the number of significantly associated variants currently identified in GWAS. The blue bar represents other as-yet undiscovered genetic variants and nongenetic factors that contribute to trait variability.

An open question remains as to what precise time points these genetic influences act during the stages of growth (fetal, infant, childhood, pubertal). Differences in final stature result from cumulative effects at different developmental stages,[1] and there is evidence that many of the same genetic signals act on body growth throughout the life course. This association tracks back to fetal growth; using GWAS summary data, both birth weight and birth length are significantly genetically correlated with adult height.[5] In addition, the fetal-specific contribution and the maternal-specific contributions are similar, meaning that neither maternal nor fetal factors are solely driving the association with stature.[6] In a recent study that built PRS based on genetic association data for various traits (using independent SNPs for each GWAS at $P<10^{-5}$), the adult height PRS was actually a better predictor of birth weight than a PRS built on birth weight itself,[7] showing that the bulk of adult height-associated genetic factors actively

Table 2
Heritability estimates for various endocrine-related traits and diseases

Trait/Disease	Approximate Sample Size	Total Heritability, %	SNP Heritability, %	No. of Independent Significant SNPs Identified	Variance Explained by Significant SNPs, %	References
Height	700,000	50–80	48.3	3290	24.5	Yengo et al,[1] 2018
BMI	700,000	31–90	22.4	941	6.0	Yengo et al,[1] 2018; Feng,[62] 2016
Age at menarche	370,000	50–80	32	389	7.4	Day et al,[40] 2017
Type 1 diabetes	15,000	40–85	79 (28 without MHC)[a]	57	NR	Aylward et al,[47] 2018; Jerram & Leslie,[63] 2017
Type 2 diabetes	898,000 (9% cases)	20–80	40	403	18	Mahajan et al,[48] 2018; Ali,[64] 2013
Bone mineral density	426,000	50–80	36	1103	20.3	Kemp et al,[28] 2017; Morris et al,[30] 2018

Abbreviations: MHC, major histocompatibility complex; NR, not reported.
[a] Unpublished, personal communication with R. Mishra, 2019.
Data from Refs.[1,28,30,40,47,48,62–64]

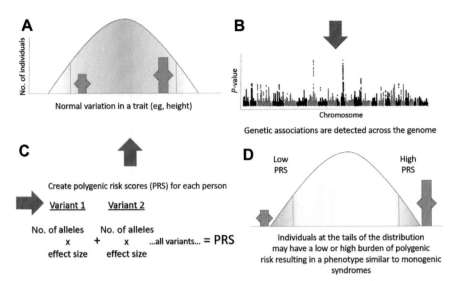

Fig. 2. PRS. (*A*) Individuals within the normal distribution of a trait, such as height, are subjected to GWAS, which detect associated variants across the genome. (*B*) The association *P* value for each tested SNP is shown across the genome to reveal associated loci. (*C*) These variants can then be combined into PRS for each individual, by summing the number of associated variants multiplied by the effect size of each variant. (*D*) Recently, studies have found that individuals with suspected monogenic syndromes at the tail ends of the normal distribution (eg, idiopathic short stature, severe obesity, or T2D) may have a relatively low or high PRS resulting in a monogenic-like phenotype.

influence body size already during gestation. These same variants also affect height later in childhood: In 2010, 16 significant loci for adult height aggregated into a PRS were significantly associated with pediatric height ($P<2 \times 10^{-16}$).[8] Similarly, in a cohort of healthy children and adolescents, the authors found that a PRS based on the 3290 near-independent adult-BMI associated SNPs reported in Yengo and colleagues was strongly associated with height Z-score adjusted for age ($P = 2.20 \times 10^{-38}$) (Cousminer DL and Mitchell JA, unpublished data, 2020).

Individual adult height-associated loci have been uncovered in GWAS efforts of body size across various growth stages. For example, 8 of 10 loci associated with pubertal growth (a period during which individuals achieve ~20% of their final height) were also associated with adult height, but individual associations with height at different ages across adolescence varied; some signals associated with height steadily from age 5 to adult (such as at *MAPK3*), whereas other signals drove height growth mostly during puberty (eg, at *LIN28B*). Other variants had patterns of influence on height that differed between boys and girls, although there was no evidence for a sexually heterogeneous effect on adult stature (eg, at *GNA12*). In general, signals that were associated with pubertal timing also had changing height effects during puberty, whereas signals that were not associated with puberty had a more steady influence on height across childhood and adolescence.[9]

For many traits, individuals who present at the tail ends of the normal distribution are considered to have clinically relevant forms of the trait, such as people who are at the lower end of the normal height distribution (ie, people considered to have idiopathic short stature) but without any comorbidities accounting for their presentation. Typically, it is thought that these individuals have rarer variants with higher phenotypic impact, but recent studies are finding that loci detected in GWAS also contribute to the trait extremes (see **Fig. 2**). For example, in a Taiwanese study, 13 height-associated common variants were also associated with familial short stature, individually and in aggregate.[10] Other studies have investigated the polygenic architecture in both extremely short and tall individuals and concluded that common variants do influence height at the tails.[11] No recent studies to the authors' knowledge have addressed this question, although the community is well equipped to gain clarity in this area with thousands of associated variants and tools to build optimized PRS even from sub-genome-wide significant signals.

A major limitation in translating GWAS findings into the clinic has been assigning the correct causal gene at each of the many loci discovered. Several methods have been used to prioritize candidate causal genes; for example, in Yengo and colleagues,[1] enrichment of pan-tissue expression quantitative trait loci among lead height signals prioritized 610 genes, which were found to be significantly enriched for skeletal growth, cartilage development, and connective tissue development. Genetic studies are also attempting to identify existing drugs that might be repurposed for treating familial short stature (eg, Wong and colleagues[12]). However, each of these putative effector genes requires in-depth functional follow-up to confirm their influence on height growth as well as their impact as a therapeutic option for height extremes.

Body Mass Index

The genetic background of BMI has been investigated in both adults and children, although the sample sizes in the pediatric setting still lag behind those in adults. In the GIANT consortium, for height, more than 700,000 adults were included in the latest metaanalysis of BMI.[1] Meanwhile, the Early Growth Genetics Consortium has carried out genetic studies of both BMI as a quantitative trait[13] and childhood obesity treated as a dichotomous trait (cases <95th percentile of BMI for age vs controls >50th percentile across all measurements).[14,15] For adults, 941 independent variants across the genome have been identified.[1] Interestingly, these signals largely point toward the brain and central regulation of appetite and food intake control rather than peripheral mechanisms.[16]

Again, the question remains of how these variants confer their effects throughout life. In general, the genetic architecture of childhood and adult BMI is highly similar, with a high genetic correlation between the traits.[5] On the other hand, in contrast to adult height-associated variants, the genetic determinants of BMI before age 5 appear to be distinct from those regulating childhood and adult BMI. A recent study investigating the genetic underpinnings of early growth traits (infant peak height velocity, infant peak weight velocity, age, and BMI at adiposity peak [AP] just before 1 year of age, and age and BMI at adiposity rebound [AR] around age 5 to 6 years) found weak genetic correlations between adult BMI and AP in infancy, but high correlations between adult BMI and AR around age 5. Furthermore, a PRS comprising 97 significantly associated adult BMI variants robustly associated with BMI and age at AR, but not with the infant traits.[17]

In general, genetic variants associated with childhood BMI/obesity have shown stronger effect sizes in children.[1,13] One exception appears to be the FTO locus, which has varying effect sizes across life, with a positive association with BMI from around 5 years old,[18] becoming stronger during childhood and adolescence, and peaking at age 20.[19] This locus is also associated with age and BMI at AR,[17] but not during infancy; indeed, a study investigating BMI in age bins across early life found that the FTO effect appeared around age 5 and increased in magnitude up to age 7.[20] Similarly, genetic variation at the LEPR locus harbored the strongest impact on infant

BMI, with a peak at age 1.5 years.[17,20] Three additional loci, near *ADCY3*, *LCORL*, and *LEP*, had more steady effects across early life BMI from birth until age 8.[20] Although the *ADCY3* and *FTO* signals also impact later-life BMI and obesity,[1,13,14] common variants at the *LEPR* signal appear to transiently impact BMI only during infancy, although mutations in the gene are also associated with severe early-onset obesity.[21]

In terms of the polygenic contribution to extreme obesity, Khera and colleagues[22] created an optimized PRS from the association landscape of BMI across the genome. They found that individuals with the highest PRS for BMI had an obesity risk similar to carriers of rare monogenic mutations in genes such as *MC4R*, which results in severe obesity.[23] As noted above, the genetic architecture of early life BMI seems to be distinct: the PRS did not predict large differences in birth weight, but by age 8, there were significant differences in BMI for individuals in the top decile versus the bottom decile of the PRS, that reached a 12.3-kg difference in weight by age 18. This weight difference was similar to the weight difference seen for older adults as well (in the UK Biobank at an average age of 57 years, there was a 13-kg difference between individuals in the top vs the bottom deciles of the PRS). It is important to keep in mind, however, that genetic and environmental influences on a trait can vary over time, such as variability in the *FTO* effect seen in older versus more contemporary cohorts,[24] and these can affect the translatability of PRS across studies.

As with height, a major challenge in translating GWAS findings is assigning the correct functional effector genes at each associated locus. Up until relatively recently, the nearest gene to the GWAS signal has been considered the most likely functional candidate. However, it is now understood that most GWAS signals are noncoding and thus unlikely to directly impact protein structure and function but rather gene regulation. Indeed, gene expression can be controlled locally or over long genomic distances via long-range interactions. As a key example, despite a large body of literature examining the FTO protein in the pathophysiology of obesity, recent studies showed that several other genes in the genomic region near *FTO* may be the principal culprits. These studies showed that the genetic variant detected in GWAS resides within an enhancer embedded in the *FTO* gene, but actually affects the expression of nearby, possibly physiologically relevant, genes, *IRX3*, *IRX5*,[25,26] and *RPGRIP1L*.[27] Much work remains to be done to identify the key effector genes at GWAS-associated loci.

Bone Mineral Density

As for adult height and BMI, pediatric studies lag far behind large-scale adult studies in both sample size and number of loci discovered, mainly because of the difficulty in ascertaining BMD data for children on a large scale. In a study of quantitative heel estimated BMD (eBMD) including ~427,000 individuals, 1106 independent genome-wide significant signals were identified. These signals collectively explained more than half of the total SNP-heritability.[28] In the GEFOS consortium, GWAS has also been carried out on adult femoral neck, lumbar spine, and radius BMD.[29] In general, effect sizes were concordant between heel eBMD and DEXA-derived BMD measures. In addition, there was a negative correlation between effect sizes for eBMD and fracture risk, suggesting that eBMD is a clinically relevant measure for osteoporosis.[30]

Meanwhile, another GEFOS study investigated the genetic effects on total body BMD across the life course by performing separate GWAS in 15-year age bins from birth to old age.[31] Seventy-eight loci were uncovered overall, with only 2 additional loci in age-specific strata, including 1 locus in children (rs72699866 near *RIN3*), which had a decreasing association with age. Meanwhile, another 2 variants had significant age-dependent effects, with both exhibiting stronger effects in older adults. In general, age-specific effects in this study were the exception rather than the norm. On the other hand, that study binned participants based on age and was unable to account for pubertal timing, which is associated with BMD. When accounting for pubertal timing among carriers of the *COLIA1* Sp1 variant associated with postmenopausal bone loss,[32] the authors found that this same variant also impacted the timing of bone accrual[33] despite only modest effects in premenopausal adults.[34] In addition, this effect was stronger in girls than in boys and had the strongest association at the lumbar spine. Therefore, such variants with effects only in periods of high bone turnover, such as at the tails of the lifespan, may only be detected when accounting for maturational stages, such as puberty and menopause, sex, and skeletal site specificity.

To address whether adult-identified BMD variants also impact pediatric BMD, 63 variants associated with DEXA-measured adult BMD were combined to create a PRS. This score was significantly associated with pediatric BMD across several skeletal sites in a longitudinal cohort of healthy children and adolescents aged 5 to 19 years at baseline,[35] with a stronger effect in girls and increasing effects with age. Furthermore, a rare variant in *EN1* was also associated with pediatric bone mass in this same cohort, but with a stronger effect in youth as compared with the larger adult GWAS.[29,36] Of clinical relevance, a PRS constructed with eBMD-associated variants was found to be lower among children with significant fracture history (having low-trauma vertebral fractures or multiple long bone fractures and excluding cases of osteogenesis imperfecta) when compared with the general population.[37] Indeed, the average PRS was −0.47 standard deviation lower than that in UK Biobank ($P = 1.1 \times 10^{-5}$), and the PRS in individuals with suspected Mendelian osteoporosis was even lower (−0.76 SD, $P = 5.3 \times 10^{-10}$), which showed that these children with significant fracture history have an increased burden of common BMD-lowering alleles.

In terms of identifying the correct effector genes at GWAS loci, strides have been made in the bone field despite the lack of relevant public resources (eg, there are no human gene expression data in the public domain for bone). For example, the authors' group developed a variant-to-gene mapping pipeline to identify interactions between GWAS signals in open chromatin and their target genes in human mesenchymal stem cell–derived osteoblasts.[38] With functional follow-up assays, the authors identified several novel target genes that impacted osteoblast activity and mineralization, providing an important advance in moving from statistical GWAS associations to target gene characterization.

Pubertal Timing

Clearly, pubertal timing is a pediatric endocrine trait in itself, but it also has implications for adult health.[39] Age at menarche (AAM) is one of the few pediatric endocrine traits that has been subjected to GWAS at a similar scale to that of recent large studies of adult traits, with 370,000 women included and 380 independent significant signals across the genome.[40] Collectively, these variants explained about a quarter of the total SNP-heritability (see **Fig. 1, Table 2**), suggesting that future studies with larger sample sizes will identify many more variants associated with puberty timing. Studies in boys of age at voice break have also yielded genome-wide significant variants, but notably, these largely overlap with the genetic architecture of pubertal timing in girls.[41] Rare variants associated with AAM have also been identified, but similar to traits mentioned above, these variants did not explain a large part of the heritability.[42] Some common and rare variants fall in or near genes known to affect monogenic aberrations of pubertal timing, including *TACR3*, *GNRH1*, *KISS1*, and *FUT2*. However, the casual target effector genes at the vast majority of common associated loci remain unsolved, and whether common variants associated with the normal distribution of pubertal timing aggregated into PRS impact idiopathic precocious or delayed puberty remains to be explored.

Diabetes

Although T1D is traditionally thought of as the childhood-onset form, the rates of both T1D and T2D in the pediatric setting are on the increase, particularly in minorities. From 2002 to 2015, the annual percentage changes in T1D and T2D were 1.9% and 4.8%, respectively, in data from the SEARCH for Diabetes in Youth Study, a population-based registry study from 5 US states.[43] Recent studies have presented diabetes subtypes as more of a spectrum of features than completely distinct types.[44–46] Using genome-wide association data, there is a genetic correlation between T1D and T2D, as well as shared genome-wide significant loci between the traits,[47] and the most recent large-scale T2D GWAS also found significant associations with traditionally T1D-specific loci.[48] These data show that studies should consider specific diabetes features rather than lumping a wide range of phenotypes together. This finding also holds for LADA, in which the significant genetic variants are shared with T1D, but a lingering genetic correlation across the genome exists with T2D.[49] Although LADA does seem to be a later-onset subtype of T1D, genetic discriminators between LADA and T1D may exist, such as the absence of some classic T1D-associated susceptibility alleles in the major histocompatibility region,[50] which itself explains half of the T1D heritability.

Overall, 403 independent significant loci have been associated with adult T2D,[48] explaining about half the total SNP-heritability of the trait. An open question remains as to how many of these act in pediatric T2D. To date, most research has focused on the leading adult T2D signal at TCF7L2. Although the role of obesity appears to be the principal driver for T2D in children, TCF7L2 has been implicated in several studies on the genetics of T2D in children. In particular, this locus was strongly associated with T2D in African American youth, again with a stronger effect size than that seen in adults.[51] No studies to date have systematically assessed other adult T2D loci or performed discovery efforts in pediatric T2D. However, in the TODAY study, ~4.5% of youths with clinically diagnosed T2D actually harbored genetic variants known to underlie Maturity Onset Diabetes of the Young, including mutations in GCK, HNF4A, HNF1A, INS, and KLF11.[52] Still, further work remains to be done to investigate the full genetic contribution to pediatric T2D.

Speaking to the overlap in genetic signals influencing diabetes types, the TCF7L2 locus also plays a role in T1D, where it influences the phenotypic heterogeneity of the disease and the progression from single to multiple autoantibody positivity in affected individuals.[53,54] However, rather than focus on commonalities, much of the drive in recent years has been in developing PRS that can help to clinically distinguish between diabetes types, such as for newborn screening,[55] distinguishing T1D from monogenic diabetes,[56] between T1D and T2D in young adults,[57] and between adult-onset T1D and T2D.[58] Furthermore, more specific PRS that are partitioned to represent specific aspects of T2D clinical heterogeneity are being developed with the aim of more accurately predicting disease progression and response to therapeutic interventions (recently reviewed in Udler and colleagues[59]).

As seen with other traits, individuals with the highest load of risk-increasing variants may also display phenotypes that recapitulate individuals with monogenic severe forms of diabetes. For example, individuals in the top 5% and 10% of the T2D PRS distribution based on common associated variants had a 2.75-fold and 2.49-fold increased risk, respectively, of developing T2D. Meanwhile, carriers of the top 0.5% of the PRS distribution had a 3.48-fold increase in T2D risk.[60]

Finally, strides have been made in identifying target effector genes at T2D-associated GWAS loci, through both fine-mapping of these loci and integration of diverse molecular data. Fine-mapping of common GWAS signals for T2D identified 8 missense coding variants in *APOE, PAM, HNF4A, RREB1, HNF1A, GCKR, PATJ,* and *CDKN1B*,[48] and missense variants in *ANKH, POC5, NEUROG3,* and *ZNF711* were also identified as likely to be causal for T2D risk. Including information on chromatin state (eg, open chromatin regions poised for transcription and enriched for markers of active transcription differ between cell types; if a GWAS signal falls into one such open region in a particular cell type, it is more likely to represent an active regulatory element in that tissue) highlighted pancreatic islet enhancer and promoter elements. Similarly, a recent study integrated multiple sources of data to assign candidate genes to GWAS loci,[61] followed by protein-protein interaction network analysis as well as tissue-specific interactome analysis. Identified networks pointed toward glucose homeostasis, regulation of the WNT signaling pathway, response to insulin, and pancreas development, and tissue-specific results highlighted the pancreatic islet as enriched for candidate genes at GWAS signals. Both known and novel genes were identified among these networks. However, further work is needed to confidently identify the target effector genes at most associated loci.

SUMMARY

Overall, genetic studies of endocrine-related traits have often shown stronger effect sizes in pediatric studies than in adult studies, with smaller sample sizes typically needed to detect these same loci in children. In general, however, pediatric studies still lag behind their better-powered adult counterparts, partly because of the lack of comparable data. Furthermore, much work remains to be done to understand how genetic variants associated with adult endocrine traits and diseases behave across life. In particular, more sophisticated longitudinal methods may reveal additional insights into the genetic underpinnings of growth trajectories. In some cases of suspected monogenic forms at the extremes of a trait, these individuals may instead have an increased burden of common risk alleles, which should increasingly be considered clinically when monogenic lesions cannot be found. Finally, the translation of GWAS findings into clinical utility has been slow, because of the need to identify the actual target effector genes at associated loci. Recent strides have been made in variant-to-gene mapping to help identify these causal genes, but much work remains to be carried out. Functional studies in appropriate cell models will aid in identifying the correct causal genes for functional investigation.

ACKNOWLEDGMENTS

D.L.C. is supported by the Eunice Kennedy Shriver National Institute of Child Health and Human Development of the National Institutes of Health (Award number K99HD099330). SFAG is supported by the Daniel B. Burke Chair for Diabetes Research and NIH Grant R01 HD058886.

DISCLOSURE

The authors have nothing to disclose.

REFERENCES

1. Yengo L, Sidorenko J, Kemper KE, et al. Meta-analysis of genome-wide association studies for height and body mass index in ~700000 individuals of European ancestry. Hum Mol Genet 2018;27(20):3641–9.

2. The EPIC-InterAct Consortium, CHD Exome+ Consortium, ExomeBP Consortium, et al. Rare and low-frequency coding variants alter human adult height. Nature 2017;542(7640):186–90.
3. Akiyama M, Ishigaki K, Sakaue S, et al. Characterizing rare and low-frequency height-associated variants in the Japanese population. Nat Commun 2019; 10(1):4393.
4. Lello L, Avery SG, Tellier L, et al. Accurate genomic prediction of human height. Genetics 2018;210(2):477–97.
5. ReproGen Consortium, Psychiatric Genomics Consortium, Genetic Consortium for Anorexia Nervosa of the Wellcome Trust Case Control Consortium 3, et al. An atlas of genetic correlations across human diseases and traits. Nat Genet 2015;47(11):1236–41.
6. EGG Consortium, Warrington NM, Beaumont RN, et al. Maternal and fetal genetic effects on birth weight and their relevance to cardio-metabolic risk factors. Nat Genet 2019;51(5):804–14.
7. Richardson TG, Harrison S, Hemani G, et al. An atlas of polygenic risk score associations to highlight putative causal relationships across the human phenome. eLife 2019;8:e43657.
8. Zhao J, Li M, Bradfield JP, et al. The role of height-associated loci identified in genome wide association studies in the determination of pediatric stature. BMC Med Genet 2010;11(1):96.
9. Cousminer DL, Berry DJ, Timpson NJ, et al. Genome-wide association and longitudinal analyses reveal genetic loci linking pubertal height growth, pubertal timing and childhood adiposity. Hum Mol Genet 2013;22(13):2735–47.
10. Lin Y-J, Liao W-L, Wang C-H, et al. Association of human height-related genetic variants with familial short stature in Han Chinese in Taiwan. Sci Rep 2017;7(1): 6372.
11. Chan Y, Holmen OL, Dauber A, et al. Common variants show predicted polygenic effects on height in the tails of the distribution, except in extremely short individuals. PLoS Genet 2011;7(12):e1002439.
12. Wong HS-C, Lin Y-J, Lu H-F, et al. Genomic interrogation of familial short stature contributes to the discovery of the pathophysiological mechanisms and pharmaceutical drug repositioning. J Biomed Sci 2019;26(1):91.
13. Felix JF, Bradfield JP, Monnereau C, et al. Genome-wide association analysis identifies three new susceptibility loci for childhood body mass index. Hum Mol Genet 2016;25(2):389–403.
14. Bradfield JP, Vogelezang S, Felix JF, et al. A trans-ancestral meta-analysis of genome-wide association studies reveals loci associated with childhood obesity. Hum Mol Genet 2019;ddz161. https://doi.org/10.1093/hmg/ddz161.
15. the Early Growth Genetics (EGG) Consortium. A genome-wide association meta-analysis identifies new childhood obesity loci. Nat Genet 2012;44(5):526–31.
16. The LifeLines Cohort Study, The ADIPOGen Consortium, The AGEN-BMI Working Group, et al. Genetic studies of body mass index yield new insights for obesity biology. Nature 2015;518(7538):197–206.
17. Couto Alves A, De Silva NMG, Karhunen V, et al. GWAS on longitudinal growth traits reveals different genetic factors influencing infant, child, and adult BMI. Sci Adv 2019;5(9):eaaw3095.
18. Sovio U, Mook-Kanamori DO, Warrington NM, et al. Association between common variation at the FTO locus and changes in body mass index from infancy to late childhood: the complex nature of genetic association through growth and development. PLoS Genet 2011;7(2):e1001307.

19. Hardy R, Wills AK, Wong A, et al. Life course variations in the associations between FTO and MC4R gene variants and body size. Hum Mol Genet 2010; 19(3):545–52.

20. Helgeland Ø, Vaudel M, Juliusson PB, et al. Genome-wide association study reveals dynamic role of genetic variation in infant and early childhood growth. Nat Commun 2019;10(1):4448.

21. Wasim M, Awan FR, Najam SS, et al. Role of leptin deficiency, inefficiency, and leptin receptors in obesity. Biochem Genet 2016;54(5):565–72.

22. Khera AV, Chaffin M, Wade KH, et al. Polygenic prediction of weight and obesity trajectories from birth to adulthood. Cell 2019;177(3):587–96.e9.

23. Yeo GSH, Farooqi IS, Aminian S, et al. A frameshift mutation in MC4R associated with dominantly inherited human obesity. Nat Genet 1998;20(2):111–2.

24. Rosenquist JN, Lehrer SF, O'Malley AJ, et al. Cohort of birth modifies the association between FTO genotype and BMI. Proc Natl Acad Sci U S A 2015;112(2): 354–9.

25. Claussnitzer M, Dankel SN, Kim K-H, et al. FTO obesity variant circuitry and adipocyte browning in humans. N Engl J Med 2015;373(10):895–907.

26. Smemo S, Tena JJ, Kim K-H, et al. Obesity-associated variants within FTO form long-range functional connections with IRX3. Nature 2014;507(7492):371–5.

27. Stratigopoulos G, Martin Carli JF, O'Day DR, et al. Hypomorphism for RPGRIP1L, a ciliary gene vicinal to the FTO locus, causes increased adiposity in mice. Cell Metab 2014;19(5):767–79.

28. Kemp JP, Morris JA, Medina-Gomez C, et al. Identification of 153 new loci associated with heel bone mineral density and functional involvement of GPC6 in osteoporosis. Nat Genet 2017;49(10):1468–75.

29. AOGC Consortium, UK10K Consortium, Zheng H, et al. Whole-genome sequencing identifies EN1 as a determinant of bone density and fracture. Nature 2015;526(7571):112–7.

30. Morris JA, Kemp JP, 23andMe Research Team, et al. An atlas of genetic influences on osteoporosis in humans and mice. Nat Genet 2018. https://doi.org/10.1038/s41588-018-0302-x.

31. Medina-Gomez C, Kemp JP, Trajanoska K, et al. Life-course genome-wide association study meta-analysis of total body BMD and assessment of age-specific effects. Am J Hum Genet 2018;102(1):88–102.

32. Grant SF, Reid DM, Blake G, et al. Reduced bone density and osteoporosis associated with a polymorphic Sp1 binding site in the collagen type I alpha 1 gene. Nat Genet 1996;14(2):203–5.

33. Cousminer DL, McCormack SE, Mitchell JA, et al. Postmenopausal osteoporotic fracture-associated COLIA1 variant impacts bone accretion in girls. Bone 2019; 121:221–6.

34. Ralston SH, Uitterlinden AG, Brandi ML, et al. Large-scale evidence for the effect of the COLIA1 Sp1 polymorphism on osteoporosis outcomes: the GENOMOS Study. PLoS Med 2006;3(4):e90.

35. Mitchell JA, Chesi A, Elci O, et al. Genetics of bone mass in childhood and adolescence: effects of sex and maturation interactions. J Bone Miner Res 2015;30(9):1676–83.

36. Mitchell JA, Chesi A, McCormack SE, et al. Rare EN1 variants and pediatric bone mass. J Bone Miner Res 2016;31(8):1513–7.

37. Manousaki D, Kämpe A, Forgetta V, et al. Increased burden of common risk alleles in children with a significant fracture history. J Bone Miner Res 2020. https://doi.org/10.1002/jbmr.3956. jbmr.3956.

38. Chesi A, Wagley Y, Johnson ME, et al. Genome-scale capture C promoter interactions implicate effector genes at GWAS loci for bone mineral density. Nat Commun 2019;10(1):1260.

39. Day FR, Elks CE, Murray A, et al. Puberty timing associated with diabetes, cardiovascular disease and also diverse health outcomes in men and women: the UK Biobank study. Sci Rep 2015;5(1). https://doi.org/10.1038/srep11208.

40. Day FR, Thompson DJ, Helgason H, et al. Genomic analyses identify hundreds of variants associated with age at menarche and support a role for puberty timing in cancer risk. Nat Genet 2017;49(6):834–41.

41. Day FR, Bulik-Sullivan B, Hinds DA, et al. Shared genetic aetiology of puberty timing between sexes and with health-related outcomes. Nat Commun 2015; 6(1). https://doi.org/10.1038/ncomms9842.

42. EPIC-InterAct Consortium, Scotland G, Lunetta KL, et al. Rare coding variants and X-linked loci associated with age at menarche. Nat Commun 2015;6(1):7756.

43. Divers J, Mayer-Davis EJ, Lawrence JM, et al. Trends in incidence of type 1 and type 2 diabetes among youths — selected counties and Indian reservations, United States, 2002–2015. MMWR Morb Mortal Wkly Rep 2020;69(6):161–5.

44. Ahlqvist E, Storm P, Käräjämäki A, et al. Novel subgroups of adult-onset diabetes and their association with outcomes: a data-driven cluster analysis of six variables. Lancet Diabetes Endocrinol 2018. https://doi.org/10.1016/S2213-8587(18)30051-2.

45. McCarthy MI. Painting a new picture of personalised medicine for diabetes. Diabetologia 2017;60(5):793–9.

46. Udler MS, Kim J, von Grotthuss M, et al. Type 2 diabetes genetic loci informed by multi-trait associations point to disease mechanisms and subtypes: a soft clustering analysis. Plos Med 2018;15(9):e1002654.

47. Aylward A, Chiou J, Okino M-L, et al. Shared genetic risk contributes to type 1 and type 2 diabetes etiology. Hum Mol Genet 2018. https://doi.org/10.1093/hmg/ddy314.

48. Mahajan A, Taliun D, Thurner M, et al. Fine-mapping type 2 diabetes loci to single-variant resolution using high-density imputation and islet-specific epigenome maps. Nat Genet 2018;50(11):1505–13.

49. Cousminer DL, Ahlqvist E, Mishra R, et al. First genome-wide association study of latent autoimmune diabetes in adults reveals novel insights linking immune and metabolic diabetes. Dia Care 2018;41(11):2396–403.

50. Mishra R, Åkerlund M, Cousminer DL, et al. Genetic discrimination between LADA and childhood-onset type 1 diabetes within the MHC. Dia Care 2020; 43(2):418–25.

51. Dabelea D, Dolan LM, D'Agostino R, et al. Association testing of TCF7L2 polymorphisms with type 2 diabetes in multi-ethnic youth. Diabetologia 2011;54(3):535–9.

52. Kleinberger JW, Copeland KC, Gandica RG, et al. Monogenic diabetes in overweight and obese youth diagnosed with type 2 diabetes: the TODAY clinical trial. Genet Med 2018;20(6):583–90.

53. Redondo MJ, Geyer S, Steck AK, et al. TCF7L2 genetic variants contribute to phenotypic heterogeneity of type 1 diabetes. Dia Care 2018;41(2):311–7.

54. Redondo MJ, Steck AK, Sosenko J, et al. Transcription factor 7-like 2 (TCF7L2) gene polymorphism and progression from single to multiple autoantibody positivity in individuals at risk for type 1 diabetes. Dia Care 2018;41(12):2480–6.

55. Sharp SA, Weedon MN, Hagopian WA, et al. Clinical and research uses of genetic risk scores in type 1 diabetes. Curr Opin Genet Dev 2018;50:96–102.

56. Patel KA, Oram RA, Flanagan SE, et al. Type 1 diabetes genetic risk score: a novel tool to discriminate monogenic and type 1 diabetes. Diabetes 2016; 65(7):2094–9.
57. Oram RA, Patel K, Hill A, et al. A type 1 diabetes genetic risk score can aid discrimination between type 1 and type 2 diabetes in young adults. Dia Care 2016;39(3):337–44.
58. Thomas NJ, Jones SE, Weedon MN, et al. Frequency and phenotype of type 1 diabetes in the first six decades of life: a cross-sectional, genetically stratified survival analysis from UK Biobank. Lancet Diabetes Endocrinol 2018;6(2):122–9.
59. Udler MS, McCarthy MI, Florez JC, et al. Genetic risk scores for diabetes diagnosis and precision medicine. Endocr Rev 2019;40(6):1500–20.
60. Khera AV, Chaffin M, Aragam KG, et al. Genome-wide polygenic scores for common diseases identify individuals with risk equivalent to monogenic mutations. Nat Genet 2018;50(9):1219–24.
61. Fernández-Tajes J, Gaulton KJ, van de Bunt M, et al. Developing a network view of type 2 diabetes risk pathways through integration of genetic, genomic and functional data. Genome Med 2019;11(1):19.
62. Feng R. How much do we know about the heritability of BMI? Am J Clin Nutr 2016; 104(2):243–4.
63. Jerram S, Leslie RD. The genetic architecture of type 1 diabetes. Genes 2017; 8(8):209.
64. Ali O. Genetics of type 2 diabetes. World J Diabetes 2013;4(4):114.

Delayed and Precocious Puberty: Genetic Underpinnings and Treatments

Anisha Gohil, DO*, Erica A. Eugster, MD

KEYWORDS

- Delayed puberty • Hypogonadotropic hypogonadism
- Hypergonadotropic hypogonadism • Central precocious puberty
- Peripheral precocious puberty

KEY POINTS

- Delayed puberty can be a common variant or be due to a defect in the hypothalamic-pituitary-gonadal axis.
- Isolated cases of hypogonadotropic hypogonadism with and without anosmia are caused by several mutations, but most cases remain idiopathic.
- Sex chromosomal aneuploidies such as Turner syndrome and Klinefelter syndrome are important causes of hypergonadotropic hypogonadism.
- Four monogenic mutations (*KISS1*, *KISS1R*, *MKRN3*, *DLK1*) are known to cause central precocious puberty (CPP).
- Genetic causes of peripheral precocious puberty include McCune-Albright Syndrome (MAS) and familial male-limited precocious puberty (FMPP).

INTRODUCTION

Great variability in timing of pubertal onset exists, with both genetic and environmental factors playing a role.[1] However, genetics is the main contributor with 50% to 80% influence over determination of pubertal timing.[1] This is particularly true for menarche, with approximately half of the variation in timing being from genetic factors.[2] Important insights into the critical role of genetics have been revealed from twin studies that have demonstrated that monozygotic compared with dizygotic twins have greater concordance in pubertal timing.[1] In the past decade, large genome-wide association studies have identified multiple loci responsible for the timing of menarche.[3,4] Although these loci explain only a small percentage of the variance and heritability of pubertal timing, they have revealed that it is highly polygenic.[3,4] The many single gene disorders

Division of Pediatric Endocrinology, Department of Pediatrics, Riley Hospital for Children at IU Health, Indiana University School of Medicine, 705 Riley Hospital Drive, Room 5960, Indianapolis, IN 46202, USA
* Corresponding author.
E-mail address: agohil@iu.edu

Endocrinol Metab Clin N Am 49 (2020) 741–757
https://doi.org/10.1016/j.ecl.2020.08.002
0889-8529/20/© 2020 Elsevier Inc. All rights reserved.

contributing to either delayed or precocious puberty also demonstrate the significant and highly complex role of genes in the regulation of puberty.[1]

This review describes the main genetic causes of delayed puberty (hypogonadotropic and hypergonadotropic) and precocious puberty (central and peripheral), as well as the available treatment options for these conditions. The full-length phrasing of acronyms for gene mutations found in this review are listed in **Table 1**.

CONTENT
Constitutional Delayed Puberty

Constitutional delay of growth and puberty is a variation of normal development in which puberty occurs at or later than the upper end of the normal range.[5] Puberty is considered delayed when there is a lack of breast development in a girl by age 13 and lack of testicular enlargement to 4 mL or more in a boy by age 14. Most delayed puberty is self-limited with two-thirds of patients having constitutional delay.[6] There is often a family history of delayed puberty. Interestingly, individuals with constitutional delay have been found to have significantly higher rates of pathogenic variants compared with unaffected family members or controls, particularly in the genes TAC3 and IL17RD, the latter thought to have a role in fate specification of gonadotropin-releasing hormone (GnRH) neurons.[7]

Hypogonadotropic Hypogonadism

Hypogonadotropic hypogonadism (HH) is caused by abnormalities within the hypothalamus or pituitary and is characterized by low gonadotropin and sex steroid levels.

Table 1
Acronyms and full titles of gene mutations associated with delayed and precocious puberty

Acronym	Full-Length Title
ANOS1	Anosmin 1
FGFR1	Fibroblast Growth Factor Receptor 1
PROK2	Prokineticin 2
PROKR2	Prokineticin Receptor 2
CHD7	Chromodomain Helicase DNA-Binding Protein 7
FGF8	Fibroblast Growth Factor 8
GNRHR	Gonadotropin-Releasing Hormone Receptor
KISS1	Kisspeptin 1 Metastasis Suppressor
KISS1R	Kisspeptin 1 Receptor
LEP	Leptin
LEPR	Leptin Receptor
TAC3	Tachykinin 3
TACR3	Tachykinin Receptor 3
NELF	Nasal Embryonic Luteinizing Hormone-Releasing Hormone Factor
IL17RD	Interleukin 17 Receptor D
PROP1	PROP Paired-Like Homeobox 1
HESX1	Homeobox Gene Expressed in Embryonic Stem Cells
LHX3	LIM Homeobox Gene 3
DAX1	Dosage-Sensitive Sex Reversal-Adrenal Hypoplasia Congenita Critical Region on the X-Chromosome, Gene 1
BBS	Bardet-Biedl Syndrome
FMR1	Fragile X Mental Retardation 1
GALT	Galactose-1-Phosphate Uridylyltransferase
MKRN3	Makorin Ring Finger Protein 3
DLK1	Delta Like Non-canonical Notch Ligand 1
GNAS1	Guanine Nucleotide-Binding Protein, Alpha-Stimulating Activity Polypeptide 1

Etiologies of HH can be congenital or acquired.[5] This review focuses on congenital forms, including gene mutations and syndromes.

Kallmann syndrome

Isolated HH (IHH) without other pituitary hormone deficiencies can occur with or without anosmia. With anosmia, the condition is called Kallmann syndrome.[8] During normal embryologic development, GnRH secreting neurons originate in the olfactory placode and migrate to the hypothalamus.[9] Certain mutations disrupt the interconnected olfactory and GnRH neuronal migration process, leading to Kallmann syndrome.[8]

Approximately 60% of individuals with IHH have anosmia (Kallmann syndrome).[10] Fifteen percent of cases are caused by a mutation in ANOS1 (also known as KAL1) or FGFR1.[10] The ANOS1 gene encodes for the neural cell adhesion protein molecule anosmin-1, which is essential for normal neuronal migration during early development.[10] ANOS1 mutations are X-linked recessive and associated findings include unilateral renal agenesis and bimanual synkinesis.[8] FGFR1 mutations demonstrate autosomal dominant transmission and can be associated with cleft palate, dental agenesis, or skeletal anomalies.[8] An additional 5% to 10% of cases are caused by PROK2 and PROKR2 mutations that exhibit an autosomal recessive form of transmission.[10] Although isolated GnRH deficiency caused by a CHD7 mutation is associated with CHARGE syndrome, there are also reports of it causing Kallmann syndrome in individuals without a CHARGE phenotype.[11] FGF8 mutations, inherited in an autosomal dominant pattern, cause fewer than 5% of cases.[10] Mutations in some genes have been found to cause both anosmic and normosmic forms and include FGFR1, PROK2, PROKR2, CHD7, and FGF8.[8]

Normosmic types

The other 40% of cases of IHH are normosmic and inherited in an autosomal recessive pattern.[10] The most common reason for normosmic IHH is a mutation in the GnRH receptor (GNRHR), which accounts for 16% to 40% of cases.[10] Kisspeptin, a hypothalamic neuropeptide, and its receptor are encoded by the genes KISS1 and KISS1R, respectively. KISS1 and KISS1R mutations in consanguineous families with normosmic IHH have been reported.[12,13] Patients with leptin (LEP) and leptin receptor (LEPR) mutations have severe obesity from a very young age and often develop HH, highlighting leptin's permissive role in the process of pubertal initiation and maturation.[14] TAC3 and TACR3 encode for neurokinin B, another hypothalamic neuropeptide, and its receptor and loss-of-function mutations in these genes are also found in families with normosmic IHH.[15]

Despite the many mutations that are known to cause IHH, the etiology in most cases remains enigmatic with 60% to 75% of anosmic and 50% of normosmic IHH cases being classified as idiopathic.[10] One of the most fascinating aspects of IHH is the potential for spontaneous recovery of the hypothalamic-pituitary-gonadal (HPG) axis later in life. Reversal of Kallmann syndrome and normosmic IHH has been seen in approximately 10% of cases, and therefore embarking on a trial-off of hormone replacement therapy in these patients is reasonable.[16] Comparable frequencies of reversible versus nonreversible IHH are reported with FGFR1, PROKR2, and GNRHR mutations.[17] In contrast, reversibility was more frequent with TAC3 and TACR3 mutations.[17] Spontaneous recovery with ANOS1 mutations is rare.[17]

Digenic mutations

Two genes acting synergistically to produce a more severe phenotype of IHH than either single gene acting alone is known as a digenic mutation.[18] FGFR1 and NELF mutations were found in one pedigree with Kallmann syndrome, and GNRHR and FGFR1 mutations were found in a second pedigree with normosmic IHH.[18] The frequency of digenic mutations in IHH is estimated at 2.5%.[19]

Mutations affecting hypothalamic-pituitary-gonadal development

Mutations in the pituitary transcription factors PROP1, HESX1, and LHX3 affect the development of the pituitary gland and cause deficiencies of multiple pituitary hormones, including gonadotropins.[14] PROP1 mutations lead to deficiencies of luteinizing hormone (LH), follicle-stimulating hormone (FSH), thyroid-stimulating hormone (TSH), growth hormone (GH), and prolactin.[20] Individuals with PROP1 mutations are noted to initially have pituitary hyperplasia that later develops into hypoplasia.[21] The hormonal profile of LHX3 mutations is similar to that seen in PROP1 with deficiencies of LH, FSH, TSH, GH, and prolactin.[22] Mutations in HESX1 are associated with septo-optic dysplasia (SOD), which is typified by the triad of pituitary hormone abnormalities, optic nerve hypoplasia, and midline brain defects, such as agenesis of the corpus callosum or septum pellucidum.[23] When HH occurs in the setting of SOD, it is often present in combination with other pituitary hormone deficiencies.[24]

Adrenal hypoplasia congenital is caused by a DAX-1 mutation and is an X-linked recessive disorder.[25] DAX-1 is an orphan nuclear receptor found in the adrenal gland, gonads, hypothalamus, and pituitary gonadotroph cells.[26] Due to its sex-linked inheritance pattern, all affected individuals are male.[26] Affected individuals tend to develop adrenal insufficiency as neonates or infants, although onset in later childhood can occur.[25,26] These boys fail to enter puberty due to HH.[25,26]

Several mutations affect various levels of the HPG axis to cause HH. Mutations in the beta-subunit of LH and FSH are very rare.[27] Female individuals with mutations in the beta-subunit of LH have normal pubertal development, but secondary amenorrhea and infertility.[27] Male individuals have immature Leydig cells, testosterone deficiency, and impaired spermatogenesis.[27] A mutation in the beta-subunit of FSH results in pubertal delay and primary amenorrhea in female individuals,[28] whereas male individuals have small testes, testosterone deficiency, and azoospermia.[29]

Syndromes

Many syndromes include HH.[6] Three of the more well-known are Prader-Willi, Bardet-Biedl, and CHARGE syndromes, each of which will be highlighted here. Prader-Willi syndrome most often occurs due to a de novo deletion of paternally inherited genes on chromosome 15q11-q13, but may also result from maternal uniparental disomy of chromosome 15.[30] Several neuroendocrine abnormalities secondary to hypothalamic-pituitary dysfunction are present including GH insufficiency with associated short stature, hypogonadism, hypothyroidism, and obesity.[30] Genital hypoplasia is present at birth in both sexes, but is more noticeable in boys, as cryptorchidism is present in more than 80% and may be seen with underdevelopment of the scrotum and small testes.[30,31] Puberty is often delayed or incomplete.[31] The hypogonadism in male individuals was historically considered centrally mediated, but primary testicular failure, or a combination of both are now recognized.[32] Ovarian function in girls appears to be normal.[33]

Features of Bardet-Biedl syndrome include retinal dystrophy, polydactyly, obesity, developmental delays, renal anomalies, genitourinary malformations in female individuals, and HH in male individuals.[34] The condition is inherited autosomal recessively, and 16 genes have been implicated, with the most common being *BBS1* and *BBS10*.[34] Mutations lead to cilia cell structure dysfunction, which is thus thought to underlie the features of this condition.[34]

CHARGE syndrome features include coloboma, heart malformations, choanal atresia, growth retardation, genital anomalies, and ear abnormalities. Most cases are de novo and caused by a *CHD7* gene mutation.[35] *CHD7* is expressed in the pituitary[36] and mutations in this gene mainly lead to HH, but GH deficiency and rarely hypopituitarism have also been described.[35]

Hypergonadotropic Hypogonadism

In contrast to HH, in which the abnormalities reside within the hypothalamus or pituitary, the defect in hypergonadotropic hypogonadism is at the level of the gonads themselves. Hence, the condition, which can be congenital or acquired, is referred to as primary hypogonadism and is characterized by elevated gonadotropin levels with low sex steroid hormone concentrations.[5] This review covers congenital causes that occur secondary to chromosomal abnormalities, genetic mutations, or syndromes.

Sex chromosomal abnormalities

Turner syndrome (TS) is defined by the presence of one intact X-chromosome with partial or complete absence of the second X-chromosome in addition to characteristic clinical features.[37] The prevalence rate is 25 to 50 per 100,000 female individuals.[37] Hypergonadotropic hypogonadism occurs secondary to primary ovarian failure, which begins in utero with accelerated oocyte atresia and a severe reduction in follicle formation.[38] Spontaneous breast development occurs in approximately one-third of girls,[37] particularly in those with mosaicism compared with those with X-monosomy.[39] Spontaneous menarche may also occur in approximately 16.1% to 19% of girls, again more likely in those with mosaicism.[39,40] Nevertheless, most girls with TS regardless of karyotype eventually require hormone replacement therapy due to lack of or arrested pubertal development.[37,39]

Other X-chromosome abnormalities can also lead to primary ovarian failure. Translocations affecting either of the 2 critical regions Xq13→q22 and Xq22→q26 on the long-arm of the X-chromosome contribute to primary ovarian failure.[41] When the deletion is distal to Xq24, female individuals often have either primary or secondary amenorrhea without short stature or other features of TS.[37] Primary hypogonadism is also a feature of other conditions of X-chromosome aneuploidy such as triple X syndrome.[42]

The most common sex chromosome aneuploidy affecting male individuals is Klinefelter syndrome with a prevalence of 1 in every ~660 male individuals.[43] Klinefelter syndrome is characterized by an extra X-chromosome, and the most common karyotype is XXY. Classic clinical features are tall stature, gynecomastia, hypergonadotropic hypogonadism, infertility, small testes, and speech and learning difficulties. The condition often goes undiagnosed in the pediatric age range, with affected men typically presenting in their mid-30s[44] with infertility or hypogonadism.[43] Although the onset of puberty is unremarkable, it does not progress normally and testicular volume typically stalls out at ~6 mL.[44] Subsequently, the testicles shrink due to hyalinization of the seminiferous tubules and loss of germ cells.[43] Leydig cell hyperplasia is also seen histologically and is likely due to elevated LH concentrations.[43]

Syndromes

Fragile X syndrome results from expansion of CGG repeats in an untranslated region of the *FMR1* gene. Greater than 200 repeats results in silencing of the gene, but a repeat length of 55 to 200 is classified as a premutation carrier. Varying degrees of ovarian dysfunction occur in female premutation carriers,[45] and range from regular menses with infertility due to primary ovarian insufficiency, to oligomenorrhea or amenorrhea before age 40 due to premature ovarian failure.[46]

Galactosemia most often occurs secondary to impaired activity of the enzyme galactose-1-phosphate uridyltransferase due to a mutation in the *GALT* gene, resulting in the inability to break down galactose. This metabolic disorder results in severe vomiting, diarrhea, failure to thrive, cataracts, hepatomegaly with jaundice, and potentially *Escherichia coli* sepsis after the introduction of milk shortly after birth.[47] Despite lifelong adherence to dietary restriction of galactose, 80% of female individuals with the condition develop primary ovarian failure.[48] Primary gonadal failure is absent in male individuals.[48] Although the etiology is not completely understood, studies suggest that the ovarian failure occurs very early in the prenatal or perinatal period due to direct toxicity of galactose or its metabolites on ovarian tissue.[47,49]

Follicle-stimulating hormone and luteinizing hormone receptor dysfunction

Mutations in the FSH and LH receptor are uncommon causes of hypergonadotropic hypogonadism in the general population. In 75 female individuals with hypergonadotropic hypogonadism from 13 Finnish families, 22 female individuals had an inactivating point mutation in the FSH receptor gene.[50,51] Female individuals with homozygous mutations were infertile, demonstrating the importance of FSH for follicular maturation.[50,51] However, some of their brothers also had homozygous mutations, but did not have complete infertility.[51] Instead they had varying degrees of oligospermia suggesting that FSH is important but not essential for spermatogenesis.[51]

Depending on the severity of the LH receptor mutation, the genital phenotype in 46XY individuals ranges from mild ambiguity to complete female-appearing external genitalia.[52] 46XX individuals with LH receptor mutations have a milder presentation with normal secondary sexual characteristics, but with anovulatory amenorrhea and low estrogen levels.[53]

Genetic etiologies of both hypogonadotropic and hypergonadotropic hypogonadism are found in **Table 2**.

Precocious Puberty

Precocious puberty refers to secondary sexual development ensuing before the norms for racial or ethnic background and traditionally has been defined as before age 8 in girls and age 9 in boys.[54,55] Central precocious puberty (CPP) involves early activation of the HPG axis and laboratory evidence of elevated random or stimulated gonadotropin and sex steroid levels. Peripheral precocious puberty (PPP) describes pubertal onset that does not originate from the HPG axis and levels of gonadotropins are suppressed in the setting of elevated sex steroid levels. Causes of both central and peripheral precocious puberty include genetic, acquired, and idiopathic conditions.[56,57] This review is limited to CPP and PPP arising from genetic mutations and observed in the context of some specific syndromes.

Central precocious puberty

The 4 known monogenic causes of CPP arise from mutations in kisspeptin (*KISS1*), the kisspeptin receptor (*KISS1R*), makorin Ring Finger protein 3 (*MKRN3*), and deltalike homolog 1 (*DLK1*).[56] Historically, most cases of CPP are idiopathic, but because 27.5% of cases have a positive family history, a genetic cause is suspected.[58] Kisspeptin, a stimulator of GnRH neurons, is considered the primary "gatekeeper" of puberty.[59] Activating mutations in the *KISS1* and *KISS1R* genes have been found thus far

Table 2
Genetic etiologies of hypogonadotropic and hypergonadotropic hypogonadism

Abnormality	Mutation or Abnormality	Important Clinical Highlights
Hypogonadotropic hypogonadism		
Isolated		
Anosmic	ANOS1, FGFR1, PROK2, PROKR2, CHD7, FGF8	ANOS1: unilateral renal agenesis, bimanual synkinesis. FGFR1: cleft palate, dental agenesis, skeletal anomalies.
Normosmic	GNRHR, KISS1, KISS1R, LEP, LEPR, TAC3, TACR3	Most common is GNRHR. LEP and LEPR with early-onset obesity.
Anosmic or normosmic	FGFR1, PROK2, PROKR2, CHD7, FGF8	CHD7 may be seen without CHARGE phenotype.
Hypothalamic-pituitary-gonadal axis		
Pituitary transcription factors	PROP1, HESX1, LHX3	PROP1 and LHX3: LH, FSH, TSH, GH, and prolactin deficiencies. HESX1: Associated with SOD.
Adrenal hypoplasia congenital	DAX-1	Adrenal insufficiency at an early age.
Gonadotropins	LH and FSH beta-subunit	LH beta-subunit: 2° amenorrhea in female individuals. Impaired spermatogenesis in male individuals. FSH beta-subunit: 1° amenorrhea in female individuals. Azoospermia in male individuals.
Syndromes		
Prader-Willi	Paternal deletion or maternal uniparental disomy of chromosome 15q11-q13	Genital hypoplasia both sexes. Cryptorchidism in 80% of male individuals.
Bardet-Biedl	BBS genes (most common BBS1 & BBS10)	Genitourinary malformations in female individuals. Hypogonadism in male individuals.
CHARGE	CHD7	Expressed in pituitary, mainly hypogonadism, may have GH deficiency.
Hypergonadotropic hypogonadism		
Sex chromosome abnormality		
Turner syndrome	Partial or complete absence of 2nd X-chromosome	Spontaneous breast development and menarche more common in mosaic genotype.

(continued on next page)

Table 2
(continued)

Abnormality	Mutation or Abnormality	Important Clinical Highlights
Klinefelter syndrome	Extra X-chromosome (most common XXY)	Testicular volume maxes ~6 mL, then shrinks down. Often men present in mid-30s with infertility.
Syndromes		
Fragile X premutation carrier	55–200 CGG repeats in *FMR1*	Premutation carriers only with infertility, oligo or amenorrhea.
Galactosemia	*GALT*	80% of female individuals with primary ovarian failure.
Gonadotropin receptors	LH and FSH receptor	LH receptor: Anovulatory amenorrhea in female individuals. Genital ambiguity in 46XY individuals. FSH receptor: Infertility in female individuals. Impaired spermatogenesis in male individuals.

Abbreviations: FSH, follicle-stimulating hormone; GH, growth hormone; LH, luteinizing hormone; TSH, thyroid-stimulating hormone.

in 1 patient with CPP each[58–61] and appear to be an uncommon cause of CPP.[62,63] Both mutations cause delayed degradation of the mutant protein resulting in prolonged intracellular signaling and subsequent amplification of their physiologic effect.[64]

MKRN3 acts as an inhibitor of pubertal initiation and therefore loss-of-function mutations result in CPP.[64] In a sample of 38 healthy girls, MKRN3 levels declined before the onset of puberty and were lower in subjects with early puberty compared with age-matched prepubertal controls.[65] Mutations in *MKRN3* are the most common cause of familial cases of CPP[64] and were originally described in 5 of 15 affected families.[66] *MKRN3* is a maternally imprinted and paternally expressed gene, and accordingly all subjects exhibiting the phenotype inherit the mutation from their fathers.[66] Sporadic MKRN3 mutations have also been described.[67]

DLK1, also known as preadipocyte factor-1, is widely expressed in several tissues prenatally, but after birth is mainly expressed in the adrenals, pituitary, and ovaries.[64] Although DLK1 is known to be a potent inhibitor of adipocyte differentiation, its relation to pubertal onset is not well understood.[68] However, it was found to be expressed in several mouse hypothalamic nuclei.[68] A loss-of-function *DLK1* mutation was found in 5 female family members and their serum DLK1 levels were undetectable.[69] Similar to *MKRN3, DLK1* is a maternally imprinted and paternally inherited gene, so only female individuals who inherited the mutation from their father had CPP.[69] In a larger sample of 60 girls with idiopathic CPP representing 23 familial cases, no mutations in *DLK1* were found, and therefore *DLK1* mutations are likely a rare cause of CPP.[70] Interestingly, adult women with a *DLK1* mutation and history of CPP exhibit a distinct metabolic phenotype marked by higher rates of obesity, dyslipidemia, and polycystic ovary syndrome compared with controls.[71] Thus, DLK1 may represent an important link between metabolism and reproduction.

CPP has been reported as part of several genetic syndromes including Temple syndrome (90% of cases), Russell-Silver syndrome (up to 25% of cases), Williams syndrome (10%–18% of cases), and Prader-Willi syndrome (4%–10% of cases).[64] Children with neurofibromatosis type 1, particular in the setting of optic pathway gliomas, are also at increased risk for CPP.[72]

Peripheral precocious puberty

McCune-Albright syndrome (MAS) is characterized by the triad of café-au-lait macules, fibrous dysplasia, and precocious puberty. Other endocrinopathies such as Cushing syndrome, GH excess, and hyperthyroidism can also occur. It is caused by a post-zygotic mutation in the guanine nucleotide binding protein alpha stimulating gene (GNAS1), which leads to constitutive activation of the adenylyl cyclase system with subsequent cell proliferation and hormone production.[73] Because it is a post-zygotic mutation, it is not inherited from an individual's parents, and therefore cannot be passed down to offspring. It is an extremely heterogenous disorder due to mosaicism. Therefore, depending on which cells are affected, the severity and clinical findings vary greatly.[57] PPP is most commonly diagnosed in girls aged 1 to 5 years, and results from autonomous production of estrogen from large unilateral ovarian cysts.[74] MAS in girls presents with sudden onset of painless vaginal bleeding and minimal breast development.[74] The breast development and other signs of MAS may be missed leading to unnecessary oophorectomy in girls mistakenly thought to have an ovarian granulosa cell tumor.[57,74,75] PPP in boys with MAS is much less common, but presents with early secondary sexual development and accelerated linear growth velocity. A Sertoli-cell only GNAS1 mutation has also been described in boys with MAS resulting in testicular enlargement without PPP.[76]

Familial male-limited precocious puberty (FMPP) has an autosomal dominant inheritance pattern and is often associated with a positive family history, but may also arise de novo.[57] The condition is caused by an activating mutation of the LH receptor that results in autonomous production of testosterone by testicular Leydig cells. Although female individuals are asymptomatic carriers due to the requirement for both LH and FSH for ovarian estrogen production, male individuals present with virilization before age 4.[77] As in other forms of PPP in boys, classic findings include virilization such as an enlarged phallus and pubic hair that is out of proportion to a smaller than expected testicular volume.[57,75]

Genetic etiologies of both CPP and PPP are summarized in **Table 3**.

Treatment of Delayed and Precocious Puberty

The primary goal of treatment in hypogonadism is to mimic normal pubertal progression using replacement of sex steroids.[5] There are a multitude of different options for sex steroid replacement and no universally accepted standard treatment algorithm exists. Representative formulations and suggested doses for estrogen and progesterone replacement in girls[5,37,78–80] and testosterone replacement in boys[5,43,78,81] are summarized in **Tables 4** and **5**, respectively. The primary goals for the management of CPP and PPP are preservation of height potential and prevention of further pubertal progression.[55,57] GnRH analogs (GnRHas) have a long history of safety and efficacy and are standard of care for the treatment of CPP.[56] The number of extended release GnRHa preparations has steadily increased and includes 3-monthly and 6-monthly injectables and a subcutaneous implant that is marketed for annual use, but provides

Table 3
Genetic etiologies of central and peripheral precocious puberty

Abnormality	Mutation or Abnormality	Important Clinical Highlights
Central precocious puberty (CPP)		
Monogenic causes	*KISS1, KISS1R, MKRN3, DLK1*	*MKRN3* most common cause of familial CPP. *KISS1, KISS1R,* and *DLK1* are very uncommon. *DLK1* associated with metabolic syndrome phenotype.
Syndromes		
Temple	Maternal uniparental disomy or paternal deletion of chromosome 14q32.2	CPP in 90% of cases Loss of DLK1 expression
Russell-Silver	Hypomethylation of chromosome 11p15 or maternal uniparental disomy of chromosome 7	CPP in up to 25% of cases
Williams	Deletion of chromosome 7q11.23	CPP in 10%–18% of cases
Prader-Willi	Paternal deletion or maternal uniparental disomy of chromosome 15q11-q13	CPP in 4%–10% of cases
Neurofibromatosis type 1	*NF1*	Increased risk particularly in setting of optic pathway glioma
Peripheral precocious puberty		
Syndromes		
McCune-Albright	Post-zygotic mutation in *GNAS1*	PPP most commonly presents in girls aged 1–5 y as sudden onset of painless vaginal bleeding
Familial male-limited precocious puberty	Activating mutation of luteinizing hormone receptor	Virilization in boys before age 4. Enlarged phallus and pubic hair out of proportion to the small testicular volume.

HPG axis suppression for at least 2 years.[82,83] Not all long-acting GnRHas result in equivalent suppression of the HPG axis, however. The 11.25 mg 3-monthly GnRHa formulation is associated with less suppression than the 30-mg dosage,[54] and none of the injectable preparations are as potent as the histrelin implant.[84] Although these observations make prescribing decisions more challenging, little comparative information is available and it is unknown whether disparities in the degree of biochemical suppression will translate into meaningful differences in clinical outcomes such as height.[85] Ongoing controversies in the treatment of CPP include whether a brain MRI is necessary in all cases,[86] when therapy should be discontinued, and which girls

Table 4
Commonly used estrogen and progesterone formulations for hypogonadism in the United States

Estrogen Formulation	Brand Name	Initiation Dose[a]	Adult Dose
Transdermal			
• Patch	Vivelle	6.25–12.5 μg twice weekly	25–100 μg twice weekly
Oral			
• Micronized 17β-estradiol	Estrace	0.25 mg daily	1–4 mg daily
Progesterone Formulation		**Notes for Clinical Care**	**Adult Dose[b]**
Oral			
• Medroxyprogesterone acetate	Provera	Progestin added after first episode of vaginal bleeding or after 2 y of estrogen treatment	10 mg daily for 10 d each mo
• Micronized progesterone	Prometrium		100–200 mg daily for 10–21 d each mo or continuously
Estrogen and Progesterone Formulation		**Notes for Clinical Care**	**Adult Dose**
Oral contraceptive pill (OCP)		Do not use OCP to initiate puberty	Multiple types with various doses of estrogen and progestin

[a] Increase estradiol dose every 6 months over 2 to 3-year period with goal of adult dosing range.
[b] Given with estradiol.

Table 5
Commonly used testosterone formulations for hypogonadism in the United States

Testosterone Formulation	Brand Name	Initiation Dose[a]	Adult Dose
Transdermal			
Testosterone patch	Androderm	Do not use transdermal route to initiate puberty.	2–6 mg daily
Testosterone gel	Androgel (1.62%)		20.25–81 mg daily
Intramuscular[b]			
Testosterone cypionate	Depot-Testosterone	50–100 mg monthly	200–250 mg every 2–4 wk
Testosterone enanthate	Delatestryl	50–100 mg monthly	200–250 mg every 2–4 wk
Subcutaneous			
Testosterone enanthate	Xyosted	Do not use Xyosted to initiate puberty.	50–100 mg once weekly

[a] Increase testosterone dose every 3 to 6 months over 3 to 4-year period with goal of adult dosing range. Follow trough serum testosterone levels and adjust adult dose accordingly to maintain testosterone in mid-normal range.
[b] Can be given via subcutaneous route with doses of 50 to 150 mg weekly.

Table 6
Gonadotropin-releasing hormone analogs used in central precocious puberty in the United States

Formulation	Frequency	Dose	Route
Leuprolide	Monthly	0.2–0.3 mg/kg every 1 mo	Intramuscular injection
	3-monthly	11.25 or 30 mg every 3 mo	Intramuscular injection
	6-monthly	45 mg every 6 mo	Subcutaneous injection
Triptorelin	6-monthly	22.5 mg every 6 mo	Intramuscular injection
Histrelin	1–2 y	50 mg every 1–2 y	Subcutaneous implant

Data from Klein KO, Freire A, Gryngarten MG, et al. Phase 3 Trial of a Small-volume Subcutaneous 6-Month Duration Leuprolide Acetate Treatment for Central Precocious Puberty. J Clin Endocrinol Metab 2020;105(10):dgaa479.

should be treated.[87] Medications for treating PPP in boys with FMPP have been largely successful.[75] In girls with MAS, treatment of PPP remains challenging and approaches often have limited success.[75] Formulations and doses of GnRH analogs[55,88]

Table 7
Therapeutic options for use in McCune-Albright syndrome and familial male-limited precocious puberty

McCune-Albright Syndrome	Mechanism of Action
Females	
Letrozole	Third-generation aromatase inhibitor
Tamoxifen	Selective estrogen receptor modulator
Fulvestrant	Estrogen receptor antagonist
Males	
Letrozole	Third-generation aromatase inhibitor
Anastrozole	Third-generation aromatase inhibitor
Bicalutamide[a]	Nonsteroidal androgen receptor antagonist
Familial Male-Limited Precocious Puberty	**Mechanism of Action**
Aromatase Inhibitor	
Letrozole	Third-generation aromatase inhibitor
Anastrozole	Third-generation aromatase inhibitor
Antiandrogen[a]	
Bicalutamide	Nonsteroidal androgen receptor antagonist
Spironolactone	Weak antiandrogenic agent

[a] Used in combination with an aromatase inhibitor.

and therapeutic options for MAS and FMPP[57,75] are shown in **Tables 6** and **7**, respectively.

SUMMARY

The genetic disorders contributing to either delayed or precocious puberty demonstrate the highly complex role of genetics in the regulation of puberty. There are numerous genetic etiologies of delayed or precocious puberty ranging from single gene mutations, digenic mutations, congenital syndromes, and chromosomal abnormalities to cases that remain idiopathic. Future research expanding our current understanding and the discovery of new mutations underlying idiopathic cases are critical for improving our diagnostic, prognostic, and therapeutic outcomes for children and adults with these conditions.

DISCLOSURE

The work was supported by NIH grant T32DK065549 to A. Gohil.

REFERENCES

1. Palmert MR, Hirschhorn JN. Genetic approaches to stature, pubertal timing, and other complex traits. Mol Genet Metab 2003;80(1–2):1–10.
2. Towne B, Czerwinski SA, Demerath EW, et al. Heritability of age at menarche in girls from the Fels Longitudinal Study. Am J Phys Anthropol 2005;128(1):210–9.
3. Day FR, Thompson DJ, Helgason H, et al. Genomic analyses identify hundreds of variants associated with age at menarche and support a role for puberty timing in cancer risk. Nat Genet 2017;49(6):834–41.
4. Perry JR, Day F, Elks CE, et al. Parent-of-origin-specific allelic associations among 106 genomic loci for age at menarche. Nature 2014;514(7520):92–7.
5. Viswanathan V, Eugster EA. Etiology and treatment of hypogonadism in adolescents. Pediatr Clin 2011;58(5):1181–200.
6. Howard SR, Dunkel L. The genetic basis of delayed puberty. Neuroendocrinology 2018;106(3):283–91.
7. Zhu J, Choa RE-Y, Guo MH, et al. A shared genetic basis for self-limited delayed puberty and idiopathic hypogonadotropic hypogonadism. J Clin Endocrinol Metab 2015;100(4):E646–54.
8. Kim S-H. Congenital hypogonadotropic hypogonadism and Kallmann syndrome: past, present, and future. Endocrinol Metab 2015;30(4):456–66.
9. Wray S, Grant P, Gainer H. Evidence that cells expressing luteinizing hormone-releasing hormone mRNA in the mouse are derived from progenitor cells in the olfactory placode. Proc Natl Acad Sci U S A 1989;86(20):8132–6.
10. Bianco SD, Kaiser UB. The genetic and molecular basis of idiopathic hypogonadotropic hypogonadism. Nat Rev Endocrinol 2009;5(10):569.
11. Balasubramanian R, Choi J-H, Francescatto L, et al. Functionally compromised CHD7 alleles in patients with isolated GnRH deficiency. Proc Natl Acad Sci U S A 2014;111(50):17953–8.
12. Nimri R, Lebenthal Y, Lazar L, et al. A novel loss-of-function mutation in GPR54/KISS1R leads to hypogonadotropic hypogonadism in a highly consanguineous family. J Clin Endocrinol Metab 2011;96(3):E536–45.
13. Topaloglu AK, Tello JA, Kotan LD, et al. Inactivating KISS1 mutation and hypogonadotropic hypogonadism. N Engl J Med 2012;366(7):629–35.

14. Gajdos ZK, Hirschhorn JN, Palmert MR. What controls the timing of puberty? An update on progress from genetic investigation. Curr Opin Endocrinol Diabetes Obes 2009;16(1):16–24.

15. Young J, Bouligand J, Francou B, et al. TAC3 and TACR3 defects cause hypothalamic congenital hypogonadotropic hypogonadism in humans. J Clin Endocrinol Metab 2010;95(5):2287–95.

16. Raivio T, Falardeau J, Dwyer A, et al. Reversal of idiopathic hypogonadotropic hypogonadism. N Engl J Med 2007;357(9):863–73.

17. Sidhoum VF, Chan Y-M, Lippincott MF, et al. Reversal and relapse of hypogonadotropic hypogonadism: resilience and fragility of the reproductive neuroendocrine system. J Clin Endocrinol Metab 2014;99(3):861–70.

18. Pitteloud N, Quinton R, Pearce S, et al. Digenic mutations account for variable phenotypes in idiopathic hypogonadotropic hypogonadism. J Clin Invest 2007; 117(2):457–63.

19. Sykiotis GP, Plummer L, Hughes VA, et al. Oligogenic basis of isolated gonadotropin-releasing hormone deficiency. Proc Natl Acad Sci U S A 2010; 107(34):15140–4.

20. Wu W, Cogan JD, Pfäffle RW, et al. Mutations in PROP 1 cause familial combined pituitary hormone deficiency. Nat Genet 1998;18(2):147–9.

21. Ward RD, Raetzman LT, Suh H, et al. Role of PROP1 in pituitary gland growth. Mol Endocrinol 2005;19(3):698–710.

22. Bhangoo AP, Hunter CS, Savage JJ, et al. A novel LHX3 mutation presenting as combined pituitary hormonal deficiency. J Clin Endocrinol Metab 2006;91(3): 747–53.

23. Dattani MT, Martinez-Barbera J-P, Thomas PQ, et al. Mutations in the homeobox gene HESX1/Hesx1 associated with septo-optic dysplasia in human and mouse. Nat Genet 1998;19(2):125–33.

24. Haddad NG, Eugster EA. Hypopituitarism and neurodevelopmental abnormalities in relation to central nervous system structural defects in children with optic nerve hypoplasia. J Pediatr Endocrinol Metab 2005;18(9):853–8.

25. Muscatelli F, Strom TM, Walker AP, et al. Mutations in the DAX-1 gene give rise to both X-linked adrenal hypoplasia congenita and hypogonadotropic hypogonadism. Nature 1994;372(6507):672–6.

26. Achermann JC, Meeks JJ, Jameson JL. Phenotypic spectrum of mutations in DAX-1 and SF-1. Mol Cell Endocrinol 2001;185(1–2):17–25.

27. Lofrano-Porto A, Barra GB, Giacomini LA, et al. Luteinizing hormone beta mutation and hypogonadism in men and women. N Engl J Med 2007;357(9):897–904.

28. Layman LC, Lee E-J, Peak DB, et al. Delayed puberty and hypogonadism caused by mutations in the follicle-stimulating hormone β-subunit gene. N Engl J Med 1997;337(9):607–11.

29. Phillip M, Arbelle JE, Segev Y, et al. Male hypogonadism due to a mutation in the gene for the β-subunit of follicle-stimulating hormone. N Engl J Med 1998; 338(24):1729–32.

30. Miller JL. Approach to the child with Prader-Willi syndrome. J Clin Endocrinol Metab 2012;97(11):3837–44.

31. Goldstone A, Holland A, Hauffa B, et al. Recommendations for the diagnosis and management of Prader-Willi syndrome. J Clin Endocrinol Metab 2008;93(11): 4183–97.

32. Radicioni A, Di Giorgio G, Grugni G, et al. Multiple forms of hypogonadism of central, peripheral or combined origin in males with Prader–Willi syndrome. Clin Endocrinol 2012;76(1):72–7.

33. Siemensma EP, Van Alfen-van der Velden A, Otten BJ, et al. Ovarian function and reproductive hormone levels in girls with Prader-Willi syndrome: a longitudinal study. J Clin Endocrinol Metab 2012;97(9):E1766–73.
34. Forsythe E, Beales PL. Bardet-Biedl syndrome. European Journal of Human Genetics 2013;21(1):8–13.
35. Gregory LC, Gevers EF, Baker J, et al. Structural pituitary abnormalities associated with CHARGE syndrome. J Clin Endocrinol Metab 2013;98(4):E737–43.
36. Sanlaville D, Etchevers HC, Gonzales M, et al. Phenotypic spectrum of CHARGE syndrome in fetuses with CHD7 truncating mutations correlates with expression during human development. J Med Genet 2006;43(3):211–317.
37. Gravholt CH, Andersen NH, Conway GS, et al. Clinical practice guidelines for the care of girls and women with Turner syndrome: proceedings from the 2016 Cincinnati International Turner Syndrome Meeting. Eur J Endocrinol 2017;177(3): G1–70.
38. Reynaud K, Cortvrindt R, Verlinde F, et al. Number of ovarian follicles in human fetuses with the 45, X karyotype. Fertil Steril 2004;81(4):1112–9.
39. Pasquino AM, Passeri F, Pucarelli I, et al. Spontaneous pubertal development in Turner's syndrome. J Clin Endocrinol Metab 1997;82(6):1810–3.
40. Folsom LJ, Slaven JE, Nabhan ZM, et al. Characterization of spontaneous and induced puberty in girls with Turner syndrome. Endocr Pract 2017;23(7):768–74.
41. Therman E, Laxova R, Susman B. The critical region on the human Xq. Hum Genet 1990;85(5):455–61.
42. Goswami R, Goswami D, Kabra M, et al. Prevalence of the triple X syndrome in phenotypically normal women with premature ovarian failure and its association with autoimmune thyroid disorders. Fertil Steril 2003;80(4):1052–4.
43. Bojesen A, Gravholt CH. Klinefelter syndrome in clinical practice. Nat Clin Pract Urol 2007;4(4):192–204.
44. Groth KA, Skakkebæk A, Høst C, et al. Klinefelter syndrome—a clinical update. J Clin Endocrinol Metab 2013;98(1):20–30.
45. Schwartz C, Dean J, Howard-Peebles P, et al. Obstetrical and gynecological complications in fragile X carriers: a multicenter study. Am J Med Genet 1994; 51(4):400–2.
46. Karimov C, Moragianni V, Cronister A, et al. Increased frequency of occult fragile X-associated primary ovarian insufficiency in infertile women with evidence of impaired ovarian function. Hum Reprod 2011;26(8):2077–83.
47. Fridovich-Keil JL, Gubbels CS, Spencer JB, et al. Ovarian function in girls and women with GALT-deficiency galactosemia. J Inherit Metab Dis 2011;34(2): 357–66.
48. Waggoner D, Buist N, Donnell G. Long-term prognosis in galactosaemia: results of a survey of 350 cases. J Inherit Metab Dis 1990;13(6):802–18.
49. Kaufman FR, Kogut MD, Donnell GN, et al. Hypergonadotropic hypogonadism in female patients with galactosemia. N Engl J Med 1981;304(17):994–8.
50. Aittomäki K, Lucena JD, Pakarinen P, et al. Mutation in the follicle-stimulating hormone receptor gene causes hereditary hypergonadotropic ovarian failure. Cell 1995;82(6):959–68.
51. Tapanainen JS, Aittomäki K, Min J, et al. Men homozygous for an inactivating mutation of the follicle-stimulating hormone (FSH) receptor gene present variable suppression of spermatogenesis and fertility. Nat Genet 1997;15(2):205–6.
52. Latronico AC, Anasti J, Arnhold IJ, et al. Testicular and ovarian resistance to luteinizing hormone caused by inactivating mutations of the luteinizing hormone–receptor gene. N Engl J Med 1996;334(8):507–12.

53. Huhtaniemi I, Alevizaki M. Gonadotrophin resistance. Best Pract Res Clin Endocrinol Metab 2006;20(4):561–76.

54. Fuqua JS. Treatment and outcomes of precocious puberty: an update. J Clin Endocrinol Metab 2013;98(6):2198–207.

55. Carel J-C, Eugster EA, Rogol A, et al. Consensus statement on the use of gonadotropin-releasing hormone analogs in children. Pediatrics 2009;123(4): e752–62.

56. Aguirre RS, Eugster EA. Central precocious puberty: From genetics to treatment. Best Pract Res Clin Endocrinol Metab 2018;32(4):343–54.

57. Eugster EA. Peripheral precocious puberty: causes and current management. Horm Res 2009;71(Suppl. 1):64–7.

58. Silveira LG, Noel S, Silveira-Neto A, et al. Mutations of the KISS1 gene in disorders of puberty. J Clin Endocrinol Metab 2010;95(5):2276–80.

59. Rhie Y-J, Lee K-H, Ko JM, et al. KISS1 gene polymorphisms in Korean girls with central precocious puberty. J Korean Med Sci 2014;29(8):1120–5.

60. Oh YJ, Rhie Y-J, Nam H-K, et al. Genetic variations of the KISS1R gene in Korean girls with central precocious puberty. J Korean Med Sci 2017;32(1):108–14.

61. Teles MG, Bianco SD, Brito VN, et al. A GPR54-activating mutation in a patient with central precocious puberty. N Engl J Med 2008;358(7):709–15.

62. Tommiska J, Sørensen K, Aksglaede L, et al. LIN28B, LIN28A, KISS1, and KISS1R in idiopathic central precocious puberty. BMC Res Notes 2011;4(1):363.

63. Krstevska-Konstantinova M, Jovanovska J, Tasic VB, et al. Mutational analysis of KISS1 and KISS1R in idiopathic central precocious puberty. J Pediatr Endocrinol Metab 2014;27(1–2):199–201.

64. Canton APM, Seraphim CE, Brito VN, et al. Pioneering studies on monogenic central precocious puberty. Arch Endocrinol Metab 2019;63(4):438–44.

65. Hagen CP, Sørensen K, Mieritz MG, et al. Circulating MKRN3 levels decline prior to pubertal onset and through puberty: a longitudinal study of healthy girls. J Clin Endocrinol Metab 2015;100(5):1920–6.

66. Abreu AP, Dauber A, Macedo DB, et al. Central precocious puberty caused by mutations in the imprinted gene MKRN3. N Engl J Med 2013;368(26):2467–75.

67. Macedo DB, Abreu AP, Reis ACS, et al. Central precocious puberty that appears to be sporadic caused by paternally inherited mutations in the imprinted gene makorin ring finger 3. J Clin Endocrinol Metab 2014;99(6):E1097–103.

68. Villanueva C, Jacquier S, de Roux N. DLK1 is a somato-dendritic protein expressed in hypothalamic arginine-vasopressin and oxytocin neurons. PLoS One 2012;7(4):e36134.

69. Dauber A, Cunha-Silva M, Macedo DB, et al. Paternally inherited DLK1 deletion associated with familial central precocious puberty. J Clin Endocrinol Metab 2017;102(5):1557–67.

70. Grandone A, Capristo C, Cirillo G, et al. Molecular screening of MKRN3, DLK1, and KCNK9 genes in girls with idiopathic central precocious puberty. Horm Res 2017;88(3–4):194–200.

71. Gomes LG, Cunha-Silva M, Crespo RP, et al. DLK1 is a novel link between reproduction and metabolism. J Clin Endocrinol Metab 2019;104(6):2112–20.

72. Habiby R, Silverman B, Listernick R, et al. Precocious puberty in children with neurofibromatosis type 1. J Pediatr 1995;126(3):364–7.

73. Wagoner HA, Steinmetz R, Bethin KE, et al. GNAS mutation detection is related to disease severity in girls with McCune-Albright syndrome and precocious puberty. Pediatr Endocrinol Rev 2007;4:395–400.

74. Nabhan ZM, West KW, Eugster EA. Oophorectomy in McCune-Albright syndrome: a case of mistaken identity. J Pediatr Surg 2007;42(9):1578–83.

75. Schoelwer M, Eugster EA. Treatment of Peripheral Precocious Puberty. Endocr Dev 2016;29:230–9. https://doi.org/10.1159/000438895.

76. Coutant RG, Lumbroso S, Rey R, et al. Macroorchidism due to autonomous hyperfunction of Sertoli cells and Gsα gene mutation: an unusual expression of McCune-Albright syndrome in a prepubertal boy. J Clin Endocrinol Metab 2001;86(4):1778–81.

77. Shenker A, Laue L, Kosugi S, et al. A constitutively activating mutation of the luteinizing hormone receptor in familial male precocious puberty. Nature 1993; 365(6447):652–4.

78. Lexicomp Online. Pediatric & neonatal lexi-drugs online. Hudson (OH): Wolters Kluwer Clinical Drug Information. Inc; 2013.

79. Klein KO, Rosenfield RL, Santen RJ, et al. Estrogen replacement in Turner syndrome: literature review and practical considerations. J Clin Endocrinol Metab 2018;103(5):1790–803.

80. Schindler A, Campagnoli C, Druckmann R, et al. Classification and pharmacology of progestins. Maturitas 2003;46 Suppl 1:S7–16.

81. Spratt DI, Stewart II, Savage C, et al. Subcutaneous injection of testosterone is an effective and preferred alternative to intramuscular injection: demonstration in female-to-male transgender patients. J Clin Endocrinol Metab 2017;102(7): 2349–55.

82. Krishna KB, Fuqua JS, Rogol AD, et al. Use of gonadotropin-releasing hormone analogs in children: update by an International Consortium. Horm Res 2019; 91(6):357–72.

83. Lewis KA, Goldyn AK, West KW, et al. A single histrelin implant is effective for 2 years for treatment of central precocious puberty. J Pediatr 2013;163(4):1214–6.

84. Silverman LA, Neely EK, Kletter GB, et al. Long-term continuous suppression with once-yearly histrelin subcutaneous implants for the treatment of central precocious puberty: a final report of a phase 3 multicenter trial. J Clin Endocrinol Metab 2015;100(6):2354–63.

85. Eugster EA. Treatment of central precocious puberty. J Endocr Soc 2019;3(5): 965–72.

86. Cantas-Orsdemir S, Garb JL, Allen HF. Prevalence of cranial MRI findings in girls with central precocious puberty: a systematic review and meta-analysis. J Pediatr Endocrinol Metab 2018;31(7):701–10.

87. Franzini I, Yamamoto FM, Bolfi F, et al. GnRH analog is ineffective in increasing adult height in girls with puberty onset after 7 years of age: a systematic review and meta-analysis. Eur J Endocrinol 2018;179(6):381–90.

88. Gohil A, Eugster EA. GnRH analogs (mechanism, past studies, drug options, use in precocious puberty, use in gender-nonconforming youth). In: Finlayson C, editor. Pubertal suppression in transgender youth. St Louis (MO): Elsevier; 2019. p. 25–32.

Phthalate Exposure, Adolescent Health, and the Need for Primary Prevention

Clara G. Sears, PhD*, Joseph M. Braun, RN, MSPH, PhD

KEYWORDS

- Phthalates • Adolescent health • Endocrine-disrupting chemicals • Obesity
- Puberty • Neurodevelopment

KEY POINTS

- Phthalates are endocrine-disrupting chemicals added to household goods and personal care products.
- Exposure to phthalates during prenatal and childhood development can disrupt the functioning of neuroendocrine axes and may alter adiposity, puberty, and neurodevelopment.
- Health care professionals can help concerned patients reduce phthalate exposure by providing them with educational resources and advocating for sensible public health policies.

INTRODUCTION

Adolescence, a critical period of development from puberty until adulthood, is a susceptible and malleable period of life.[1,2] Development during adolescence, like gestation and childhood, is orchestrated in part by endogenous hormones. During adolescence, a surge in gonadal hormones activates downstream biological pathways to drive development of secondary sexual characteristics, changes in body size and composition, and neurodevelopmental maturation. The successful completion of these processes is essential to health in adulthood.

Chemicals that are capable of disrupting hormone homeostasis during gestation and childhood can impede adolescent maturation and are often referred to as endocrine-disrupting chemicals.[3,4] Phthalates are a class of compounds considered to be endocrine-disrupting chemicals because of their ability to disrupt androgen homeostasis (**Table 1**). Phthalates are commonly used as scent retainers, emollients, and plasticizers in some personal care products, food packaging, and building

Department of Epidemiology, Brown University School of Public Health, Box G-S121-2, 121 South Main Street, Providence, RI 02912, USA
* Corresponding author.
E-mail address: clara_sears@brown.edu
Twitter: @JosephMBraun1 (J.M.B.)

Endocrinol Metab Clin N Am 49 (2020) 759–770
https://doi.org/10.1016/j.ecl.2020.08.004
0889-8529/20/© 2020 Elsevier Inc. All rights reserved.

endo.theclinics.com

Table 1
Metabolites and common uses of phthalate diesters and their replacements

Phthalate Esters	Metabolites	Common Uses[100,101]

DEHP	Mono-2-ethylhexyl phthalate
	Mono-2-ethyl-5-
	  carboxypentyl phthalate
	Mono-2-ethyl-5-
	  hydroxyhexyl phthalate
	Mono-2-ethyl-5-
	  oxohexyl phthalate
		PVC plastics, food packaging,
		  plastic medical tubing
		  and bags

1,2-Cyclo-hexane
  dicarboxylic acid,
  diisononyl ester
	Cyclohexane-1,
	  2-dicarboxylic acid
	  monohydroxy isononyl ester
		DEHP replacements: PVC plastics,
		  food packaging,
		  medical tubing/bags

Bis(2-ethylhexyl)
  terephthalate
	Mono-2-ethylhydroxyhexyl
	  terephthalate
	Mono-2-ethyl-5-carboxypentyl
	  terephthalate
		DEHP replacement: PVC plastics,
		  food packaging,
		  medical tubing/bags

Butylbenzyl phthalate	Mono-benzyl phthalate	Vinyl flooring, adhesives,
		  food packaging,
		  synthetic leather, toys

Diethyl phthalate	Monoethyl phthalate	Scent retainer in
		  personal care products and
		  medication excipient

Di-n/i-butyl phthalate	Mono-n/i-butyl phthalate	Scent retainer in
		  personal care products,
		  medication excipient,
		  cellulose plastics, adhesives

Di-isodecyl phthalate
Di-isononyl phthalate
	Monocarboxynonyl phthalate
	Monocarboxyoctyl phthalate
		Plastics, flooring, shoes,
		  restricted use in toys,
		  synthetic leather,
		  building materials

Abbreviations: DEHP, di-2-ethylhexyl phthalate; PVC, polyvinyl chloride.
Data from Sathyanarayana S. Phthalates and Children's Health. Curr Probl Pediatr Adolesc Health Care. 2008;38(2):34-49; and Bui TT, Giovanoulis G, Cousins AP, et al. Human exposure, hazard and risk of alternative plasticizers to phthalate esters. Sci Total Environ. 2016;541:451-467.

materials.[5–9] Phthalates are not covalently bound to these products and therefore can be ingested after leaching from plastic packaging, dermally absorbed after use of products, and inhaled after release into indoor air or dust.

After entering the body, phthalates are metabolized into biologically active mono-ester metabolites, which are excreted in the urine (half-life <24 hours).[10–12] Biomonitoring studies around the world indicate ubiquitous exposure to phthalates during pregnancy and childhood.[13–17]

HORMONAL MECHANISMS OF PHTHALATE ACTION

Phthalate exposure during gestation and childhood may interfere with neuroendocrine axes and disrupt the actions of gonadal hormones, glucocorticoids, and thyroid hormones in adolescence.[18–24] Furthermore, these disruptions may vary by sex because of sex-specific differentiation in the organization of the nervous system.[25]

Numerous studies in animals and humans show that some phthalates are antiandrogenic and exposure may contribute to reduced fetal testis and testosterone production in humans and rats, shorter anogenital distance in humans and rats, and decreased sperm concentration in humans.[24,26–28] Furthermore, in vitro and in vivo studies indicate that some phthalates interfere with the activity of androgen receptors, as well as estrogen receptors α and β.[29] Results from human studies are less conclusive than those in animal models but suggest that these alterations in gonadal hormone homeostasis may subsequently affect the timing and progression of puberty.[30–33]

Phthalate exposure during gestation and early childhood may inhibit 11-β-hydroxysteroid dehydrogenase-2, the enzyme responsible for deactivating cortisol, which could contribute to sex-specific disruptions of glucocorticoid homeostasis.[18,23,34–36] For example, higher concentrations of some phthalates during gestation were positively associated with cortisol levels among female infants, whereas inverse associations were observed among male infants. Prolonged increase in cortisol levels may adversely affect neurodevelopment and growth given the importance of this hormonal axis to these end points and known effects of clinically increased cortisol levels (e.g., Cushing syndrome).[18,37]

Studies in both animal models and humans suggest that exposure to some phthalates also alters thyroid function. Higher concentrations of some phthalates have been associated with decreased free and total thyroxine (T4) as well as total triiodothyronine (T3) levels.[19,38–41] In addition, some phthalates may reduce cellular T3 uptake and antagonize T3 binding to thyroid receptor β, as well as interfere with the transcription of the sodium-iodine transporter.[39,42,43] However, studies of the association between phthalate exposure during different periods and thyroid-stimulating hormone are less conclusive.[44,45] Alterations in thyroid hormone levels can contribute to impaired growth, disruptions in energy metabolism, and adverse neurobehavioral outcomes. For example, a study in mice reports that di-2-ethylhexyl phthalate (DEHP) induces hypothyroidism, contributing to increased weight gain and adipogenesis.[46]

PHTHALATES AND ADIPOSITY

Environmental exposures during early life that interfere with neuroendocrine axes could alter energy metabolism, appetite, and adipogenesis.[47,48] Several epidemiologic studies have evaluated whether phthalate exposure during gestation and childhood is associated with excess adiposity or risk of obesity/overweight throughout childhood.[49–62] However, only a few prospective studies have evaluated these associations during adolescence.

Two studies of adolescents reported that phthalate exposure during gestation and childhood were associated with higher body mass index, larger waist circumference, or increased risk of being overweight or obese.[53,54] For example, a doubling of several prenatal urinary phthalate metabolite concentrations was associated with a 20% to 30% increase in odds of being overweight or obese at age 12 years among both boys and girls.[54] In contrast, a different study of adolescents aged 8 to 14 years found that prenatal urinary concentrations of one of the same phthalate metabolites was associated with lower body mass index.[62] Furthermore, several other studies in younger populations have reported inconsistent associations between phthalate exposure and measures of adiposity, such as body mass index, percentage fat mass, or waist circumference.[51,52,56,59]

PHTHALATES AND PUBERTAL DEVELOPMENT

Disruptions to gonadal hormone homeostasis caused by phthalate exposure could act independently of, or in combination with, childhood adiposity to interfere with the timing and progression of puberty. However, epidemiologic studies evaluating the association between phthalate exposure and pubertal timing are few and inconclusive.[30,31,33,63]

Results from epidemiologic studies suggest that prenatal or childhood exposure to various phthalates is associated with both delayed and earlier pubertal onset, whereas others suggest no association with pubertal development.[30,31,33,63–66] These inconsistencies could be caused by differences in the timing and assessment of phthalate exposure and the measurement of pubertal development (i.e., self-reported measures or clinician-assessed Tanner staging by trained professionals). Perhaps the strongest evidence indicating an effect of phthalate exposure on pubertal development is from two studies reporting a younger age of menarche associated with prenatal and childhood diethyl phthalate (DEP) exposure. Watkins and colleagues[30] (2017) found that girls born to women with higher prenatal urinary concentrations of monoethyl phthalate (DEP metabolite) had higher odds of menarche before the study visit at 8 to 13 years (mean age = 10.0 years; standard deviation = 1.5). Another study suggested that higher urinary concentrations of monoethyl phthalate at ages 6 to 8 years were associated with an earlier reported age of menarche.[67]

PHTHALATES AND NEURODEVELOPMENT

Given the role of the hypothalamic-pituitary-adrenal, hypothalamic-pituitary-gonad, and hypothalamic-pituitary-thyroid axes in neurodevelopment, phthalate exposure could have adverse effects on cognition or behavior.[24,26,27,37]

Prenatal phthalate exposure has been associated with more autistic behaviors, reduced mental and psychomotor development, poorer language development, emotional problems, and attention-deficit/hyperactivity disorder (ADHD)–related behaviors.[68–77] For example, Engel and colleagues[74] (2018) found that children of women in the highest quintile of urinary DEHP metabolites during pregnancy had three times the odds of being diagnosed with ADHD compared with children of women in the lowest quintile. In addition, some studies report that childhood phthalate exposure is associated with reduced cognitive abilities and behavioral problems.[78–82] However, other studies have not found associations between prenatal or childhood phthalate exposure and neurobehavioral outcomes.[71,80,83–85]

REDUCING PHTHALATE EXPOSURES

In the United States, manufactured chemical substances, such as phthalates, can be used in industrial processes and consumer products without comprehensive research on the long-term health effects of exposure. Chemicals are usually identified as potentially hazardous to human health only after a substantial body of experimental and/or observational evidence is accumulated. Typically, by that point, exposure is already pervasive in the pediatric population and their environment, making it difficult to identify and remove significant exposure sources. Moreover, when hazardous chemicals are identified and removed from consumer goods, they are often replaced by chemicals that are structurally similar and have unknown long-term health effects.

For example, because of concerns about health effects and ubiquitous exposure in populations worldwide, bis(2-ethylhexyl) terephthalate (DEHTP) and diisononyl ester (DINCH) are replacing DEHP in polymers, adhesives, toys, flooring, medical devices, food packaging, and more (**Fig. 1**). Since the late 2000s, increases in urinary concentrations of DEHTP and DINCH metabolites have been observed in populations across

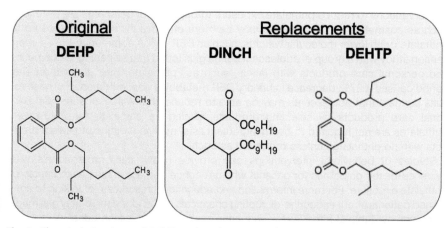

Fig. 1. Chemical structure of DEHP and replacements. (*From* National Center for Biotechnology Information. PubChem Database. Bis(2-ethylhexyl) phthalate, CID=8343, https://pubchem.ncbi.nlm.nih.gov/compound/8343#section=2D-Structure, PubChem Database. H26MNT7GT7, Source=ChemIDplus, SID=135261294, https://pubchem.ncbi.nlm.nih.gov/substance/135261294, and National Center for Biotechnology Information. PubChem Database. CID=22932, https://pubchem.ncbi.nlm.nih.gov/compound/22932#section=2D-Structure (accessed on July 20, 2020); with permission.)

the US and Europe.[86–91] Recent studies of the effects of DINCH on hormone homeostasis suggest that this phthalate replacement could have similar effects to the phthalate that it replaced.[92–94]

While waiting for regulatory or policy interventions, some studies have evaluated behavioral interventions to reduce phthalate exposure.[8,95,96] The capacity of behavioral interventions to reduce exposure varies by the specific phthalate. In addition, the effectiveness of interventions may vary over childhood and adolescence because changing behaviors could alter the relative contribution of different exposure routes to an individual's overall exposure level (e.g., dust from hand-to-mouth activity). In addition to identifying actions that individuals can take to reduce exposure, these studies can also inform regulatory decisions by identifying exposure routes.

Interventions targeting dietary sources of phthalates may be more effective in reducing childhood exposure to phthalates with high molecular weights, such as DEHP, which are commonly used as plastic additives in food processing.[8,97] Rudel and colleagues[8] (2011) found that a three-day intervention that provided families with fresh food for all meals caused an ~50% decrease in the levels of DEHP metabolites. However, a separate study by Sathyanarayana and colleagues[95] (2013) observed a 2377% increase in DEHP metabolites among families receiving fresh foods for a five-day complete dietary replacement intervention. The significant increase in DEHP metabolites among participants receiving the dietary intervention was likely caused by high concentrations of DEHP in coriander (21,400 ng/g) and milk (673 ng/g).[95] On average, they estimated that children ingested 183 μg DEHP/kg/d during this intervention. This amount is nine times (183 μg/kg/d) the quantity that regulatory agencies determine to be safe based on toxicologic data (US Environmental Protection Agency [EPA] oral reference dose = 20 μg/kg/d for increased liver weight). This study shows that, even with professional knowledge and extensive effort, it can be difficult, if not impossible, to identify and eliminate all significant dietary sources of phthalates.

Interventions to reduce phthalate exposure through use of personal care products, such as cosmetics and fragrances, may be more effective in reducing exposure to phthalates with lower molecular weights, such as DEP.[16,98] A community-based intervention study with a group of adolescent Latina girls found that switching to cosmetics and personal care products with labels, such as "phthalate free," for a three-day period caused a 27% decrease in urinary DEP metabolite concentrations.[96] These results suggest that adolescents may be able to reduce chemical exposure from personal care products by selecting products labeled as phthalate free. However, phthalates are not required to be on ingredient lists, making it difficult to select products with no phthalates unless promoted as such.

Studies of behavioral interventions can provide health care professionals with evidence-based guidelines for patients who are concerned about the health effects of phthalate exposure. For more information and educational resources for talking to concerned patients about endocrine-disrupting chemicals, the Endocrine Society has made resources available at https://www.endocrine.org/topics/edc/talking-edcs/.

However, relying on behavioral interventions is onerous and ineffective in eliminating pervasive exposure to phthalates across all stages of life. Therefore, it is critical that health care professionals are also engaged in health policy that promotes primary prevention and furthers children's environmental health research. Health professionals can be patient advocates by submitting public comments when the EPA conducts assessments of the health risks of endocrine-disrupting chemicals. In December 2019, the EPA released a list of 20 high-priority chemicals that will undergo risk evaluation per the Frank R. Lautenberg Chemical Safety for the 21st Century Act, an amendment to the Toxic Substances Control Act (TSCA). Of the 20 chemicals that will be assessed, six are phthalates.[99] The outcome of these risk evaluations will dictate how manufacturers can use these chemicals.

SUMMARY

Epidemiologic and experimental studies have shown that exposure to phthalates can disrupt hormone homeostasis. The research into how these disruptions across the lifespan alter adiposity, puberty, and neurodevelopment during adolescence is still ongoing. However, given scientific evidence showing pervasive exposure and potential health impacts of phthalates and other endocrine-disrupting chemicals, public health researchers are already investigating strategies to prevent childhood and adolescent exposure to phthalates in the absence of regulatory action. Health care professionals play an integral role in preventing phthalate exposure by providing resources to concerned patients and advocating for sensible public health policies.

DISCLOSURE

Dr J.M. Braun was financially compensated for serving as an expert witness for plaintiffs in litigation related to tobacco smoke exposures and received an honorarium for serving on an advisory board to Quest Diagnostics. Dr J.M. Braun served as an expert witness in litigation related to perfluorooctanoic acid contamination in drinking water in New Hampshire. Funds received from this arrangement are paid to Brown University and are not used for direct personal benefit (e.g., salary/fringe, travel).

REFERENCE

1. Dahl RE. Adolescent brain development: a period of vulnerabilities and opportunities. keynote address. Ann N Y Acad Sci 2004;1021(1):1–22.

2. Dahl RE, Allen NB, Wilbrecht L, et al. Importance of investing in adolescence from a developmental science perspective. Nature 2018;554(7693):441–50.
3. Braun JM. Early-life exposure to EDCs: role in childhood obesity and neurodevelopment. Nat Rev Endocrinol 2017;13(3):161–73.
4. Gore AC, Krishnan K, Reilly MP. Endocrine-disrupting chemicals: Effects on neuroendocrine systems and the neurobiology of social behavior. Horm Behav 2019;111:7–22.
5. Cirillo T, Fasano E, Esposito F, et al. Study on the influence of temperature, storage time and packaging type on di- n -butylphthalate and di(2-ethylhexyl) phthalate release into packed meals. Food Addit Contam 2013;30(2):403–11.
6. Duty SM, Ackerman RM, Calafat AM, et al. Personal care product use predicts urinary concentrations of some phthalate monoesters. Environ Health Perspect 2005;113(11):1530–5.
7. Just AC, Adibi JJ, Rundle AG, et al. Urinary and air phthalate concentrations and self-reported use of personal care products among minority pregnant women in New York city. J Expo Sci Environ Epidemiol 2010;20(7):625–33.
8. Rudel RA, Gray JM, Engel CL, et al. Food packaging and bisphenol a and bis(2-ethyhexyl) phthalate exposure: findings from a dietary intervention. Environ Health Perspect 2011;119(7):914–20.
9. Wormuth M, Scheringer M, Vollenweider M, et al. What are the sources of exposure to eight frequently used phthalic acid esters in Europeans? Risk Anal 2006; 26(3):803–24.
10. Kao ML, Ruoff B, Bower N, et al. Pharmacokinetics, metabolism and excretion of 14C-monoethyl phthalate (MEP) and 14C-diethyl phthalate (DEP) after single oral and IV administration in the juvenile dog. Xenobiotica 2012;42(4):389–97.
11. Koch HM, Preuss R, Angerer J. Di(2-ethylhexyl)phthalate (DEHP): human metabolism and internal exposure - an update and latest results1. Int J Androl 2006; 29(1):155–65.
12. Koch HM, Christensen KLY, Harth V, et al. Di-n-butyl phthalate (DnBP) and diisobutyl phthalate (DiBP) metabolism in a human volunteer after single oral doses. Arch Toxicol 2012;86(12):1829–39.
13. Casas L, Fernández MF, Llop S, et al. Urinary concentrations of phthalates and phenols in a population of Spanish pregnant women and children. Environ Int 2011;37(5):858–66.
14. Kasper-Sonnenberg M, Koch HM, Wittsiepe J, et al. Levels of phthalate metabolites in urine among mother-child-pairs - results from the Duisburg birth cohort study, Germany. Int J Hyg Environ Health 2012;215(3):373–82.
15. Teitelbaum SL, Britton JA, Calafat AM, et al. Temporal variability in urinary concentrations of phthalate metabolites, phytoestrogens and phenols among minority children in the United States. Environ Res 2008;106(2):257–69.
16. Watkins DJ, Eliot M, Sathyanarayana S, et al. Variability and Predictors of Urinary Concentrations of Phthalate Metabolites during Early Childhood. Environ Sci Technol 2014;48(15):8881–90.
17. Woodruff TJ, Zota AR, Schwartz JM. Environmental Chemicals in Pregnant Women in the United States: NHANES 2003–2004. Environ Health Perspect 2011;119(6):878–85.
18. Kim JH, Lee J, Moon H-B, et al. Association of phthalate exposures with urinary free cortisol and 8-hydroxy-2′-deoxyguanosine in early childhood. Sci Total Environ 2018;627:506–13.
19. Kim MJ, Moon S, Oh B-C, et al. Association between diethylhexyl phthalate exposure and thyroid function: a meta-analysis. Thyroid 2019;29(2):183–92.

20. Meeker JD, Ferguson KK. Urinary phthalate metabolites are associated with decreased serum testosterone in men, women, and children from NHANES 2011–2012. J Clin Endocrinol Metab 2014;99(11):4346–52.

21. Sathyanarayana S, Barrett E, Butts S, et al. Phthalate exposure and reproductive hormone concentrations in pregnancy. Reproduction 2014;147(4):401–9.

22. Sathyanarayana S, Butts S, Wang C, et al. Early prenatal phthalate exposure, sex steroid hormones, and birth outcomes. J Clin Endocrinol Metab 2017; 102(6):1870–8.

23. Sun X, Li J, Jin S, et al. Associations between repeated measures of maternal urinary phthalate metabolites during pregnancy and cord blood glucocorticoids. Environ Int 2018;121:471–9.

24. Committee on Endocrine-Related Low-Dose Toxicity, Board on Environmental Studies and Toxicology, Division on Earth and Life Studies, National Academies of Sciences, Engineering, and Medicine. Application of systematic review methods in an overall strategy for evaluating low-dose toxicity from endocrine active chemicals. Washington, DC: National Academies Press; 2017. https:// doi.org/10.17226/24758.

25. Juraska JM, Sisk CL, DonCarlos LL. Sexual differentiation of the adolescent rodent brain: Hormonal influences and developmental mechanisms. Horm Behav 2013;64(2):203–10.

26. Hannas BR, Lambright CS, Furr J, et al. Dose-response assessment of fetal testosterone production and gene expression levels in rat testes following in utero exposure to diethylhexyl phthalate, diisobutyl phthalate, diisoheptyl phthalate, and diisononyl phthalate. Toxicol Sci 2011;123(1):206–16.

27. Howdeshell KL, Wilson VS, Furr J, et al. A mixture of five phthalate esters inhibits fetal testicular testosterone production in the sprague-dawley rat in a cumulative, dose-additive manner. Toxicol Sci 2008;105(1):153–65.

28. Radke EG, Braun JM, Meeker JD, et al. Phthalate exposure and male reproductive outcomes: A systematic review of the human epidemiological evidence. Environ Int 2018;121:764–93.

29. Engel A, Buhrke T, Imber F, et al. Agonistic and antagonistic effects of phthalates and their urinary metabolites on the steroid hormone receptors ERα, ERβ, and AR. Toxicol Lett 2017;277:54–63.

30. Watkins DJ, Sánchez BN, Téllez-Rojo MM, et al. Phthalate and bisphenol A exposure during in utero windows of susceptibility in relation to reproductive hormones and pubertal development in girls. Environ Res 2017;159:143–51.

31. Watkins DJ, Téllez-Rojo MM, Ferguson KK, et al. In utero and peripubertal exposure to phthalates and BPA in relation to female sexual maturation. Environ Res 2014;134:233–41.

32. Berger K, Eskenazi B, Kogut K, et al. Association of prenatal urinary concentrations of phthalates and bisphenol a and pubertal timing in boys and girls. Environ Health Perspect 2018;126(9):097004.

33. Wolff MS, Teitelbaum SL, McGovern K, et al. Phthalate exposure and pubertal development in a longitudinal study of US girls. Hum Reprod 2014;29(7): 1558–66.

34. Zhao B, Chu Y, Huang Y, et al. Structure-dependent inhibition of human and rat 11β-hydroxysteroid dehydrogenase 2 activities by phthalates. Chem Biol Interact 2010;183(1):79–84.

35. Ma X, Lian Q-Q, Dong Q, et al. Environmental inhibitors of 11β-hydroxysteroid dehydrogenase type 2. Toxicology 2011;285(3):83–9.

36. Ye L, Guo J, Ge R-S. Environmental pollutants and hydroxysteroid dehydrogenases. In: Litwack G, editor. Vitamins & hormones, vol. 94. Elsevier; 2014. p. 349–90. https://doi.org/10.1016/B978-0-12-800095-3.00013-4.

37. Lechan RM. Neuroendocrinology. In: Melmed S, Koenig R, Rosen C, et al, editors. Williams textbook of endocrinology. 14th edition. Philadelphia: Elsevier; 2019. p. 114–83.

38. Boas M, Frederiksen H, Feldt-Rasmussen U, et al. Childhood exposure to phthalates: associations with thyroid function, insulin-like growth factor i, and growth. Environ Health Perspect 2010;118(10):1458–64.

39. Ghisari M, Bonefeld-Jorgensen EC. Effects of plasticizers and their mixtures on estrogen receptor and thyroid hormone functions. Toxicol Lett 2009;189(1): 67–77.

40. Huang H-B, Pan W-H, Chang J-W, et al. Does exposure to phthalates influence thyroid function and growth hormone homeostasis? The Taiwan Environmental Survey for Toxicants (TEST) 2013. Environ Res 2017;153:63–72.

41. Meeker JD, Calafat AM, Hauser R. Di(2-ethylhexyl) phthalate metabolites may alter thyroid hormone levels in men. Environ Health Perspect 2007;115(7): 1029–34.

42. Breous E, Wenzel A, Loos U. The promoter of the human sodium/iodide symporter responds to certain phthalate plasticisers. Mol Cell Endocrinol 2005; 244(1–2):75–8.

43. Shimada N. Characteristics of 3,5,3'-triiodothyronine (T3)-uptake system of tadpole red blood cells: effect of endocrine-disrupting chemicals on cellular T3 response. J Endocrinol 2004;183(3):627–37.

44. Romano ME, Eliot MN, Zoeller RT, et al. Maternal urinary phthalate metabolites during pregnancy and thyroid hormone concentrations in maternal and cord sera: The HOME Study. Int J Hyg Environ Health 2018;221(4):623–31.

45. Meeker JD, Ferguson KK. Relationship between urinary phthalate and Bisphenol A concentrations and serum thyroid measures in U.S. adults and adolescents from the National Health and Nutrition Examination Survey (NHANES) 2007–2008. Environ Health Perspect 2011;119(10):1396–402.

46. Lv Z, Cheng J, Huang S, et al. DEHP induces obesity and hypothyroidism through both central and peripheral pathways in C3H/He mice: DEHP-Induced Obesity and Hypothyroidism. Obesity 2016;24(2):368–78.

47. Barker DJP. Developmental origins of chronic disease. Public Health 2012; 126(3):185–9.

48. Ornoy A. Prenatal origin of obesity and their complications: Gestational diabetes, maternal overweight and the paradoxical effects of fetal growth restriction and macrosomia. Reprod Toxicol 2011;32(2):205–12.

49. Botton J, Philippat C, Calafat AM, et al. Phthalate pregnancy exposure and male offspring growth from the intra-uterine period to five years of age. Environ Res 2016;151:601–9.

50. Bowman A, Peterson KE, Dolinoy DC, et al. Phthalate exposures, DNA methylation and adiposity in mexican children through adolescence. Front Public Health 2019;7:162.

51. Buckley JP, Engel SM, Mendez MA, et al. Prenatal phthalate exposures and childhood fat mass in a New York City Cohort. Environ Health Perspect 2016; 124(4):507–13.

52. Buckley JP, Engel SM, Braun JM, et al. Prenatal phthalate exposures and body mass index among 4- to 7-year-old children: a pooled analysis. Epidemiology 2016;27(3):449–58.

53. Deierlein AL, Wolff MS, Pajak A, et al. Longitudinal associations of phthalate exposures during childhood and body size measurements in young girls. Epidemiology 2016;27(4):492–9.

54. Harley KG, Berger K, Rauch S, et al. Association of prenatal urinary phthalate metabolite concentrations and childhood BMI and obesity. Pediatr Res 2017; 82(3):405–15.

55. Heggeseth BC, Holland N, Eskenazi B, et al. Heterogeneity in childhood body mass trajectories in relation to prenatal phthalate exposure. Environ Res 2019; 175:22–33.

56. Maresca MM, Hoepner LA, Hassoun A, et al. Prenatal exposure to phthalates and childhood body size in an urban cohort. Environ Health Perspect 2016; 124(4):514–20.

57. Shoaff J, Papandonatos GD, Calafat AM, et al. Early-life phthalate exposure and adiposity at 8 years of age. Environ Health Perspect 2017;125(9):097008.

58. Vafeiadi M, Myridakis A, Roumeliotaki T, et al. Association of early life exposure to phthalates with obesity and cardiometabolic traits in childhood: sex specific associations. Front Public Health 2018;6:327.

59. Valvi D, Casas M, Romaguera D, et al. Prenatal phthalate exposure and childhood growth and blood pressure: evidence from the Spanish INMA-Sabadell Birth Cohort Study. Environ Health Perspect 2015;123(10):1022–9.

60. Wang H, Zhou Y, Tang C, et al. Urinary phthalate metabolites are associated with body mass index and waist circumference in chinese school children. PLoS One 2013;8(2):e56800.

61. Xia B, Zhu Q, Zhao Y, et al. Phthalate exposure and childhood overweight and obesity: Urinary metabolomic evidence. Environ Int 2018;121:159–68.

62. Yang TC, Peterson KE, Meeker JD, et al. Bisphenol A and phthalates in utero and in childhood: association with child BMI z-score and adiposity. Environ Res 2017;156:326–33.

63. Radke EG, Glenn BS, Braun JM, et al. Phthalate exposure and female reproductive and developmental outcomes: a systematic review of the human epidemiological evidence. Environ Int 2019;130:104580.

64. Wolff MS, Teitelbaum SL, Pinney SM, et al. Investigation of relationships between urinary biomarkers of phytoestrogens, phthalates, and phenols and pubertal stages in girls. Environ Health Perspect 2010;118(7):1039–46.

65. Hart R, Doherty DA, Frederiksen H, et al. The influence of antenatal exposure to phthalates on subsequent female reproductive development in adolescence: a pilot study. REPRODUCTION 2014;147(4):379–90.

66. Su P-H, Chen J-Y, Lin C-Y, et al. Sex steroid hormone levels and reproductive development of eight-year-old children following in utero and environmental exposure to phthalates. PLoS One 2014;9(9):e102788.

67. Wolff MS, Pajak A, Pinney SM, et al. Associations of urinary phthalate and phenol biomarkers with menarche in a multiethnic cohort of young girls. Reprod Toxicol 2017;67:56–64.

68. Miodovnik A, Engel SM, Zhu C, et al. Endocrine disruptors and childhood social impairment. NeuroToxicology 2011;32(2):261–7.

69. Olesen TS, Bleses D, Andersen HR, et al. Prenatal phthalate exposure and language development in toddlers from the Odense Child Cohort. Neurotoxicol Teratol 2018;65:34–41.

70. Whyatt RM, Liu X, Rauh VA, et al. Maternal prenatal urinary phthalate metabolite concentrations and child mental, psychomotor, and behavioral development at 3 years of age. Environ Health Perspect 2012;120(2):290–5.

71. Factor-Litvak P, Insel B, Calafat AM, et al. Persistent associations between maternal prenatal exposure to phthalates on child IQ at age 7 years. PLoS One 2014;9(12):e114003.

72. Li N, Papandonatos GD, Calafat AM, et al. Identifying periods of susceptibility to the impact of phthalates on children's cognitive abilities. Environ Res 2019;172: 604–14.

73. Engel SM, Miodovnik A, Canfield RL, et al. Prenatal phthalate exposure is associated with childhood behavior and executive functioning. Environ Health Perspect 2010;118(4):565–71.

74. Engel SM, Villanger GD, Nethery RC, et al. Prenatal phthalates, maternal thyroid function, and risk of attention-deficit hyperactivity disorder in the norwegian mother and child cohort. Environ Health Perspect 2018;126(5):057004.

75. Kobrosly RW, Evans S, Miodovnik A, et al. Prenatal phthalate exposures and neurobehavioral development scores in boys and girls at 6–10 years of age. Environ Health Perspect 2014;122(5):521–8.

76. Lien Y-J, Ku H-Y, Su P-H, et al. Prenatal exposure to phthalate esters and behavioral syndromes in children at 8 years of age: taiwan maternal and infant cohort study. Environ Health Perspect 2015;123(1):95–100.

77. Kim Y, Ha E, Kim E, et al. Prenatal exposure to phthalates and infant development at 6 months: prospective mothers and children's environmental health (MOCEH) study. Environ Health Perspect 2011;119(10):1495–500.

78. Arbuckle TE, Davis K, Boylan K, et al. Bisphenol A, phthalates and lead and learning and behavioral problems in Canadian children 6–11 years of age: CHMS 2007–2009. NeuroToxicology 2016;54:89–98.

79. Hu D, Wang Y-X, Chen W-J, et al. Associations of phthalates exposure with attention deficits hyperactivity disorder: A case-control study among Chinese children. Environ Pollut 2017;229:375–85.

80. Huang H-B, Chen H-Y, Su P-H, et al. Fetal and childhood exposure to phthalate diesters and cognitive function in children up to 12 years of age: taiwanese maternal and infant cohort study. PLoS One 2015;10(6):e0131910.

81. Kim B-N, Cho S-C, Kim Y, et al. Phthalates exposure and attention-deficit/hyperactivity disorder in school-age children. Biol Psychiatry 2009;66(10): 958–63.

82. Kim JI, Hong Y-C, Shin CH, et al. The effects of maternal and children phthalate exposure on the neurocognitive function of 6-year-old children. Environ Res 2017;156:519–25.

83. Braun JM, Kalkbrenner AE, Just AC, et al. Gestational exposure to endocrine-disrupting chemicals and reciprocal social, repetitive, and stereotypic behaviors in 4- and 5-year-old children: the HOME study. Environ Health Perspect 2014;122(5):513–20.

84. Gascon M, Valvi D, Forns J, et al. Prenatal exposure to phthalates and neuropsychological development during childhood. Int J Hyg Environ Health 2015; 218(6):550–8.

85. Polanska K, Ligocka D, Sobala W, et al. Phthalate exposure and child development: The Polish Mother and Child Cohort Study. Early Hum Dev 2014;90(9): 477–85.

86. Centers for Disease Control and Prevention. National Report on Human Exposure to Environmental Chemicals. 2019. Available at: https://www.cdc.gov/exposurereport/. Accessed February 3, 2020.

87. Correia-Sá L, Schütze A, Norberto S, et al. Exposure of Portuguese children to the novel non-phthalate plasticizer di-(iso-nonyl)-cyclohexane-1,2-dicarboxylate (DINCH). Environ Int 2017;102:79–86.
88. Giovanoulis G, Alves A, Papadopoulou E, et al. Evaluation of exposure to phthalate esters and DINCH in urine and nails from a Norwegian study population. Environ Res 2016;151:80–90.
89. Lessmann F, Correia-Sá L, Calhau C, et al. Exposure to the plasticizer di(2-ethylhexyl) terephthalate (DEHTP) in Portuguese children – Urinary metabolite levels and estimated daily intakes. Environ Int 2017;104:25–32.
90. Machtinger R, Berman T, Adir M, et al. Urinary concentrations of phthalate metabolites, bisphenols and personal care product chemical biomarkers in pregnant women in Israel. Environ Int 2018;116:319–25.
91. Silva MJ, Wong L-Y, Samandar E, et al. Exposure to di-2-ethylhexyl terephthalate in the U.S. general population from the 2015–2016 National Health and Nutrition Examination Survey. Environ Int 2019;123:141–7.
92. Albert O, Nardelli TC, Lalancette C, et al. Effects of in utero and lactational exposure to new generation green plasticizers on adult male rats: a comparative study with di(2-Ethylhexyl) phthalate. Toxicol Sci 2018;164(1):129–41.
93. Engel A, Buhrke T, Kasper S, et al. The urinary metabolites of DINCH ® have an impact on the activities of the human nuclear receptors ERα, ERβ, AR, PPARα and PPARγ. Toxicol Lett 2018;287:83–91.
94. Campioli E, Lee S, Lau M, et al. Effect of prenatal DINCH plasticizer exposure on rat offspring testicular function and metabolism. Sci Rep 2017;7(1):11072.
95. Sathyanarayana S, Alcedo G, Saelens BE, et al. Unexpected results in a randomized dietary trial to reduce phthalate and bisphenol A exposures. J Expo Sci Environ Epidemiol 2013;23(4):378–84.
96. Harley KG, Kogut K, Madrigal DS, et al. Reducing phthalate, paraben, and phenol exposure from personal care products in adolescent girls: findings from the HERMOSA intervention study. Environ Health Perspect 2016;124(10):1600–7.
97. Serrano SE, Braun J, Trasande L, et al. Phthalates and diet: a review of the food monitoring and epidemiology data. Environ Health 2014;13(1):43.
98. Philippat C, Bennett D, Calafat AM, et al. Exposure to select phthalates and phenols through use of personal care products among Californian adults and their children. Environ Res 2015;140:369–76.
99. United States Environmental Protection Agency. EPA Finalizes List of Next 20 Chemicals to Undergo Risk Evaluation under TSCA. 2019. Available at: https://www.epa.gov/newsreleases/epa-finalizes-list-next-20-chemicals-undergo-risk-evaluation-under-tsca. Accessed February 3, 2020.
100. Sathyanarayana S. Phthalates and Children's Health. Curr Probl Pediatr Adolesc Health Care 2008;38(2):34–49.
101. Bui TT, Giovanoulis G, Cousins AP, et al. Human exposure, hazard and risk of alternative plasticizers to phthalate esters. Sci Total Environ 2016;541:451–67.

UNITED STATES POSTAL SERVICE ®

Statement of Ownership, Management, and Circulation
(All Periodicals Publications Except Requester Publications)

1. Publication Title	2. Publication Number	3. Filing Date
ENDOCRINOLOGY AND METABOLISM CLINICS OF NORTH AMERICA	000 – 275	9/18/2020

4. Issue Frequency	5. Number of Issues Published Annually	6. Annual Subscription Price
MAR, JUN, SEP, DEC	4	$375.00

7. Complete Mailing Address of Known Office of Publication (Not printer) (Street, city, county, state, and ZIP+4®)

ELSEVIER INC.
230 Park Avenue, Suite 800
New York, NY 10169

Contact Person: Malathi Samayan
Telephone (Include area code): 91-44-4299-4507

8. Complete Mailing Address of Headquarters or General Business Office of Publisher (Not printer)

ELSEVIER INC.
230 Park Avenue, Suite 800
New York, NY 10169

9. Full Names and Complete Mailing Addresses of Publisher, Editor, and Managing Editor (Do not leave blank)

Publisher (Name and complete mailing address)

DOLORES MELONI, ELSEVIER INC.
1600 JOHN F KENNEDY BLVD. SUITE 1800
PHILADELPHIA, PA 19103-2899

Editor (Name and complete mailing address)

KATERINA HEIDHAUSEN, ELSEVIER INC.
1600 JOHN F KENNEDY BLVD. SUITE 1800
PHILADELPHIA, PA 19103-2899

Managing Editor (Name and complete mailing address)

PATRICK MANLEY, ELSEVIER INC.
1600 JOHN F KENNEDY BLVD. SUITE 1800
PHILADELPHIA, PA 19103-2899

10. Owner (Do not leave blank. If the publication is owned by a corporation, give the name and address of the corporation immediately followed by the names and addresses of all stockholders owning or holding 1 percent or more of the total amount of stock. If not owned by a corporation, give the names and addresses of the individual owners. If owned by a partnership or other unincorporated firm, give its name and address as well as those of each individual owner. If the publication is published by a nonprofit organization, give its name and address.)

Full Name	Complete Mailing Address
WHOLLY OWNED SUBSIDIARY OF REED/ELSEVIER, US HOLDINGS	1600 JOHN F KENNEDY BLVD. SUITE 1800 PHILADELPHIA, PA 19103-2899

11. Known Bondholders, Mortgagees, and Other Security Holders Owning or Holding 1 Percent or More of Total Amount of Bonds, Mortgages, or Other Securities. If none, check box ▶ ☐ None

Full Name	Complete Mailing Address
N/A	

12. Tax Status (For completion by nonprofit organizations authorized to mail at nonprofit rates) (Check one)
The purpose, function, and nonprofit status of this organization and the exempt status for federal income tax purposes:
☒ Has Not Changed During Preceding 12 Months
☐ Has Changed During Preceding 12 Months (Publisher must submit explanation of change with this statement)

PS Form **3526**, July 2014 [Page 1 of 4 (see instructions page 4)] PSN: 7530-01-000-9931 PRIVACY NOTICE: See our privacy policy on www.usps.com.

13. Publication Title	14. Issue Date for Circulation Data Below
ENDOCRINOLOGY AND METABOLISM CLINICS OF NORTH AMERICA	JUNE 2020

15. Extent and Nature of Circulation			Average No. Copies Each Issue During Preceding 12 Months	No. Copies of Single Issue Published Nearest to Filing Date
a. Total Number of Copies (Net press run)			225	179
b. Paid Circulation (By Mail and Outside the Mail)	(1)	Mailed Outside-County Paid Subscriptions Stated on PS Form 3541 (Include paid distribution above nominal rate, advertiser's proof copies, and exchange copies)	103	84
	(2)	Mailed In-County Paid Subscriptions Stated on PS Form 3541 (Include paid distribution above nominal rate, advertiser's proof copies, and exchange copies)	0	0
	(3)	Paid Distribution Outside the Mails Including Sales Through Dealers and Carriers, Street Vendors, Counter Sales, and Other Paid Distribution Outside USPS®	71	60
	(4)	Paid Distribution by Other Classes of Mail Through the USPS (e.g. First-Class Mail®)	0	0
c. Total Paid Distribution [Sum of 15b (1), (2), (3), and (4)]		▶	174	144
d. Free or Nominal Rate Distribution (By Mail and Outside the Mail)	(1)	Free or Nominal Rate Outside-County Copies included on PS Form 3541	32	18
	(2)	Free or Nominal Rate In-County Copies Included on PS Form 3541	0	0
	(3)	Free or Nominal Rate Copies Mailed at Other Classes Through the USPS (e.g. First-Class Mail)	0	0
	(4)	Free or Nominal Rate Distribution Outside the Mail (Carriers or other means)	0	0
e. Total Free or Nominal Rate Distribution (Sum of 15d (1), (2), (3) and (4))		▶	32	18
f. Total Distribution (Sum of 15c and 15e)		▶	206	162
g. Copies not Distributed (See Instructions to Publishers #4 (page #3))		▶	19	17
h. Total (Sum of 15f and g)		▶	225	179
i. Percent Paid (15c divided by 15f times 100)			84.46%	88.88%

* If you are claiming electronic copies, go to line 16 on page 3. If you are not claiming electronic copies, skip to line 17 on page 3.

16. Electronic Copy Circulation		Average No. Copies Each Issue During Preceding 12 Months	No. Copies of Single Issue Published Nearest to Filing Date
a. Paid Electronic Copies	▶		
b. Total Paid Print Copies (Line 15c) + Paid Electronic Copies (Line 16a)	▶		
c. Total Print Distribution (Line 15f) + Paid Electronic Copies (Line 16a)	▶		
d. Percent Paid (Both Print & Electronic Copies) (16b divided by 16c × 100)	▶		

☒ I certify that 50% of all my distributed copies (electronic and print) are paid above a nominal price.

17. Publication of Statement of Ownership
☒ If the publication is a general publication, publication of this statement is required. Will be printed in the DECEMBER 2020 issue of this publication.   ☐ Publication not required.

18. Signature and Title of Editor, Publisher, Business Manager, or Owner	Date
Malathi Samayan - Distribution Controller *Malathi Samayan*	9/18/2020

I certify that all information furnished on this form is true and complete. I understand that anyone who furnishes false or misleading information on this form or who omits material or information requested on the form may be subject to criminal sanctions (including fines and imprisonment) and/or civil sanctions (including civil penalties).

PS Form **3526**, July 2014 (Page 3 of 4)   PRIVACY NOTICE: See our privacy policy on www.usps.com

Moving?

Make sure your subscription moves with you!

To notify us of your new address, find your **Clinics Account Number** (located on your mailing label above your name), and contact customer service at:

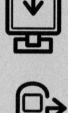

Email: journalscustomerservice-usa@elsevier.com

800-654-2452 (subscribers in the U.S. & Canada)
314-447-8871 (subscribers outside of the U.S. & Canada)

Fax number: 314-447-8029

Elsevier Health Sciences Division
Subscription Customer Service
3251 Riverport Lane
Maryland Heights, MO 63043

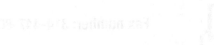

Printed and bound by CPI Group (UK) Ltd, Croydon, CR0 4YY

08/05/2025

01864692-0001